QUICK LOOK
PHARMACOLOGY

QUICK LOOK
PHARMACOLOGY

Edited by

Robert B. Raffa, Ph.D.

Associate Professor of Pharmacology
Department of Pharmaceutical Sciences
Temple University School of Pharmacy
Research Associate Professor
Department of Pharmacology
Temple University School of Medicine
Philadelphia, Pennsylvania

**Fence Creek
Publishing**

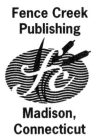

**Madison,
Connecticut**

Typesetter: Pagesetters, Brattleboro, VT
Printer: Port City Press, Baltimore, MD
Illustrations by Visible Productions, Fort Collins, CO
Distributors:

United States and Canada
Blackwell Science, Inc.
Commerce Place
350 Main Street
Malden, MA 02148
Telephone orders: 800-215-1000 or 781-388-8250
Fax orders: 781-388-8270

Australia
Blackwell Science, PTY LTD.
54 University Street
Carlton, Victoria 3053
Telephone orders: 61-39-347-0300
Fax orders: 61-39-347-5001

Outside North America and Australia
Blackwell Science, LTD.
c/o Marston Book Service, LTD.
P.O. Box 269
Abingdon Oxon, OX 14 4XN England
Telephone orders: 44-1-235-465500
Fax orders: 44-1-235-465555

1 2 3 4 5 6 7 8 9 10

Table of Contents

Contributors

Paul Actor, Ph.D.

President
Paul Actor Associates
Phoenixville, Pennsylvania

Tai Akera, M.D., Ph.D.

Vice President
MSD Research Laboratories
Tokyo, Japan

Barrie Ashby, Ph.D.

Professor of Pharmacology
Department of Pharmacology
Temple University School of Medicine
Philadelphia, Pennsylvania

Daniel D. Bikle, M.D., Ph.D.

Professor of Medicine and Dermatology
Department of Medicine
University of California, San Francisco
Co-Director, Special Diagnostic and Treatment Center
Veterans Affairs Medical Center
San Francisco, California

Thomas F. Burks, Ph.D.

Professor of Pharmacology
Department of Pharmacology
University of Texas–Houston Medical School
Executive Vice President
Office of Research and Academic Affairs
University of Texas Health Science Center–Houston
Houston, Texas

David B. Bylund, Ph.D.

Professor and Chair
Department of Pharmacology
University of Nebraska College of Medicine
Omaha, Nebraska

Ellen E. Codd, M.S.

Principal Scientist
The R. W. Johnson Pharmaceutical Research Institute
Spring House, Pennsylvania

Stephen A. Cooper, D.M.D., Ph.D.

Vice President
Clinical and Medical Affairs
Whitehall Robins Health Care
Madison, New Jersey

Charles R. Craig, Ph.D.

Professor of Pharmacology and Toxicology
Departments of Pharmacology and Toxicology
Director, M.D./Ph.D. Medical Scientist Program
West Virginia School of Medicine
Morgantown, West Virginia

Ian A. Critchley, Ph.D.

Director of Laboratory Services
MRL Pharmaceutical Services
Herndon, Virginia

Michael J. Davies, M.S.

Research Associate
Department of Physiological Sciences
Eastern Virginia Medical School
Norfolk, Virginia

Stephen N. Davis, M.D.

Associate Professor of Medicine
Division of Diabetes and Endocrinology
Vanderbilt University School of Medicine
Nashville, Tennessee

Peter H. Doukas, Ph.D.

Dean
Temple University School of Pharmacy
Philadelphia, Pennsylvania

Toby K. Eisenstein, Ph.D.

Professor of Immunology
Departments of Microbiology and Immunology
Temple University School of Medicine
Philadelphia, Pennsylvania

William S. Evans, M.D.

Professor of Medicine
Department of Medicine
University of Virginia School of Medicine
Charlottesville, Virginia

Herbert Faleck, M.D.

Department of Nervous System Clinical Research
Novartis Pharmaceutical Corporation
East Hanover, New Jersey

Alan P. Farwell, M.D.

Associate Professor of Medicine
Division of Endocrinology and Metabolism
University of Massachusetts School of Medicine
Worcester, Massachusetts

Steven P. Gelone, Pharm.D.

Associate Professor of Pharmacology
Temple University School of Pharmacy
Assistant Professor of Medicine
Clinical Pharmacist in Infectious Diseases
Temple University School of Medicine
Philadelphia, Pennsylvania

Philip D. Hansten, Pharm.D.

Professor of Pharmacology
Department of Pharmacology
University of Washington School of Pharmacy
Seattle, Washington

Daniel H. Havlichek, Jr., M.D.

Associate Professor of Medicine
Division of Infectious Diseases
Michigan State University College of Medicine
East Lansing, Michigan

J. Paul Hieble, Ph.D.

Director, Cardiovascular Pharmacology
SmithKline Beecham Pharmaceuticals
King of Prussia, Pennsylvania

Christopher D. Huston, M.D.

Fellow in Infectious Diseases
Department of Medicine
University of Virginia School of Medicine
Charlottesville, Virginia

Paul A. Insel, M.D.

Professor of Pharmacology and Medicine
Departments of Pharmacology and Medicine
University of California School of Medicine
La Jolla, California

Edwin K. Jackson, Ph.D.

Professor of Pharmacology and Medicine
Departments of Pharmacology and Medicine
Associate Director, Center for Clinical Pharmacology
University of Pittsburgh School of Medicine
Pittsburgh, Pennsylvania

Henry I. Jacoby, Ph.D.

Vice President
Discovery Research Consultants
Brigantine, New Jersey

Marie C. Kerbeshian, Ph.D.

Postdoctoral Fellow
NSF Center for Biological Timing
University of Virginia Health Sciences Center
Charlottesville, Virginia

Cherng-ju Kim, Ph.D.

Associate Professor of Pharmaceutics
Department of Pharmaceutical Sciences
Temple University School of Pharmacy
Philadelphia, Pennsylvania

Jan M. Kitzen, R.Ph., Ph.D.

Adjunct Associate Professor of Pharmacology
Temple University School of Medicine
Philadelphia, Pennsylvania
Scientific Writer, Special Projects
Wyeth-Ayerst Research
Radnor, Pennsylvania

Sandra Knowles, B.Sci.Phm.

Department of Clinical Pharmacology
Sunnybrook Medical Center
Toronto, Ontario, Canada

Lynn D. Kramer, M.D.

Vice President and Global Head
CNS Clinical Development and Regulatory Affairs
Novartis Pharmaceutical Corporation
East Hanover, New Jersey

James M. Larner, M.D.

Associate Professor of Radiation Oncology
and Medicine
Department of Internal Medicine
University of Virginia School of Medicine
Charlottesville, Virginia

Thomas J. Lauterio, Ph.D.

Professor of Physiology
Departments of Physiology and Internal Medicine
Eastern Virginia Medical School
Norfolk, Virginia

T. Philip Malan, Jr., Ph.D., M.D.

Associate Professor of Anesthesiology
Department of Anesthesiology
University of Arizona School of Medicine
Tucson, Arizona

Sabri Markabi, M.D.

Department of Nervous System Clinical Research
Novarits Pharmaceutical Corporation
East Hanover, New Jersey

Robert B. McCall, Ph.D.

Distinguished Scientist
CNS Research
Pharmacia and Upjohn
Kalamazoo, Michigan

Sayoko E. Moroi, M.D., Ph.D.

Assistant Professor of Ophthalmology
W. K. Kellogg Eye Center
University of Michigan School of Medicine
Ann Arbor, Michigan

Rachael L. Neve, Ph.D.

Associate Professor of Genetics
Department of Genetics
Harvard University Medical School
Cambridge, Massachusetts
Director, Neurogenics Laboratory
McLean Hospital
Belmont, Massachusetts

John J. O'Neill, Ph.D.

Professor Emeritus
Department of Pharmacology
Temple University School of Medicine
Philadelphia, Pennsylvania

Mercedes Perusquía, Ph.D.

Professor of Cell Biology
National Autonomous University of Mexico
Mexico City, Mexico

William A. Petrie, Jr., M.D., Ph.D.

Professor of Medicine, Microbiology, and Pathology
Departments of Medicine, Microbiology, and Pathology
University of Virginia School of Medicine
Charlottesville, Virginia

Robert B. Raffa, Ph.D.

Associate Professor of Pharmacology
Department of Pharmaceutical Sciences
Temple University School of Pharmacy
Research Associate Professor
Department of Pharmacology
Temple University School of Medicine
Philadelphia, Pennsylvania

Richard H. Rech, Ph.D.

Professor of Pharmacology
Department of Pharmacology and Toxicology
Michigan State University College of Human Medicine
East Lansing, Michigan

Ross A. Reife, M.D.

Director, CNS Clinical Research
The R. W. Johnson Pharmaceutical Research Institute
Raritan, New Jersey

Sandra C. Roerig, Ph.D.

Associate Professor of Pharmacology
Department of Pharmacology
Louisiana State University School of Medicine
Shreveport, Louisiana

Richard P. Shank, Ph.D.

Senior Research Fellow
The R. W. Johnson Pharmaceutical Research Institute
Spring House, Pennsylvania

Neal Shear, M.D.

Professor of Medicine, Pediatrics, and Pharmacology
Departments of Medicine and Pharmacology
Sunnybrook Medical Center
Toronto, Ontario, Canada

J. Bryan Smith, Ph.D.

Professor of Pharmacology
Chair, Department of Pharmacology
Temple University School of Medicine
Philadelphia, Pennsylvania

Paul L. Stahle, M.S.

Senior Associate Scientist
Metabolism Department
The R. W. Johnson Pharmaceutical Research Institute
Spring House, Pennsylvania

Gary E. Stein, Pharm.D.

Professor of Medicine and Pharmacology
Departments of Medicine and Pharmacology
Michigan State University College of Human Medicine
East Lansing, Michigan

Ronald J. Tallarida, Ph.D.

Professor of Pharmacology
Department of Pharmacology
Temple University School of Medicine
Philadelphia, Pennsylvania

J. Andrew Wasserstrom, Ph.D.

Associate Professor of Medicine
Department of Medicine
Northwestern University School of Medicine
Chicago, Illinois

Cynthia L. Williams, Ph.D.

Adjunct Assistant Professor of Pharmacology
Department of Integrative Biology and Pharmacology
University of Texas–Houston Medical School
Houston, Texas

Michael Williams, Ph.D., D.Sc.

Divisional Vice President
Neurological and Urological Diseases
Abbott Laboratories
Abbott Park, Illinois

Stephen J. Winters, M.D.

Professor of Medicine
Department of Medicine
University of Pittsburgh School of Medicine
Pittsburgh, Pennsylvania

Preface

This book was designed to assist those students who are preparing for course or professional tests that require an understanding of the basic principles of pharmacology. The intended readers include students in pharmacology, pharmacy, medicine, nursing, dentistry, physical therapy, and other health care professions, as well as students taking introductory courses in pharmacology at the undergraduate level. It is intended to present the most relevant material in a concise and clear manner. Each topic is presented in a two-page format. One page consists of an illustration or table that succinctly gives an overview of the topic, and the other page consists of reading material that supplements and expands upon the topic.

To present the most authoritative and up-to-date material on each topic, recognized experts in each field were chosen as authors. The author of each chapter was instructed to distill the most relevant information on his or her topic and to follow general guidelines on the style of presentation of material. However, each author was free to choose the optimum manner of presentation of this material. Hence, each topic is presented in a form intended both for ease of use and quality of content. In addition, each author has supplied sample test questions as a guide and for the reader's self-evaluation of progress and comprehension of the material. All of the authors are familiar with the common test questions in pharmacology examinations. However, none of the questions are to be construed as taken directly from past or future tests. In some instances, it was necessary to edit material to meet space constraints. Every effort was made to do so without negative impact on content or style.

This book is intended solely as a review of pharmacology concepts, not as a guide to the practice of medicine, pharmacy, or other health profession. Drugs are listed as prototypes and some more commonly known trade names are used. The use or exclusion of a trade name is not intended to indicate product preference or to indicate relative efficacy or safety. Likewise, statements regarding clinical efficacy or safety are based on reference materials, not personal experience. The absence of mention of an adverse effect is not to be understood as the absence of such an adverse effect. The selection of representative agents is based on reference material and is not intended to imply superiority over other agents, and exclusion is not intended to imply lack of efficacy or excess adverse effects. All statements are to be viewed as generalities (exceptions might exist). The mention of specific drugs is not to be viewed as condoning, recommending, or supporting the clinical use of these substances without a thorough review of the appropriate prescribing information by qualified professionals and the informed and qualified weighing of perceived benefits versus possible risks in an individual patient.

It is hoped that by taking a "quick look" at this book the reader can efficiently preview, learn, or review the basic concepts and applications of the 74 topics in pharmacology that are presented. Any feedback about the success of this approach or suggestions for enhancing the attainment of this goal would be greatly appreciated.

Robert B. Raffa, Ph.D.

Acknowledgments

I wish to give special thanks to Jeanne Coughlin, my Administrative Assistant, whose efforts on behalf of this book—as on previous projects—made the endeavor possible and pleasant. It is no exaggeration to state that without her contributions, and particularly her skills in interacting with the authors, this book would not have been accomplished. I also wish to thank each and every author for taking the time to share their expertise with students in the early stages of their careers, who will use this book. I would also like to thank Matt Harris of Fence Creek for suggesting the project and Jane Edwards and Nancy G. Lucas for seeing it to completion. Dr. Ron Tallarida gets the award for being the first author to submit his chapter.

This book is dedicated to my family and to the patients who might benefit from the students who use it.

Pharmacologic Abbreviations

aa	of each	gtt	a drop	OS	left eye	qod	every other day
ac	before meals	h	hour	os	mouth	s	without
ad lib	freely, as desired	hs	hour of sleep,	OU	both eyes	SC	subcutaneous
bid	two times a day		bedtime	oz	ounce	sos	one dose if necessary
c̄	with	IM	intramuscular	pc	after meals	sp	spirits
cap	capsule	IV	intravenous	po	by mouth	ss	one-half
d	day	m	minim	pr	by rectum	stat	immediately
dr	dram	mL	milliliter	PRN	when required	tab	tablet
elix or el	elixir	od	every day	q	every	tid	three times a day
ext	extract	OD	right eye	qd	every day	tr	tinct., tincture
g	gram	oh	every hour	qh	every hour	ung	ointment
gr	grain	on	every night	qid	four times daily		

Abbreviations Used in *Quick Look Pharmacology*

A

ACE	angiotensin-converting enzyme
ACh	acetylcholine
ACTH	adrenocorticotropic hormone
ADP	adenosine diphosphate
ADH	antidiuretic hormone (vasopressin)
AEDs	antiepileptic drugs
AIDS	acquired immunodeficiency syndrome
AMA	American Medical Association
Am B	amphotericin B
AMIPA	α-Amino-3-hydroxy-5-methyl-4-isoxazole proprionic acid
ANF	antinuclear factor
Apo E	apolipoprotein E
ANS	autonomic nervous system
ATP	adenosine triphosphate
ATPase	adenosine triphosphatase
AV	atrioventricular
AVP	arginine vasopressin

B

BBB	blood–brain barrier
BD2	benzodiazepine

C

Ca^{2+}	calcium ion
cAMP	cyclic adenosine monophosphate
CCK	cholecystokinin
cGMP	cyclic guanosine monophosphate
CGRP	calcitonin gene-related peptide
CHF	congestive heart failure
Cl^-	chloride ion
CNS	central nervous system
CO	carbon monoxide
CoA	coenzyme A
COPD	chronic obstructive pulmonary disease
CRF	corticotropin-releasing factor
CRH	corticotropin-releasing hormone
CSF	cerebrospinal fluid

D

DA	dopamine
DAG	diacylglycerol
DPT	diphtheria, pertussis, and tetanus vaccine
dTTP	deoxythymidine triphosphate

E

ECG	electrocardiogram
EC50	estimated concentration to produce 50% effect
ED50	estimated dose to produce 50% effect
EPI	epinephrine
ER	endoplasmic reticulum

F

FAD	flavin adenine dinucleotide
FDA	Food and Drug Administration
5-FU	5-fluorouracil

G

GABA	γ-aminobutyric acid
GDP	guanosine diphosphate
GH	growth hormone
GHRH	growth hormone–releasing hormone
GI	gastrointestinal
Glu	glutamic acid
Gly	glycine
GMP	guanosine monophosphate
GnRH	gonadotropin-releasing hormone
G6PD	glucose-6-phosphate-dehydrogenase
GSH	growth-stimulating hormone
GTP	guanosine triphosphate
GU	genitourinary

H

H_1	histamine
HDL	high-density lipoprotein
Hep B	hepatitis B vaccine
5-HT	5-hydroxytryptamine (serotonin)
HIV	human immunodeficiency virus
HRT	hormone replacement therapy

I

IA	intra-arterial
Ig	immunoglobulin
IGF-1	insulin-like growth factor 1
IM	intramuscular
IND	investigational new drug
INH	isoniazid (isonicotinic acid hydrazide)
IP	intraperitoneal
IP_3	inositol triphosphate
IRB	Institutional Review Board
IRR	infusion-related reactions
IV	intravenous

J

JPET	*Journal of Pharmacology and Experimental Therapeutics*

K

K^+	potassium ion
"Kat"	methcathinone

L

LD_{50}	median lethal dose
LDL	low-density lipoprotein
LH	luteinizing hormone
LSD	lysergic acid diethylamide
LTA	lymphocytic toxicity assay
LTC	leukotriene C

M

M_1	muscarinic
MAO	monoamine oxidase
MAOI	monoamine oxidase inhibitors
mRNA	messenger RNA
MSH	melanocyte-stimulating hormone

N

Na^+	sodium ion
NAD	nicotinamide adenine dinucleotide
NAD^+	oxidized NAD
NADH	reduced NAD
NADP	NAD phosphate
NDA	new-drug application
NE	norepinephrine
NK	natural killer (cells)
NMDA	*N*-methyl-D-aspartate
NO	nitric oxide
NPY	neuropeptide Y
NSAIDs	nonsteroidal anti-inflammatory drugs
NTE	neuropathy target esterase

O

OTC	over the counter

P

PAS	p-aminosalicyclic acid
PBPs	penicillin-binding proteins
PCP	phencyclidine
PDR	*Physicians' Desk Reference*
PG	prostaglandin
PI	phosphatidylinositol
PIP_2	phosphatidylinositol 4,5-biphosphate
PLC	phospholipase C

PNS	peripheral nervous system	t-PA	tissue plasminogen activator
po	oral route	TCA	tricyclic antidepressant
PPD	purified protein derivative	TI	therapeutic index
PTH	parathyroid hormone	7-TM GPCRs	7-transmembrane G-protein–coupled receptors
PZA	pyrazinamide	*TiPS*	*Trends in Pharmacological Sciences*

R

TRH thyrotropin-releasing hormone

RAST	radioallergosorbent test	tRNA	transfer RNA
RBC	red blood cell	TSH	thyroid-stimulating hormone (thyrotropin)
REM	rapid eye movement	$T_{1/2}$	half-life

S

U

SA	sinoatrial	u-PA	urokinase
SAR	structure activity relationship	USAN	U. S. Adopted Name
SC	subcutaneous		
SNRI	selective norepinephrine reuptake inhibitor		

V

SRIF	somatotropin release-inhibiting hormone	VIP	vasoactive intestinal peptide
SSRI	selective serotonin reuptake inhibitor		

T

W

T_3	triiodothyronine	WBC	white blood cell
T_4	thyroxine	WHO	World Health Organization

PART I
General Principles

1 Pharmacology; Drug Names; Sources of Information
Robert B. Raffa, Ph.D.

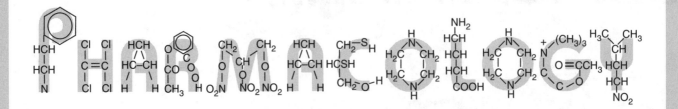

P	Phenethylamine	Endogenous amine related structurally to amphetamine
		Present in urine
		Produces similar pharmacologic effects as amphetamine
		Elevated in urine in some forms of psychosis
H	Tetrachloroethylene	Antihelminthic against nematodes (e.g., roundworms)
		Antihelminthic against trematodes (e.g., flatworms)
A	Cyclopropane	Flammable gas
		Inhalational anesthetic
R	Aspirin	Cyclooxygenase inhibitor
		Analgesic (NSAID)
		Antipyretic (fever reduction)
		Anti-inflammatory
		Anticoagulant
M	Nitroglycerin	Vasodilator
		Releases NO in smooth muscle
		Used to treat angina
		Veterinary use for asthma
A	Cyclopropane	Flammable gas
		Inhalational anesthetic
C	Dimercaprol	BAL (British antilewisite)
		Chelating agent
		Used to treat heavy-metal poisoning
O	Piperazine	Antihelminthic against nematodes
		Building block of several drug classes
L	GABA	γ-Aminobutyric acid
		Inhibitory CNS neurotransmitter
O	Piperazine	Antihelminthic against nematodes
		Building block of several drug classes
G	Acetylcholine	Neurotransmitter in parts of the autonomic nervous system
		Neurotransmitter at the skeletal neuromuscular junction
		Neurotransmitter in the CNS
		Ophthalmic
Y	Amyl nitrate	Vasodilator
		Used to treat anginal pain

OVERVIEW

- Life on earth evolved from simple molecules, and organisms were constructed with those chemical building blocks.
- As a result, chemicals can modify physiologic processes.
- *Pharmacology* is the study of the biologic actions of such agents, specifically, the study of therapeutic agents.
- An approved drug has several names: chemical, pharmaceutical company designation, nonproprietary (generic), and proprietary (trade).
- Sources of information about all aspects of drug use and abuse include: compendiums that serve as approved references; primary literature; review articles on basic science; desk references on therapeutic application and drug interactions; and numerous books, pamphlets, and letters, and other sources of news and views on drug topics, economics, and related issues.

Pharmacology

Pharmacology grew from mysticism and haphazard informalism into a science based on the study of the biochemical nature of the organization and communication networks of living organisms and the modulation of these systems for therapeutic purposes. The anatomic organization of the human nervous system, particularly the chemical component of neurocommunication (neurotransmitters), allows for the targeting of specific organs or functions. For example, in the periphery, the major neurotransmitters are ACh and NE. Compounds that enhance or antagonize these neurotransmitters (i.e., act as mimics [agonists] or antagonists at their receptors) can likewise mimic or antagonize the physiologic processes normally mediated by the neurotransmitters. Hence such compounds can predictably enhance or inhibit the normal physiologic processes and restore their level of activity to normal homeostatic conditions. Knowing the anatomic distribution of the neurotransmitters also allows prediction of many of the so-called side effects of drugs. A similar strategy is applied to the CNS, but the complexity of the anatomy and physiology makes the process more difficult. When applied to invading organisms or aberrant cells (cancer), selective targeting of biochemical processes permits therapeutic destruction. Advances in all areas of science have improved the design and development of new drugs. Molecular biology input and genetic engineering coupled with traditional pharmacologic approaches offers new possibilities for treating and curing illness and disease.

Medicinal Chemistry

The enzymes that catalyze biochemical reactions and the receptors that transduce the effects of neurotransmitters impose a strict three-dimensional constraint on the types of molecules that can influence their activity. The drug must have the requisite three-dimensional "lock-and-key" fit. Designing exogenous molecules that meet such requisites is the realm of medicinal chemistry. The fact that most enzymes and receptors allow some "wiggle room" for substrate or ligand means that compounds can possess and display different degrees of fit. In pharmacologic terms, the ligand's shape and chemical composition influence its affinity for a receptor or binding site and its level of intrinsic activity (efficacy). The three-dimensional shape of a drug molecule determines whether it is a full or partial agonist, an antagonist, or even an inverse agonist.

Drug Names

- The chemical name describes the atoms and the functional groups of the molecule (e.g., [5α,6α]-7,8-didehydro-4,5-epoxy-17-methyl-morphinan-3,6-diol for morphine).

- The pharmaceutical company designation denotes the company and the company's own internal tracking system (e.g., MK-801 for a Merck compound).
- The nonproprietary or generic name is an approved pharmacologic designation (e.g., propranolol for a particular antihypertensive). The nonproprietary name is approved by the United States Adopted Name Council with input from the United States Pharmacopeial Convention Inc., American Pharmaceutical Association, AMA, FDA, and sometimes WHO.
- The trade name is owned by the holder of the trademark (e.g., Inderal for the drug propranolol). If there is no patent on a drug or if the patent has expired, a drug can have more than one trade name, each owned by different manufacturers.

SOME DESCRIPTIVE TERMINOLOGY

Pharmacokinetics is the study of the movement of drug substance through body components, from the site of administration, to the site of action, and to elimination.

Pharmacodynamics is the study of the mechanism of action of drugs.

Pharmacotherapeutics is the application of pharmacologic principles to clinical practice.

Pharmacognosy is the study of therapeutic plant and animal extracts.

Pharmacy involves the compounding and the proper and safe distribution and use of drugs.

Toxicology is the study of the biologic damage caused by substances, including drugs.

SOME SPECIFIC SOURCES OF INFORMATION ABOUT DRUGS

- *United States Pharmacopeia* (officially sanctioned in the United States)
- *National Formulary* (officially sanctioned in the United States)
- *American Drug Index*
- *Drug Evaluations Annual* (AMA publication)
- *Modern Drug Encyclopedia*
- *Physician's Desk Reference* (*PDR*) and associated publications
- *Medical Letter on Drugs and Therapeutics*
- *Merck Index*
- *Annual Review of Pharmacology and Toxicology*
- *Journal of Pharmacology and Experimental Therapeutics*
- *Trends in Pharmacological Sciences*

2 Routes of Drug Administration

Robert B. Raffa, Ph.D.

From application to distribution

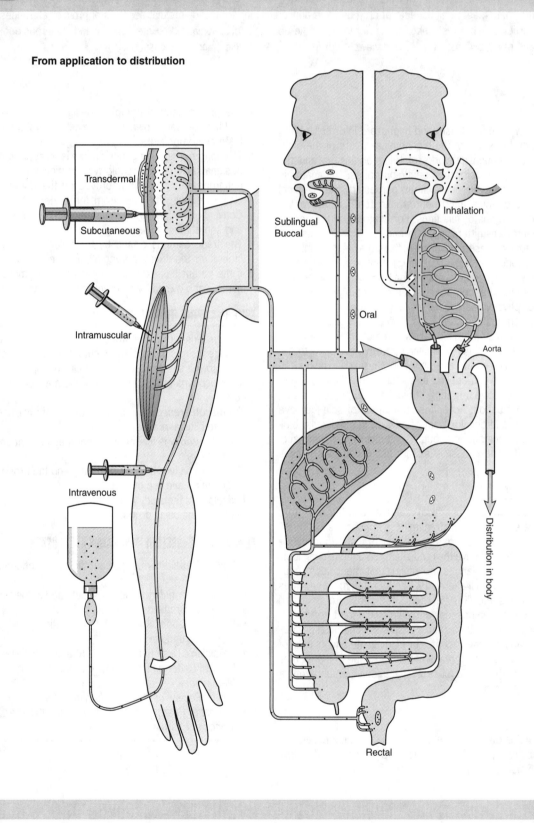

Transdermal

Subcutaneous

Intramuscular

Intravenous

Sublingual
Buccal

Oral

Inhalation

Aorta

Distribution in body

Rectal

OVERVIEW

- The choice of the route of administration of a particular drug is sometimes an option.
- In such cases, the oral route often is the most convenient, but other routes may be preferable in specific circumstances (such as direct injection of an analgesic into the spinal cord for postsurgical pain relief).
- Sometimes the options are limited, such as when the patient is unconscious or uncooperative, or when the drug is available in limited formulations.
- In all cases, the selected route of administration affects the rate and extent of absorption, the rate of metabolism and elimination, and the maximal achievable effect per dose.

Topical Routes

Skin. Undamaged skin is normally impermeable to hydrophilic (water-soluble) drugs; lipophilic (lipid-soluble = hydrophobic) drugs do penetrate; either kind can be formulated to aid penetration. Damaged skin (e.g., burns, wounds) loses its protective barrier and systemic absorption may occur, leading to toxicity. Uses include treatment of acne, psoriasis, topical infections, and others.

Transdermal. Patches or other devices contain "reservoirs" of drug substance. Advantages include convenience, avoidance of injections, and the maintenance of a constant or prolonged release. Disadvantages include possible immune reaction at site of application, difficulty in reversing effect of the reservoir once established, and the danger of accidental ingestion by small children. Uses include administration of analgesics, cardiovascular drugs, and other agents.

Mucous Membranes. The mucous membranes provide a thin, highly vascularized surface for drug absorption. It is also a convenient substitute for oral route in unconscious, uncooperative, or vomiting patients. Uses include antiseptic (e.g., oral lozenges, sprays, mouthwashes), antibacterial or antifungal action (e.g., vaginal creams and suppositories), decongestant (e.g., nasal sprays, drops), antihemorrhoidal (e.g., suppositories), systemic effect as contraceptive (e.g., vaginal foams, tablets, lotions), antianginal (e.g., sublingual vasodilators), plus others.

Ophthalmic Route

Direct application to the eye is possible using various formulations of drops, ointments, and washes. Sterile technique is required. Uses include facilitation of eye examination (e.g., production of mydriasis) or the treatment of glaucoma, inflammation, infection, and other conditions (mechanisms are described in applicable chapters).

Otic Route

Direct application is made to the ear, generally as drops, for local effect(s). Uses include treatment of inflammation (e.g., corticosteroids), infections (e.g., antibiotics), pain (e.g., local anesthetics), wax obstruction (e.g., hydrogen peroxide), and other conditions.

Systemic Routes

The term *parenteral* is used for systemic routes other than oral, sublingual, or rectal.

Oral (PO). Advantages of using the oral route are: simplest, most convenient, generally safest, most economical; drugs can be taken as tablets, capsules, or liquids; most drugs well absorbed from GI tract; can be administered with food (those that irritate GI tract); and can be taken on an empty stomach (those that are inactivated by digestive enzymes, such as penicillins). The disadvantages are: slower than IV for emergent care; some drugs inactivated in GI tract (e.g., insulin) or not well absorbed (e.g., tubocurarine); some drugs have objectionable odor or taste; nausea and vomiting may result; may cause stomach irritation (e.g., aspirin); and may stain teeth.

Intravenous (IV). The advantages of the IV route are: bypasses problems of absorption from GI tract; fast, dose can be quickly adjusted to effect; maintains constant blood levels; avoids first-pass effect (see Chap. 3); and can be administered to unconscious patient. The disadvantages are: difficult to reverse, toxicity if injection too rapid, and pain or infection at site of injection.

Intraarterial (IA). Although not common, this route has the advantage of allowing a specific target to be infused at high concentration (e.g., tumors, vasoconstriction in Raynaud's syndrome).

Subcutaneous (SC). This route involves injection into the tissue beneath the skin. Absorption is generally rapid; the effect is increased by local heating and vasodilators or enzymes that break down connective tissue; it is decreased by suspension in colloid, gelatin, or other medium. Pellets can be implanted for slow release.

Intramuscular (IM). Absorption is rapid because of high vascularity. Depot form possible (e.g., hormones in oil suspension).

Inhalation. The advantage of this route is rapid absorption resulting from large surface area and high vascularity. Uses include administration of general anesthesia, treatment of acute angina pectoris (e.g., with amyl nitrate), treatment of asthma and other pulmonary disorders (e.g., with corticosteroids, bronchodilators, antibiotics), provision of respiratory aid (e.g., O_2), as well as other applications.

Special Cases

Insufflation. Snuff of fine powder provides rapid absorption. There exists the potential problem of excess vasoconstriction (necrosis) of intranasal septum (e.g., with cocaine).

Intraneural. This route is direct injection into a nerve in order to block conduction (e.g., alcohol to block intractable trigeminal nerve pain).

Intraperitoneal (IP). This route is rapid, convenient, and reproducible because of the warm, moist environment and the extensive vascularity of the peritoneum (it is particularly useful for administration to small animals). There is a danger of puncturing intestines.

Epidural, Intrathecal, and Intracerebroventricular. These routes involve direct administration into the CNS to target the site of action of a drug and to diminish its adverse systemic effects. Epidural is commonly used for administration of analgesics (e.g., during labor, postsurgically)

3 Absorption and Distribution

Robert B. Raffa, Ph.D.

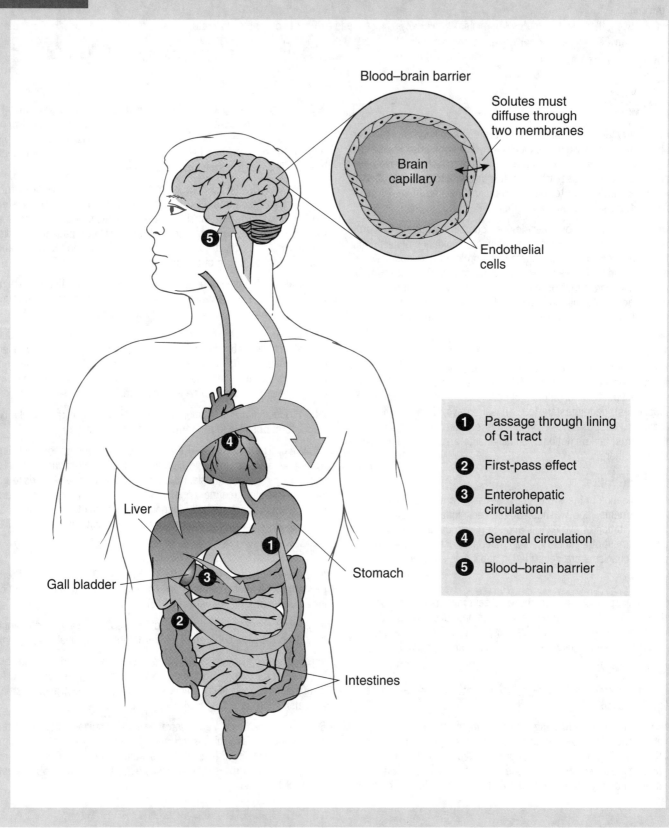

Blood–brain barrier

Solutes must diffuse through two membranes

Brain capillary

Endothelial cells

1 Passage through lining of GI tract

2 First-pass effect

3 Enterohepatic circulation

4 General circulation

5 Blood–brain barrier

Liver

Stomach

Gall bladder

Intestines

Passage through Biologic Membranes

For drug molecules to pass into the bloodstream from the common sites of administration (e.g., oral, subcutaneous, intramuscular), they must pass across the formidable barriers imposed by the biologic membrane. Consisting of a phospholipid bilayer, the membrane imposes special requirements for passage. The phosphate external layers of the "sandwich" are compatible with the aqueous surroundings, but the lipid interior restricts passage only to those substances that are at least to some extent lipid soluble, that is, lipophilic (hydrophobic).

Proteins. Generally these are too large to pass through healthy membranes without active transport process or pinocytosis.

Small Molecules. Water-soluble and lipid-soluble substances have difficulty passing across one or another of the "sandwich" layers of membranes. Weak acids ($HA \leftrightarrow H^+ + A^-$) and weak bases ($BH^+ \leftrightarrow H^+ + B$) exist in ionized and nonionized forms, depending on the pH of the surroundings. The nonionized forms are lipid soluble and more apt to pass across the membrane. The low pH of the stomach favors absorption of weak acids. In an emergency, administration of a base delays passage of overdose of a weak-acid drug.

Ions. Their small size permits some passage through membrane pores, but polarized cells (e.g., cardiac, neuronal) tightly control passage to maintain a proper degree of polarization and are sensitive to variations.

First-Pass Effect

The venous drainage of the stomach and intestines, unlike that of other organs, sends blood through the portal system to the liver rather than directly to the heart. Because significant drug biotransformation (metabolism) occurs within the liver, the amount of drug that passes into the general circulation after administration by oral or other route involving absorption by the GI tract is significantly less than would be the case after administration by routes not involving intestinal absorption (e.g., intravenous). The significant reduction is termed the "first-pass" effect, because subsequent circulatory passes are equivalent to other routes of administration.

Enterohepatic Circulation

From the liver, uncharged drug molecules or metabolites (e.g., glucuronides) can be concentrated in the gallbladder and released with bile into the intestine, where enzymes (e.g., glucuronidases) can release free drug. The quantity of recirculated drug represents an additional source for drug action. The enterohepatic recirculation cycle can establish a virtual reservoir that results in the prolongation of drug action.

Plasma-Protein Binding

Drug molecules form reversible (weak) bonds with plasma protein molecules. While bound, drug molecules are inactive and also are less likely to pass into the kidney nephron. Hence plasma-protein binding influences the magnitude (decreases) and duration (increases) of a drug's effect. The percentage of drug that is plasma-protein bound is different (and measurable) for each drug. Drugs with high percentage of plasma-protein binding are susceptible to drug–drug interactions with other drugs having high binding capability as a result of displacement and release of now unbound, active drug molecules. Plasma-protein binding is saturable; hence, drug concentration in plasma is a nonlinear function of dose at high doses and can lead to unanticipated toxicity.

Blood–Brain Barrier

The endothelial cells of capillaries within the CNS lack pores and are tightly abutted, yielding little opportunity for drug molecules to pass between the cells. Hence, drug molecules must pass through the cells, a process that requires either special properties of the drug molecule (e.g., lipid solubility) or specialized transport processes such as carrier-facilitated diffusion or receptor-mediated internalization.

4 Drug Metabolism

Paul L. Stahle, M.S.

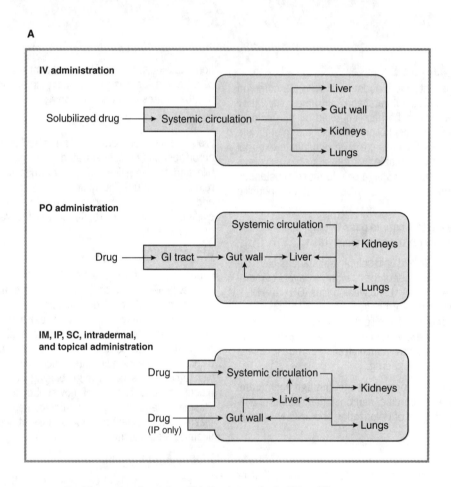

A

IV administration

Solubilized drug → Systemic circulation →
- Liver
- Gut wall
- Kidneys
- Lungs

PO administration

Drug → GI tract → Gut wall → Liver → Systemic circulation, Kidneys, Lungs

IM, IP, SC, intradermal, and topical administration

Drug → Systemic circulation → Kidneys, Lungs

Drug (IP only) → Gut wall → Liver

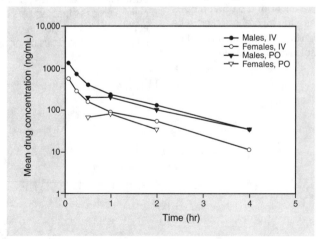

B Plasma levels of drug X following a single PO or IV administration to male and female beagle dogs

- Males, IV
- Females, IV
- Males, PO
- Females, PO

Mean drug concentration (ng/mL)

Time (hr)

OVERVIEW

- Metabolism (biotransformation) of a compound can inactivate it, detoxify it, increase its polarity, or make it more active or toxic.
- The ultimate goal of metabolism is to eliminate the compound.
- The following list of biotransformations applies to chemical compounds with low molecular weights; peptide and protein drugs are usually handled by the enzymes and binding proteins that are involved with endogenous proteins.

Phase 1 Metabolism

Phase 1 metabolism increases polarity to facilitate elimination in the urine or feces (via biliary excretion). This can produce a more active or toxic metabolite. Two large systems of enzymes that have been identified are the cytochrome P-450 mixed-function oxidase system and the flavin mixed-function oxidase system, although many other enzymes can be involved. Phase 1 metabolism usually occurs most extensively in the liver, gut wall, lungs, kidneys, or in the blood, but many other organs or tissues can be involved. The primary reactions are oxidation, reduction, and hydrolysis.

Phase 2 Metabolism

Phase 2 metabolism conjugates the polar substrates produced by phase 1 metabolism, if they are not already present in the molecule, and increases solubility in water to facilitate elimination. Conjugation reactions can occur in the kidneys, liver, and gut wall. The primary conjugates formed are glucuronides, glutathiones, sulfates, methylates, and acetylates.

Other Factors

First-pass Effect. The first-pass effect is the metabolism of a drug by the liver or gut wall following oral administration. This effect is due to the passing of blood from the GI tract through the liver prior to entering the systemic circulation. Some drugs undergo an extensive first-pass effect, which leads to decreased bioavailability.

Protein Binding. Many drugs bind extensively to plasma proteins (e.g., albumin and α_1-acid glycoprotein), which can markedly influence the distribution of the drug throughout the body.

Bioavailability. Bioavailability is the amount of drug available in the systemic circulation following an extravascular route of administration relative to IV administration.

Enterohepatic Circulation. Enterohepatic circulation occurs when a nonpolar compound is absorbed from the intestine, carried to the liver, conjugated, secreted into the bile, hydrolyzed back to the nonpolar compound in the intestine, and reabsorbed into the portal blood returning to the liver. This phenomenon can prolong the biologic half-life of a compound and extend the time course of adverse effects.

Half-life. Half-life is the amount of time it takes for the body to reduce the amount of drug in the systemic circulation by 50%. For zero-order elimination, the drug is fully eliminated (theoretically) after 2 half-lives. For the more common case of first-order elimination, after approximately 3.3 half-lives, 90% of the drug has been eliminated. Half-life can also be used to predict the time needed for a drug to reach a target blood concentration, especially during constant-rate IV infusion where the drug reaches 90% of steady-state concentration after 3.3 half-lives (for first-order kinetics).

Enzyme Induction or Inhibition. Enzymes that metabolize compounds can be affected by several factors. These factors can increase the level of enzyme present (induction) or decrease the activity (inhibition). When more than one drug that is metabolized by the same enzyme is present, one is metabolized faster than the other. This could increase the biologic half-life of the second compound, leading to toxic events. If an enzyme is induced, the level of drug present is lower than anticipated as a result of increased enzyme activity.

5 Elimination

Robert B. Raffa, Ph.D.

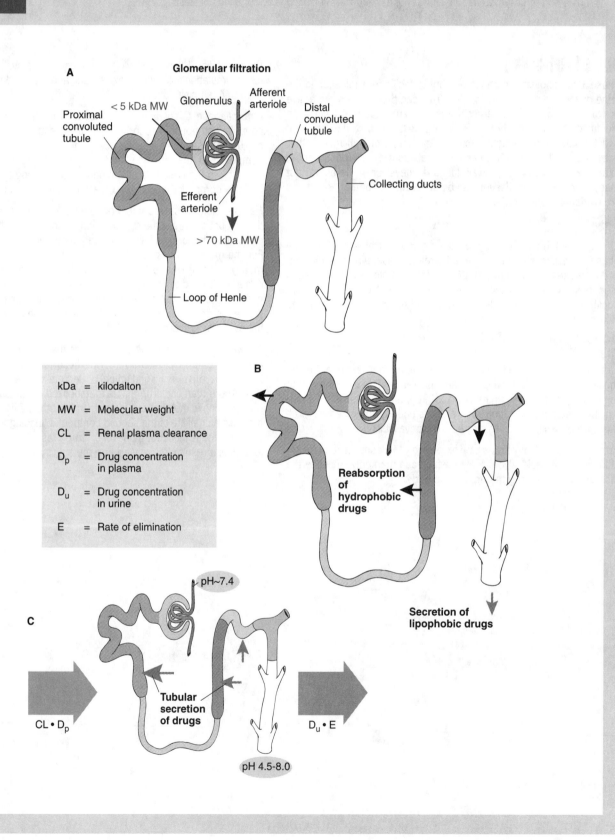

A — Glomerular filtration

Proximal convoluted tubule — < 5 kDa MW — Glomerulus — Afferent arteriole — Distal convoluted tubule — Collecting ducts — Efferent arteriole — > 70 kDa MW — Loop of Henle

kDa	=	kilodalton
MW	=	Molecular weight
CL	=	Renal plasma clearance
D_p	=	Drug concentration in plasma
D_u	=	Drug concentration in urine
E	=	Rate of elimination

B — Reabsorption of hydrophobic drugs — Secretion of lipophobic drugs

C — pH~7.4 — Tubular secretion of drugs — $CL \cdot D_p$ — $D_u \cdot E$ — pH 4.5-8.0

OVERVIEW

- The actions of drugs are terminated by the combined processes of biotransformation (i.e., metabolism), elimination, and redistribution.
- Elimination is the process by which drugs are removed from the body.
- The rate of elimination of most drugs from the blood is described by first-order kinetics (i.e., the rate is proportional to the remaining amount). Notable exceptions include ethanol, which is eliminated by zero-order kinetics (the rate is independent of the concentration).
- The major site of drug elimination in humans is the kidney.
- Drug elimination is a factor of the characteristics of the drug molecule and the state of health or disease of the kidney.
- Some drugs are actively secreted into, or removed from, the kidney tubules.
- The "renal plasma clearance" relates the elimination rate to the concentration of drug.
- If the rate of absorption and distribution of a drug exceeds its rate of elimination, accumulation may occur. Controlled levels of drugs can be achieved by loading and maintenance doses.

Rates of Elimination

For most drugs, the rate of elimination from blood is described by first-order kinetics (exponential decay): the rate of elimination is proportional to the amount of drug remaining. The equation that relates the concentration of drug in the plasma at any time T to the initial drug concentration in plasma $[D_0]$ is: $[D_T] = [D_0] \cdot e^{-kT}$. The time that the drug concentration is reduced to half its original concentration is the "half-life" or $T_{1/2}$ of the drug. The $T_{1/2}$ is a function of the drug and the characteristics and conditions of the patient. For first-order kinetics, the drug concentration is reduced by the same *fraction* in the same length of time. For example, if the $T_{1/2}$ is 2 h, the drug concentration will be one-half the original concentration after 2 h, one-quarter the original concentration after 4 h (i.e., after another half-life), one-eighth the original concentration after 6 h, and so on. For other drugs (the minority, but including ethanol), the rate of elimination is described by zero-order kinetics: the rate of elimination is constant (and thus is independent of the drug concentration). The drug concentration is always reduced by the same *amount* in the same length of time. For example, if the $T_{1/2}$ is 2 h the drug concentration will be one-half the original concentration after 2 h and zero (theoretically) after 4 h.

Routes of Elimination

The most common route of elimination of drugs in humans without renal damage is the kidney, partly because the kidney receives between one-quarter and one-fifth of the blood pumped out of the heart every beat. Other sites include the lungs (particularly for gaseous anesthetics), feces, sweat, saliva, blood loss, vomit, breast milk, and so on.

Excretion via the Kidney. The rate of elimination is the net result of glomerular filtration, secretion, and reabsorption. Plasma proteins (and drug molecules bound to them) do not pass through the glomerulus of a healthy kidney. Lipophobic drug molecules tend to pass through the tubule and are excreted in the urine, whereas lipophilic drug molecules can cross the membrane at various portions along the tubule and are reabsorbed into the plasma. For drugs that are weak acids or weak bases, the degree of ionization of the drug (and hence its lipid solubility) is a function of the pH of the tubule contents. This phenomenon is exploited in treating cases of poisoning by a weak acid (by administration of a base such as sodium bicarbonate). Some drugs (organic acids and bases) are actively transported from the plasma into the tubule. The capacity of such transport processes is limited, giving rise to drug interactions and the well-known interference with uric acid excretion by aspirin and chemically related compounds.

SOME DRUGS AND DRUG CLASSES ACTIVELY SECRETED INTO TUBULES

Acetazolamide (Diamox, generic)
Amiloride (Midamor, generic)
Chlorothiazide (Diuril, others, generic)
Ethacrynic acid (Edecrin)
Furosemide (Lasix, others, generic)
Indomethacin (Indocin, others, generic)
Penicillins
Phenylbutazone
Probenecid (Benemid, generic)
Quinine
Salicyclic acid

In addition: quaternary ammonium compounds and glucuronide, glycine, and sulfate conjugate metabolites of drugs.

Clearance

The rate of elimination of a drug (units of mass per unit time) is equal to the drug concentration (mass per unit volume) times clearance (volume per unit time). Total body clearance is equal to the sum of the individual clearances from kidneys, liver, and so on. Renal plasma clearance is defined as the volume of plasma needed to supply the amount of a drug excreted in the urine in 1 minute. From a simple mass-balance (amount *in* per unit time equals amount *out* in unit time), the equation relating renal plasma clearance (Cl), rate of excretion (E), drug concentration in plasma (D_p), and drug concentration in urine (D_u) is: $Cl \cdot D_p = D_u \cdot E$.

Effect of Multiple Dosing

If the drug is administered according to a fixed-interval schedule, the rate of accumulation is predictable from the dose (D) and the half-life of the drug. For the case of repeated IV injections of a drug that has first-order elimination kinetics, if F is the fraction of drug remaining at the time of each injection, the upper bound (U) is given by $U = D/(1 - F)$, the lower bound (L) by $L = F \cdot U$; and the mean level (M) by $M = -D/\ln(F)$. For example, if 100 mg of a drug with a $T_{1/2}$ of 2 h was administered IV every 4 h, it would attain an upper bound of 133 mg, a lower bound of about 33 mg, and a mean of about 72 mg. If the time to reach a therapeutic range is too long, an initial "loading" or "priming" dose might be administered prior to the "maintenance" dosing schedule. The patient's individual characteristics determine the exact clinical results. For example, drug elimination can be accelerated by enzyme induction, by increase in urine flow, or by change in urine pH and can be slowed by renal impairment or by change in pH or other factors.

6 Pharmacokinetic Calculations

Cherng-ju Kim, Ph.D.

A Single dose (bolus) IV injection

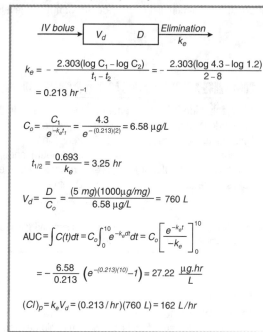

$$k_e = -\frac{2.303(\log C_1 - \log C_2)}{t_1 - t_2} = -\frac{2.303(\log 4.3 - \log 1.2)}{2 - 8}$$

$$= 0.213 \ hr^{-1}$$

$$C_o = \frac{C_1}{e^{-k_e t_1}} = \frac{4.3}{e^{-(0.213)(2)}} = 6.58 \ \mu g/L$$

$$t_{1/2} = \frac{0.693}{k_e} = 3.25 \ hr$$

$$V_d = \frac{D}{C_o} = \frac{(5 \ mg)(1000 \mu g/mg)}{6.58 \ \mu g/L} = 760 \ L$$

$$AUC = \int C(t)dt = C_o \int_0^{10} e^{-k_e t} dt = C_o \left[\frac{e^{-k_e t}}{-k_e} \right]_0^{10}$$

$$= -\frac{6.58}{0.213} \left(e^{-(0.213)(10)} - 1 \right) = 27.22 \ \frac{\mu g.hr}{L}$$

$$(Cl)_p = k_e V_d = (0.213 / hr)(760 \ L) = 162 \ L/hr$$

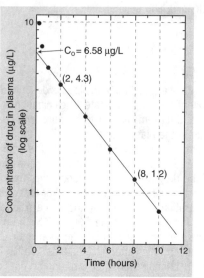

Plasma concentration of a drug as a function of time after IV injection of a single bolus (5 mg)

B Continuous IV infusion

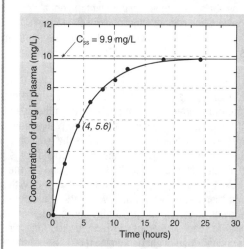

Plasma concentration of a drug for an IV infusion at 14 mg/hr for 24 hours

$$C(t) = \frac{k_o}{k_e V_d} (1 - e^{-k_e t}) = C_{ss}(1 - e^{-k_e t})$$

From the plot, $C_{ss} = 9.9 \ mg/L$

$$\frac{C(t_1)}{C_{ss}} = 1 - e^{-k_e t_1} = 1 - e^{-k_e(4)} = \frac{5.6}{9.9} = 0.57$$

$$k_e = \frac{2.303 \log(1 - 0.57)}{-4} = 0.21 \ hr^{-1}$$

$$t_{1/2} = \frac{0.693}{k_e} = \frac{0.693}{0.21 \ hr^{-1}} = 3.30 \ hr$$

$$V_d = \frac{k_o}{k_e C_{ss}} = \frac{14 \ mg/hr}{(0.21/hr)(9.9 \ mg/L)} = 6.73 \ L$$

Loading dose = $V_d C_{ss}$ = (67.3 L)(9.9 mg/L) = 67.0 mg
The concentration at 5 hours after the infusion is
stopped = $C_{ss} e^{-k_e t}$ = (9.9 mg/L)$e^{-(0.21)(5)}$ = 3.5 mg/L

OVERVIEW

- Pharmacokinetics is the study and quantitative description of the passage of a drug through the body and body compartments.
- The plasma concentration of drugs can be modeled (and predicted).
- The concentration-time profile is a function of the characteristics of the drug and the frequency of administration.

Pharmacokinetics

Pharmacokinetics is the study of the fate of a drug passing through the body and includes drug absorption, distribution, and elimination (i.e., metabolism and excretion). Factors that influence drug concentration in body fluids and tissues with time (plasma concentration–time curve) are considered here.

Single-dose IV Injection (Bolus). When a drug is administered as an IV bolus, the drug enters the body immediately and rapidly distributes throughout the circulatory system. The drug is eliminated from the plasma through excretion or biotransformation. The rate of decline of drug concentration in body fluids for most drugs is directly proportional to drug concentration remaining in the plasma expressed as:

$$\frac{dC(t)}{dt} = -k_e C(t) \tag{1}$$

where $C(t)$ is the drug concentration at time t, and k_e is the elimination rate constant. Integration of equation (1) yields:

$$C(t) = C_0 e^{-k_e t} \quad \text{or} \quad \log C(t) = \log C_0 - \frac{k_e t}{2.303} \tag{2}$$

From a plot of log $C(t)$ versus t, the slope ($-k_e/2.303$) and concentration intercept (log C_0) are obtained. The amount of drug distributed in the body cannot be measured directly because the actual volume of distribution is not known. Instead, an *apparent volume of distribution* (V_d) is used and can be calculated with the following equation:

$$V_d = \frac{D}{C_0} \tag{3}$$

where D is the dose. *Area under the curve* (AUC) represents the summation of the area under the plasma concentration–time curve from $t = 0$ to $t = \infty$

$$AUC = \int C(t)dt = C_0 \int_0^\infty e^{-k_e t} \, dt = \frac{C_0}{k_e} \tag{4}$$

Substituting equation (4) to equation (3) yields

$$V_d = \frac{D}{k_e AUC} \tag{5}$$

Amount of drug removed from the plasma for a given time interval ($dX(t)/dt$) is assumed to be proportional to the plasma concentration of drug:

$$\frac{dX(t)}{dt} = Cl_p C(t) \tag{6}$$

where Cl_p is the *total body clearance*. The rate of amount of drug removed ($dX(t)/dt$) is $k_e V_d C(t)$. The total body clearance can be determined by:

$$Cl_p = \frac{k_e V_d C(t)}{C(t)} = k_e V_d \tag{7}$$

Equation (7) shows that clearance is constant even though the plasma drug concentration and the rate of elimination decrease with time as long as the rate of elimination follows first-order kinetics.

Continuous IV Infusion. When the drug is administered by IV infusion, the plasma drug concentration versus time curve is obtained:

$$C(t) = \frac{k_0}{k_e V_d} (1 - e^{-k_e t}) \tag{8}$$

where k_0 is the infusion rate. At $t = \infty$, the steady-state concentration (C_{ss}) is expressed as:

$$C_{ss} = \frac{k_0}{k_e V_d} \tag{9}$$

When infusion and initial bolus are administered to achieve steady-state concentrations rapidly, one can determine the immediate loading dose (D_L) as:

$$D_L = \frac{k_0}{k_e}, \quad \text{or} \quad D_L = C_{ss} V_d \tag{10}$$

Mechanisms of Drug Action
Robert B. Raffa, Ph.D.

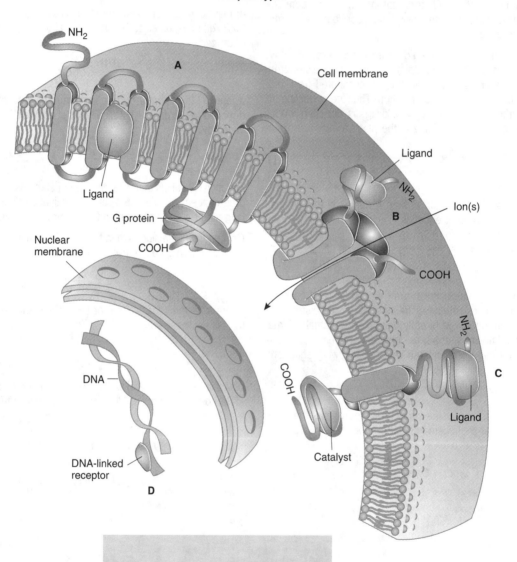

Receptor types

NH₂

A

Cell membrane

Ligand

Ligand

NH₂

G protein

Ion(s)

COOH

B

Nuclear
membrane

COOH

NH₂

DNA

C

Ligand

DNA-linked
receptor

COOH

D

Catalyst

A	G-protein–coupled receptor
B	Receptor-operated ion channel
C	Receptor that is an enzyme
D	DNA-linked receptor

OVERVIEW

- Drugs can be directed at external threats (invading organisms), internal threats (neoplasms), or at normal physiologic processes.
- Sites of drug action can be relatively nonspecific or directed at precise molecular targets (e.g., enzymes, DNA molecules, or receptors).
- Receptors transduce the signal from drug molecule to intracellular biochemical reactions (thus mimicking or antagonizing the action of an endogenous substance).
- The mechanisms by which receptors transduce the signal form the basis of classification of receptors into inotropic (related to changes in conductance of ion channels) or metabotropic (related to activation of biochemical second messengers).
- The degree of selectivity for a particular mechanism (site of action) determines a drug's therapeutic and side-effect profile.

Destruction of Invading Organisms

The goal is to target some aspect of the invading organism's anatomy or physiology that renders it susceptible but at the same time does not affect a critical component of human physiology. The greater this separation, the greater is the safety margin of the drug. Typical targets include the invading organism's cell walls or organism-specific biochemical reactions. In addition, drugs can enhance the body's immune defense mechanisms against such organisms.

Destruction of Own Cells

As in the case of invading organisms, the strategy involves targeting some aspect of the aberrant (cancer) cells that differentiates them from healthy ones. Among the many techniques used is interference with rapidly dividing cells (such as those in some tumors). Typical side effects of such drugs (or radiation) involve effects on rapidly dividing normal cells, such as hair and the GI tract (resulting in hair loss and GI upset). Another technique involves targeted delivery of drug to the tumor mass (such as intraarterial injection near the tumor site) or exploitation of differences in molecules expressed on the cell surface to produce polyclonal or monoclonal antibody drugs or drug carriers. The requirement of neoplasms for growth of new blood supplies renders them susceptible to drugs that inhibit the development of new blood vessels (angioneogenesis). In the absence of very high selectivity, drug doses must be large, with concomitant toxicity and side effects.

Modifiers of Ongoing Physiologic Processes

The chemical nature of cellular function and intra- and intercellular communication allows for intervention with drug molecules that supply substrate material or that mimic or antagonize the normal ongoing physiologic processes. The targets of such intervention include enzymes, DNA molecules, and other cellular components. Perhaps the simplest agents of drug therapy are those that counteract high acidity (large H^+ concentration) in the stomach and upper GI tract by chemically neutralizing the acid (antacids).

Major sites of the selective interaction between drug molecule and cell are specialized molecules that stereoselectively recognize signal molecules and transduce the signal into the cell interior by a series of coupled biochemical reactions. These molecules possess a three-dimensional structure sufficiently similar to the endogenous material to allow the drug molecule to "fit" into the same receptor molecule as the endogenous material and to either mimic its effects by activating the receptor or to antagonize its action by impeding the access of the endogenous substance to the receptor site.

Receptor Classification (Receptor Superfamilies)

Ligands (drugs) bind to (have affinity for) and activate (agonists) or inhibit (antagonists) receptor function to a degree that depends on the compounds' intrinsic activity (efficacy). The overall effect depends on whether the drug is an antagonist (has affinity, but zero efficacy), is a "full" or "partial" agonist (has affinity and efficacy), or is a direct (same) or inverse (opposite effect to the endogenous ligand) agonist. The effect is a function of the drug's concentration, affinity, and efficacy.

Multiple receptor types exist on most cells, and cells are usually under the influence of multiple endogenous ligands. Likewise, there is extensive intracellular cross talk among the various receptor systems and second-messenger pathways. Chronic administration of a drug can alter the control system's "set-point."

Ion-channel–linked. These receptors consist of transmembrane portions that form pores of sufficient size to allow passage of ions. The receptor is normally selective for a particular ion (typically Na^+, K^+, Cl^-, or Ca^{2+}). Ion flux results in hypo- or hyperpolarization of the cell (e.g., cardiac or neuronal tissue). The receptor can be composed of subunits that are expressed or coupled in different ways and hence mediate multiple effects. Ligands that have affinity for these receptors can modify the degree of opening of the ion pore.

G-protein–linked. These receptors consist of seven membrane-spanning (transmembrane) regions with an N-terminal extracellular region and a C-terminal intracellular one. The ligand recognition site can be in one or more of the extracellular, transmembrane, or intracellular regions. Receptor activation results in conformational change, GDP-GTP exchange, modulation of adenylate cyclase activity (conversion of ATP to cAMP), and other intracellular actions, such as activation of the DAG and IP_3 pathways. There are multiple G-protein subtypes.

Enzyme-linked. These receptors span the membrane and possess an intracellular catalytic domain that functions as an enzyme. Examples include receptors for growth factors and insulin (tyrosine kinases).

DNA-linked. These receptors consist of portions of the DNA molecule, and activation or inhibition influences protein (enzyme, receptor, etc.) production and regulation.

Other Mechanisms

- Chelating agents contain metal atoms that form chemical bonds with toxins or drugs. The complex is generally inactive.
- Antimetabolites masquerade as endogenous substances and are incorporated into biosynthetic pathways but result in end products that are inactive or less active than the endogenous substrate.
- Irritants alleviate local pain associated with aching muscles.
- Replacement therapy is used to correct deficiencies in essential biochemical substances (e.g., vitamins, minerals, hormones).

Drug Receptors and Signaling

Sandra C. Roerig, Ph.D.

A Two signaling pathways regulated by G-protein-coupled receptors

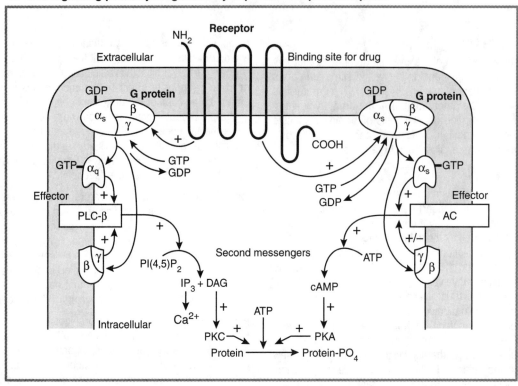

B Signaling regulated by ion channels

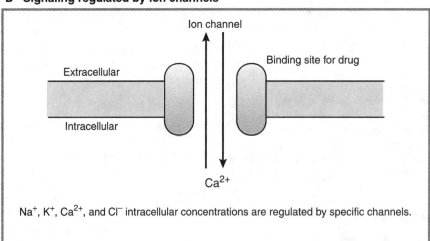

Na^+, K^+, Ca^{2+}, and Cl^- intracellular concentrations are regulated by specific channels.

G-Protein–Coupled Receptors

Some drug and endogenous transmitter ligands bind to specific *receptor proteins* found in the cell plasma membrane. Some of these receptors are composed of seven transmembrane regions, a glycosylated extracellular amino terminal region, and an intracellular carboxy-terminal region. Drugs that bind to the same receptors as the endogenous ligands mimic the effects of those ligands (e.g., morphine activates μ opioid receptors).

Receptor Structure. This family includes receptors for *nonpeptides*: norepinephrine and epinephrine ($\alpha_{1,2}$- and β_{1-3}-adrenergic receptors), dopamine (DA_{1-5}), serotonin ($5\text{-}HT_{1-5}$), acetylcholine (muscarinic, $M_{1,2}$), histamine (H_{1-3}), adenosine (A_{1-3}), purines ($P2Y_{1-6}$), γ-amino butyric acid ($GABA_B$), glutamate ($mGlu_{1-8}$), melatonin, leukotrienes ($LT_{B,D}$), and 11-*cis*-retinol (rhodopsin and other opsins); and *peptides*: opioids (μ,δ,κ), somatostatin (SS_{1-4}), cholecystokinin ($CCK_{A,B}$), angiotensin ($AT_{1A,B}$), bradykinin (B_{1-3}), tachykinins (NK_{1-3}), interleukin-8 ($IL8R_{A,B}$), thyroid and parathyroid hormones, neurotensin, thrombin, follicle-stimulating hormone (FSH), leutinizing hormone (LH), glucagon, neuropeptide Y ($Y_{1,2}$), vasopressin ($V_{1,2}$), adrenocorticotropic hormone (ACTH), and many others.

G-protein Structure. These receptors associate with heterotrimeric (α-, β-, and γ-subunits) guanine-nucleotide-binding proteins (*G proteins*). Binding of an agonist ligand to its receptor initiates activation of the associated G proteins by GTP-GDP exchange, which then stimulates the dissociation of the α- from the $\beta\gamma$-subunits. GTPase activity of the α-subunit promotes reassociation of the heterotrimer and terminates the reaction. Subunits in the G-protein family are classified according to the amino acid sequence and activity of the free α-subunit. Subunits include $\alpha_{t1,2}$, α_s, α_{i1-3}, $\alpha_{oA,B}$, α_q, α_{olf}, $\alpha_{x/z}$, α_g, and α_{11-16}. The $\beta\gamma$-subunits (β_{1-4} and γ_{1-7}) also have activity that is separate from that of the α-subunits. A single receptor can activate more than one type of G protein.

Effector Targets of G Proteins. The activated G-protein subunits transduce the agonist-induced signal from the receptor to a variety of *effector proteins* that are located in the plasma membrane or intracellularly. Effectors include:

- adenylyl cyclase (AC)
- phospholipase Cβ and γ (PLCβ,γ)
- cGMP-dependent phosphodiesterase (cGMP-PDE)
- phospholipase D (PLD)
- phospholipase A_2 (PLA$_2$)
- Na^+, K^+, and Ca^{2+} channels.

Specific G proteins affect specific effectors; for example, α_S stimulates AC, α_q stimulates PLCβ (see Fig.).

Role of Second Messengers. The effectors change the concentration of intracellular *second messengers* that activate specific *target proteins* such as cAMP-dependent protein kinase (PKA) and protein kinase C (PKC), which in turn catalyze the *phosphorylation* of numerous intracellular proteins, thereby altering their activity. Alteration of ion channel activity changes the intracellular ion concentrations to alter the cell *membrane potential* and *activity of intracellular enzymes*. Intracellular messengers include cAMP, IP_3, DAG, and leukotrienes; ions include Na^+, K^+, and Ca^{2+}.

These events constitute cascades of signal amplification; that is, activation of one receptor can produce multiple intracellular signaling events that can, in turn, regulate each other's actions.

Ion Channels

Some drugs and endogenous transmitters bind to transmembrane proteins that form a pore, which allows passage of specific mono- and divalent ions. Each pore consists of multiple, separate, subunit proteins assembled in defined patterns. Ions regulated by these receptors include Na^+, K^+, Ca^{2+}, and Cl^-. Binding of a ligand produces a conformational change in the target protein that changes the conformation of the pore to either increase or decrease ion transport 3 (see Fig.). Changes in intracellular ion concentrations alter the membrane potential to either increase or decrease the excitability of the cell.

Extracellular Ion Channels

These channels are expressed in the plasma membrane.

Ligand-gated Ion Channels. These ion channels are regulated by binding of certain transmitters and drugs. This family of channels includes nicotinic, cholinergic, ionotropic glutamate (*N*-methyl D-aspartate, AMPA, kainate), $GABA_A$, serotonin ($5\text{-}HT_3$), purine ($P2x_{1-7}$,z), and glycine receptors and channels that are activated by cyclic nucleotides, cAMP and cGMP. Drugs bind to sites on these channels to affect channel activity; for example, barbiturates bind to a site on the $GABA_A$ receptor to enhance Cl^- transport and decrease cellular excitability.

Voltage-gated Ion Channels. These ion channels are normally regulated by the membrane potential of the cell. This family includes Ca^{2+}, Na^+, K^+, and Cl^- channels, each of which has multiple subtypes with defined properties. Drugs such as nifedipine block the activity of voltage-gated Ca^{2+} channels.

Intracellular Ion Channels

These ion channels are expressed in intracellular organelles such as sarcoplasmic reticulum, endoplasmic reticulum, mitochondria, and others. Intracellular Ca^{2+} is regulated by Ca^{2+} channels that are sensitive to IP_3, ryanodine, and LTC_4. Intracellular K^+ channels are regulated by arachidonic acid and Na^+. Other intracellular cation channels are regulated by cyclic nucleotides cAMP and cGMP. An example of an agent that affects activity of intracellular Ca^{2+} channels is caffeine.

Tyrosine Kinase Receptors

Some hormones and drugs bind to receptors that contain an extracellular ligand-binding domain, a single transmembrane domain, and an intracellular domain that has tyrosine kinase activity. When activated by ligands such as insulin, nerve growth factor, platelet-derived growth factor, or other growth factors, these receptors catalyze the *phosphorylation of target proteins* important in cellular growth and differentiation.

Steroid Hormone Receptors

Steroid hormones, thyroid hormone, corticosteroids, vitamin D, and retinoids diffuse through the plasma membrane and bind to their respective intracellular receptors. These receptors act as transcription factors by binding to DNA hormone response elements in the nucleus, thus regulating *gene transcription*. Drugs can bind to and modulate the activity of these same receptors. For example, tamoxifen binds to the estrogen receptor and acts as an estrogen antagonist.

Dose-Response Curves:
Efficacy, Potency, and Therapeutic Index   Ronald J. Tallarida, Ph.D.

9

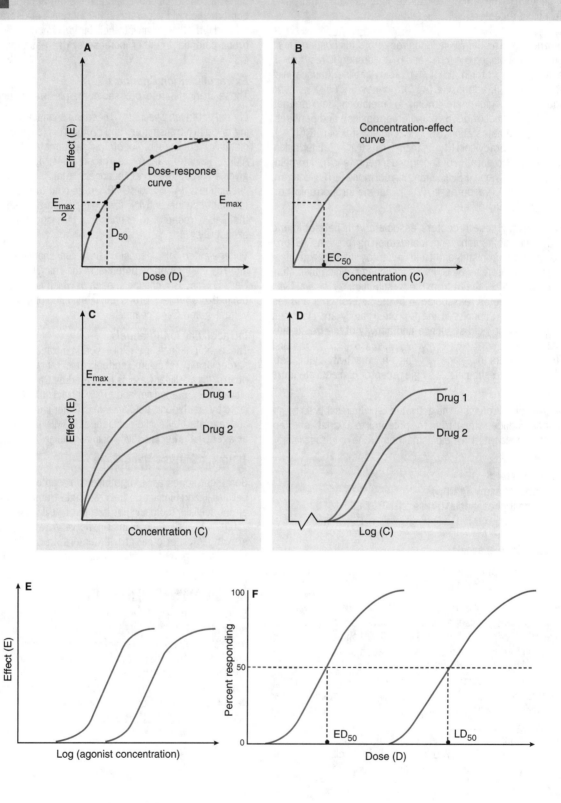

Main Ideas

Drug effects occur over time after administration and usually reach a dose-dependent peak level. These effects fade in time because the drug leaves the body. The peak (equilibrium) effect (E) is often associated with the dose (D) that produced it. The relation between E and D is illustrated in Fig. A. The smooth curve representing the plotted points is the dose-response curve. If plasma concentration (C) instead of dose, is plotted on the horizontal axis, a concentration–effect curve is obtained (Fig. B). The increase in the magnitude of the effect with increasing drug dosage or concentration indicates that the effect is graded. Fig. A, shows a graded dose–effect curve. A point (P) denotes the equilibrium effect produced by dose (D). In Fig. B, each dose results in a concentration (e.g., in plasma), which may be plotted on the horizontal axis to yield a concentration–effect curve. The drug concentration that produces an effect equal to 50% of the maximum (E_{max}) is an indicator of the drug's potency. A drug capable of producing E_{max} is termed a *full agonist*.

Efficacy

An effect refers to a change in some characteristic (e.g., blood pressure, heart rate) that is altered by the drug. In general, the magnitude of the drug-induced effect increases as the dose or concentration increases and ultimately approaches a maximum. The maximum effect of the drug is a measure of its efficacy. Usually there is an upper limit of effect (E_{max}), a limit not attained by all drugs even at their highest doses. Accordingly, different drugs with overtly similar actions may differ in efficacy. Drugs achieving E_{max} are termed *full agonists*, while those agonists whose maximal effect is detectable but less than E_{max} are termed *partial agonists* (Fig. C). Viewed as a receptor phenomenon, a partial agonist does not give the system a maximal effect even with full occupation of its cellular receptors. In contrast, a full agonist may achieve the maximal effect with only a fraction of its receptors occupied, that is, there are spare receptors. Fig. C shows a graded concentration–effect curve of drug 1 and drug 2. With sufficiently high concentrations, drug 1 attains level E_{max} and is a full agonist, whereas drug 2, which cannot produce E_{max} at any concentration, is a partial agonist; drug 2 has lower efficacy than drug 1. When the horizontal axis is calibrated in units of log (concentration), the shape of the curve changes to sigmoidal (Fig. D). Concentrations such as 10^{-7}, 10^{-6}, and 10^{-5} become -7, -6, -5, on the logarithmic scale.

Potency

The concentration–effect curve indicates the concentration at which a specific level of effect (at equilibrium) is obtained. Potency refers to how much (dose or concentration) is needed to attain the effect specified. Often the focus is on an effect level equal to 50% of the maximum. The concentration for a drug with sufficient efficacy to reach the 50% effect level is denoted by *EC50* (see Figs. A and B). This value is therefore an indication of the drug's potency. A low value of EC50 means high potency.

Antagonists

An antagonist is a drug that reduces or abolishes the effect of an active drug or endogenous substance. Different mechanisms may account for the antagonism. For example, ACh (and drugs that mimic it) slow the heart rate by acting on the SA node, whereas norepinephrine (and similar drugs) increase the heart rate. Each drug is efficacious after combination with its receptor, but the expression of these effects is in opposite directions so that administration of either one reduces the effect of the other. This type of antagonism is often termed *functional* or *physiologic*. In contrast, an antagonist drug that lacks efficacy exerts its antagonism by competing for the same receptor that is stimulated by the active drug or compound. In this case, termed *pharmacologic* or *competitive* antagonism, both compounds have affinity for a single receptor site. When the antagonist and an agonist are present together, the magnitude of the effect depends on the degree of receptor occupancy of the agonist, which in turn depends on the concentration or dose of the antagonist (Fig. E). In Fig. E the log (concentration)–effect curve of an agonist (curve 1) is displaced to the right (curve 2) in the presence of a fixed concentration of a competitive antagonist. The degree of rightward shift depends on the antagonist concentration but still reaches the same maximum as curve 1 with sufficiently high agonist concentration; thus the antagonism is reversible. Beta-blockers, such as propranolol, are competitive antagonists of norepinephrine and epinephrine at cardiac beta-receptors and thus slow the heart rate.

Quantal Dose–Effect Relations

Drug action may be expressed by specifying a particular level of effect and determining, by experiment, the percentage of subjects that achieve this effect level as a function of dose. In illustrating this relation ("quantal" or "all-or-none") the vertical axis is percent and horizontal axis represents the dose (Fig. F). The dose that is effective in 50% of subjects is termed *ED50*. When death is the effect, the dose that is lethal in 50% of subjects is termed *LD50*. The ratio, LD50:ED50, is commonly termed the *therapeutic index*, though other ratios, such as LD1:ED50, may also be used. In Fig. F the quantal dose–effect curve indicates the percentage of subjects that experience a specified level of effect (curve 1) as a function of dose and the percentage in whom the drug action is lethal (curve 2). The common therapeutic index is the ratio LD50:ED50.

PART I: QUESTIONS

Directions: For each of the following questions, choose the **one best** answer.

1. At which step in the following sequence of drug names is United States Adopted Name (USAN) Council approval needed?

(A) Chemical name

(B) Nonproprietary (generic) name

(C) First proprietary (trade) name

(D) Second trade name

2. Of the following mechanisms by which drugs produce toxic or other adverse effects, which one requires substitution for endogenous substances?

(A) Cytotoxicity

(B) Receptor activation

(C) Antimetabolite

(D) Chelation

3. Which of the following statements concerning zero-order kinetics of elmination of a drug from plasma is true?

(A) It is more common than those showing first-order kinetics.

(B) Plasma concentration decreases in proportion to its concentration in plasma.

(C) The half-life is independent of initial dose.

(D) The relationship between drug concentration and time is exponential.

(E) A constant amount of drug is eliminated per unit time.

4. Phase 1 metabolism of drugs is carried out by enzymes throughout the body. The primary sites of phase 1 metabolism are the kidneys, gut wall, liver, and

(A) adrenal glands

(B) pancreas

(C) skin

(D) bone marrow

(E) lungs

5. Which of the following terms is used to describe a type of dose–response curve?

(A) Pharmacologic

(B) Physiologic

(C) Quantal

(D) Chemical

(E) Functional

6. An example of an enteral route of drug administration is

(A) intramuscular

(B) intravenous

(C) subcutaneous

(D) transdermal patch

(E) rectal suppository

7. Official sources of information about drugs and drug use that are recognized in the United States include the

(A) *Medical Letter* and *American Drug Index*

(B) *Physician's Desk Reference* (*PDR*) and *National Formulary*

(C) *United States Pharmacopeia* and *National Formulary*

(D) *United States Pharmacopeia* and *PDR*

8. Drugs given by IV infusion attain 90% of the steady state concentrations by

(A) $3.3 \times$ half-life

(B) one half-life

(C) $0.693 \div$ half-life

(D) bioavailability $\div$ half-life

9. If a drug with a half-life of 4 hours has a plasma level of 12.5 ng/mL 12 hours after administration of a single dose, the initial plasma level was

(A) 25 ng/mL

(B) 37.5 ng/mL

(C) 50 ng/mL

(D) 100 ng/mL

10. The equation for apparent volume of distribution is

(A) $V_d = D + C_0$

(B) $V_d = D - C_0$

(C) $V_d = D \cdot C_0$

(D) $V_d = D \div C_0$

11. The bioavailability of a drug that is administered orally can be decreased by

(A) increased blood flow to GI tract

(B) delayed gastric emptying

(C) unscarred damage to stomach lining

(D) food in the stomach

12. The mechanism of action of barbiturates to decrease neuronal excitability is through

(A) stimulation of a G-protein–coupled receptor to decrease intracellular cAMP

(B) direct stimulation of an inhibitory G protein

(C) binding to a site on the $GABA_A$ receptor

(D) inhibition of a Ca^{2+} channel

13. Which of the following statements about the total body clearance of a drug that follows first-order kinetics of elimination is true?

(A) It decreases as drug concentration in plasma decreases.

(B) It decreases as the rate of elimination decreases.

(C) It remains constant.

(D) It increases as drug concentration in plasma decreases.

14. Which EC50 represents the most potent drug?

(A) EC50 = 1

(B) EC50 = 10

(C) EC50 = log (100)

(D) EC50 = 10^{-1}

15. Plasma proteins that extensively bind many drugs include

(A) hemoglobin and cytochrome P-450

(B) albumin and α_1-acid glycoprotein

(C) α_2-macroglobulin and transcortin

(D) fibrinogen and thrombin

(E) insulin and growth hormone

16. Which mechanism of drug action most closely mimics neurotransmitter or hormone action?

(A) Cytotoxicity

(B) Receptor activation

(C) Neutralization of acid

(D) Chelation

17. Oral bioavailability is a relative measure of systemic exposure comparing oral administration to

(A) intravenous administration

(B) intraperitoneal administration

(C) intramuscular administration

(D) subcutaneous administration

(E) topical administration

18. Alkalinization of the stomach decreases gastric absorption of

(A) weak acid

(B) weak base

(C) uncharged drug

19. Propranolol, a β-adrenergic receptor antagonist used therapeutically for its actions in the cardiovascular system, acts by

(A) blocking the actions of epinephrine and norepinephrine at a G-protein–coupled receptor

(B) stimulating a ligand-gated ion channel to decrease intracellular Ca^{2+}

(C) directly inhibiting the stimulatory G protein, G_s

(D) selectively blocking β_1-adrenergic receptors

20. Which of the following statements concerning first-order kinetics of elimination of a drug from plasma is true?

(A) The half-life is proportional to the concentration in the plasma.

(B) The fraction of drug eliminated per unit time is constant.

(C) The rate of elimination is constant.

(D) A drug with a $T_{1/2}$ of 2 hours is eliminated more slowly than a drug with a $T_{1/2}$ of 4 hours.

(E) A plot of drug concentration in plasma versus time is a straight line.

21. Drugs administered by the oral route may undergo extensive metabolism by the liver or gut wall prior to entering the systemic circulation. This process can significantly decrease the bioavailability of the drug relative to IV administration. This is called

(A) phase 1 metabolism

(B) phase 2 metabolism

(C) enterohepatic circulation

(D) first-pass effect

(E) biotransformation

PART I: ANSWERS AND EXPLANATIONS

1. The answer is B.

A drug's chemical name is determined by convention of an international committee; the nonproprietary name (sometimes called the generic name) and the one or more proprietary (trade) names require approval by the USAN Council, which consists of, or receives input from, the United States Pharmacopeial Convention, the American Pharmaceutical Association, the AMA, the FDA, and sometimes the WHO.

2. The answer is C.

All of the choices in the questions represent possible mechanisms by which drugs might produce deleterious effects. Receptor activation can modulate the system away from the normal homeostasis in a detrimental direction. Antimetabolites substitute for endogenous substances and become incorporated into biosynthetic pathways but can result in end-products that are less active than the endogenous substrate. Chelating agents can bind to beneficial or necessary cell components. Cytotoxic agents selectively perform destructive action on cells.

3. The answer is E.

In the case of zero-order kinetics, the drug concentration is always reduced by the same amount in the same length of time. For example, if the drug concentration decreases by one-quarter in 2 hours, then it will decrease by the same amount (not fraction) in each subsequent 2-hour interval. Zero-order elimination of drugs is less common than first-order elimination. In zero-order kinetics the rate of elimination is a constant and, thus, a plot of drug concentration versus time is linear, not exponential. A half-life ($T_{1/2}$) can be designated, but it is a function of the initial drug dose.

4. The answer is E.

The lungs are a primary site of phase 1 metabolism. Drugs administered by inhalation or in the blood may be metabolized and expired from the lungs. Once the drug has become more polar, via phase 1 metabolism, it can be excreted into the bile or urine and expelled from the body. No phase 1 metabolism has been found in the skin, bone marrow, adrenal glands, or pancreas.

5. The answer is C.

Quantal, or "all-or-none," refers to a particular way of measuring drug effect. The other terms listed in the question are types of drug antagonism. An antagonist reduces the effect of a drug or endogenous substance. The reduction can be produced by blocking a receptor, eliciting an opposite effect, or by chemical neutralization.

6. The answer is E.

The enteral routes of administration include oral, sublingual, and rectal. The other choices listed in the question (i.e., intramuscular, intravenous, subcutaneous, and transdermal routes) are all parenteral routes of drug administration.

7. The answer is C.

Both the *United States Pharmacopeia* and the *National Formulary* were given official status in 1906 as part of the Federal Food, Drug, and Cosmetics Act. The *Medical Letter on Drugs and Therapeutics*, the *American Drug Index*, and the *PDR* are excellent sources of information about drugs and drug use, but they do not have the same official status as the *United States Pharmacopeia* and the *National Formulary*.

8. The answer is A.

It takes 3.3 half-lives for a drug to reach 90% of the concentration at steady state during an IV infusion. It is also possible to predict the amount of time it takes to eliminate 90% of the drug (3.3 times half-life). The half-life increases or decreases depending on several factors including enzyme induction, enzyme inhibition, coadministration of other drugs. One half-life is the amount of time required for 50% of the drug in the systemic circulation to be reduced by the body. The elimination constant is derived from 0.693 divided by half-life. Half-life is determined by renal function and the levels of drug-metabolizing enzymes.

9. The answer is D.

The initial dose is reduced by one-half (to 50 ng/mL) at the end of 4 hours (its plasma half-life). It is reduced by another one-half (to 25 ng/mL) at the end of 8 hours and another one-half (to 12.5 ng/mL) at the end of 12 hours.

10. The answer is D.

The amount of drug that is distributed in the body cannot be measured directly because the actual volume of distribution is not known. An estimate, known as the apparent volume of distribution (V_d), is calculated as the ratio of the dose (D) to concentration (C_0). Options A, B, and C cannot be correct because in these equations the units (mass and volume) do not balance.

11. The answer is D.

Drug molecules can be sequestered by foodstuffs and delayed from entering the bloodstream. Increased blood flow to the GI tract, delayed gastric emptying (increased contact time), and injury to the stomach lining (unimpeded passage of drug) would accelerate passage into the systemic circulation and, hence, increase bioavailability of an orally administered drug.

12. The answer is C.

The $GABA_A$ receptor is a ligand-gated Cl^- channel. Stimulation of this receptor by GABA increases Cl^- conductance to decrease neuronal excitability. Barbiturates bind to an allosteric site on the $GABA_A$ receptor to potentiate the actions of GABA, thereby further decreasing neuronal excitability. Barbiturates do not directly stimulate G-protein–coupled receptors or G proteins. Barbiturates do not affect the activity of Ca^{2+} channels.

13. The answer is C.

The total body clearance (Cl_p) of a drug that follows first-order kinetics of elimination is the product of the elimination rate constant (k_e) and the apparent volume of distribution (V_d): $Cl_p = k_e \cdot V_d$. Hence, Cl_p remains constant despite the decrease in plasma concentration and the decrease in rate of elimination.

14. The answer is D.

The potency of a drug is the amount of drug required to produce some specified level of effect. The smaller the amount required, the greater the potency. 10^{-1} (= 0.1) is the smallest amount (dose or concentration). Choices A, B, and C cannot be correct because all of these numbers are greater than 0.1.

15. The answer is B.

Albumin and α_1-acid glycoprotein are the main proteins that extensively bind drugs in the plasma. This binding can decrease the unbound drug available to act pharmacologically and to be metabolized. Highly protein-bound drugs may require higher doses to achieve the desired blood levels of free drug. The remaining proteins listed have little or no binding capacity.

16. The answer is B.

All of the choices represent possible mechanisms of action of drugs. Receptor activation is the mechanism of action of a variety of drugs that mimic normal homeostatic processes mediated by neurotransmitter and hormone action. Cytotoxicity is the mechanism of action of drugs that are directed either against invading organisms, such as bacteria, viruses, protozoa, fungi, and worms (helminths), or against aberrant internal cells, such as neoplasms. Neutralization of acid is the mechanism of action shared by the more common antacids (but not the histamine H_2 receptor antagonists). Chelating agents contain metal atoms that can form chemical bonds with other molecules, such as toxins, generally inactivating the toxin.

17. The answer is A.

Bioavailability relates an extravascular dose to an IV dose. This is a way to select the best method of dose administration. The amount of the extravascular dose required to attain a similar blood level is directly proportional to the bioavailability. Intramuscular, intraperitoneal, subcutaneous, and topical are all extravascular routes; therefore, they would be related to an IV dose to calculate bioavailability.

18. **The answer is A.**

A weak acid is described by the equation HA $\leftrightarrow$ H$^+$ + A$^-$. Alkalinization (decreasing H$^+$) would shift the equilibrium of a weak acid to the right, that is, to the ionized form. The ionized form is less lipid soluble and, hence, less readily passes through the stomach lining (membranes).

19. **The answer is A.**

Propranolol binds to the β-adrenergic receptor and prevents binding of epinephrine and norepinephrine to the receptor. Because propranolol is an antagonist, it does not activate the receptor; thus, it blocks the actions of the neurotransmitters. Propranolol does not directly stimulate a ligand-gated ion channel, nor does it inhibit a G protein. Propranolol is nonselective; that is, it blocks both β$_1$ and β$_2$ receptors.

20. **The answer is B.**

In first-order elimination kinetics, the half-life of a drug is a constant for that particular drug and for the conditions of the patient at the time of drug administration, the fraction eliminated per time is constant, the rate of drug elimination is proportional to the amount of drug remaining, and the plot of drug concentration versus time would be an exponential decay, not a straight line.

21. **The answer is D.**

This is the first-pass effect of the liver or gut wall on drugs that enter the portal circulation prior to entering the systemic circulation. The liver or gut wall metabolizes the drug from the portal circulation and reduces the amount systemically available. This is a significant point with drugs administered orally. Phase 1 metabolism increases thte polarity of the molecule. Phase 2 metabolism conjugates polar molecules. Enterohepatic circulation involves drugs being metabolized in the liver, excreted in the bile, and reabsolved in the gut following hydrolysis. Any changes made to a molecule by an organism (e.g., oxidation, reduction, conjugation) is biotransformation.

PART II
Autonomic and Somatic Nervous Systems Pharmacology

10 Central Neurotransmitters

Robert B. McCall, Ph.D.

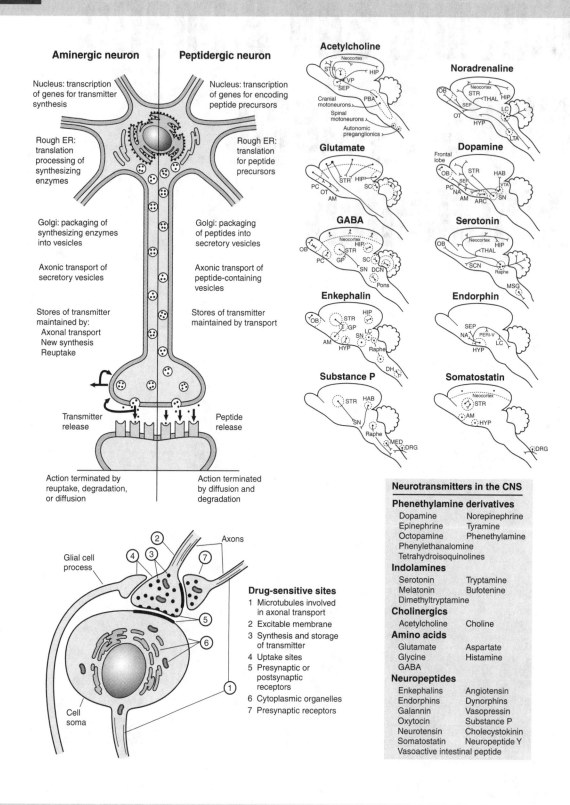

Aminergic neuron

Nucleus: transcription of genes for transmitter synthesis

Rough ER: translation processing of synthesizing enzymes

Golgi: packaging of synthesizing enzymes into vesicles

Axonic transport of secretory vesicles

Stores of transmitter maintained by:
Axonal transport
New synthesis
Reuptake

Transmitter release

Action terminated by reuptake, degradation, or diffusion

Peptidergic neuron

Nucleus: transcription of genes for encoding peptide precursors

Rough ER: translation for peptide precursors

Golgi: packaging of peptides into secretory vesicles

Axonic transport of peptide-containing vesicles

Stores of transmitter maintained by transport

Peptide release

Action terminated by diffusion and degradation

Acetylcholine
Noradrenaline
Glutamate
Dopamine
GABA
Serotonin
Enkephalin
Endorphin
Substance P
Somatostatin

Glial cell process

Axons

Cell soma

Drug-sensitive sites
1. Microtubules involved in axonal transport
2. Excitable membrane
3. Synthesis and storage of transmitter
4. Uptake sites
5. Presynaptic or postsynaptic receptors
6. Cytoplasmic organelles
7. Presynaptic receptors

Neurotransmitters in the CNS

Phenethylamine derivatives
Dopamine	Norepinephrine
Epinephrine	Tyramine
Octopamine	Phenethylamine
Phenylethanalomine	
Tetrahydroisoquinolines	

Indolamines
Serotonin	Tryptamine
Melatonin	Bufotenine
Dimethyltryptamine	

Cholinergics
Acetylcholine	Choline

Amino acids
Glutamate	Aspartate
Glycine	Histamine
GABA	

Neuropeptides
Enkephalins	Angiotensin
Endorphins	Dynorphins
Galannin	Vasopressin
Oxytocin	Substance P
Neurotensin	Cholecystokinin
Somatostatin	Neuropeptide Y
Vasoactive intestinal peptide	

- Criteria for establishing a substance as a neurotransmitter include: (1) presence of the chemical and its synthetic enzymes or transport system in the neuron, (2) stimulation of afferents releases the chemical, (3) direct application of the putative neurotransmitter at a synapse mimics the effects of physiologic stimulation, and (4) inactivating mechanisms exist to terminate action at a synapse.
- Neurotransmitters can be divided arbitrarily into three groups: amino acids, acetylcholine and the monoamines, and peptides.

Amino Acid Neurotransmitters

Amino acid neurotransmitters include GABA, glycine, glutamate, aspartate, and taurine. GABA-containing neurons constitute approximately 50% of neurons in the CNS and GABA is the primary inhibitory neurotransmitter in the brain. GABA is found in small interneurons (e.g., dorsal horn and cerebellar interneurons) and long-projecting neurons such as those projecting from the striatum to the substantia nigra. GABA's inhibitory action is fast, mediated via changes in chloride conductance. Glycine is also an inhibitory transmitter found primarily in the brainstem and spinal cord. Glutamate and aspartate are excitatory neurotransmitters. Glutamate receptors are classified as either NMDA or non-NMDA receptors depending on their responsiveness to the glutamate agonist N-methyl-D-aspartate. Non-NMDA receptors allow sodium and potassium to flow down their electrochemical gradient and mediate a fast, rapidly decaying current. NMDA receptors carry little current unless the membrane is depolarized and provide a means for calcium entry to the neuron. NMDA receptors play an important role in cortical processes of learning and memory.

Acetylcholine and the Monoamines

Acetylcholine. ACh was the first compound identified as a central neurotransmitter. Responses to ACh are mediated via nicotinic and muscarinic receptors and include an increase in nonspecific cation conductance, increases or decreases in potassium conductance, and a decrease in calcium conductance. Cholinergic neurons are scattered throughout the brain and innervate most regions of the CNS. Cholinergic neurons are important in learning, memory, and cognition, and agents that increase ACh enhance learning and memory.

Monoamines. The monoamine neurotransmitters include dopamine, norepinephrine, epinephrine, serotonin, and histamine. Monoamine neurons are relatively few in number and their cell bodies are clustered in discrete brainstem nuclei. However, monoamine neurons are characterized by extensive arborization so that their axons supply virtually all areas of the brain. These characteristics allow monoaminergic neurons to modulate synaptic activity simultaneously in widespread areas of the brain. Norepinephrine neurons are located primarily in the ventrolateral medulla and the locus caeruleus and regulate attention, arousal, and the sleep-wake cycle. Serotonin neurons are localized to raphe nuclei found along the midline of the brainstem. These neurons project to all areas of the brain and spinal cord and are involved in arousal, the sleep-wake cycle, autonomic regulation, and motor control. Dopaminergic neurons are located in the brainstem and project primarily to the basal ganglia and to cortical areas. Progressive degeneration of dopamine neurons in substantia nigra is the most prominent feature of Parkinson's disease. Alteration in dopaminergic function has also been associated with schizophrenia.

Peptide Neurotransmitters

Peptides, originally identified in the enteric nervous system of the gut, are widely distributed in brain and spinal cord neurons. Unlike classical neurotransmitters, peptides are synthesized from large polypeptide prehormones in the rough endoplasmic reticulum and transported in secretory granules to nerve terminals. Some neuropeptides, such as somatostatin, are widely distributed in the CNS, while others have a restricted distribution. Most neuropeptides have been shown to have effects on neurons in the CNS but their functional roles are not well understood. Substance P is found in sensory afferents mediating pain. Opioid peptides are concentrated in regions of the brain involved in the perception of pain and may mediate antinociceptive effects.

Coexistence of Neurotransmitters

Many neurons contain more than one neurotransmitter. Peptides and amino acid transmitters have been shown to coexist with monoaminergic neurons. The functional significance of coexistence is unclear, although it is likely that the neuropeptide is responsible for slow-onset, long-duration effects, while the classic transmitter mediates rapid, short-duration actions.

11 Cholinergic Receptors

John J. O'Neill, Ph.D.

A Muscarinic receptor

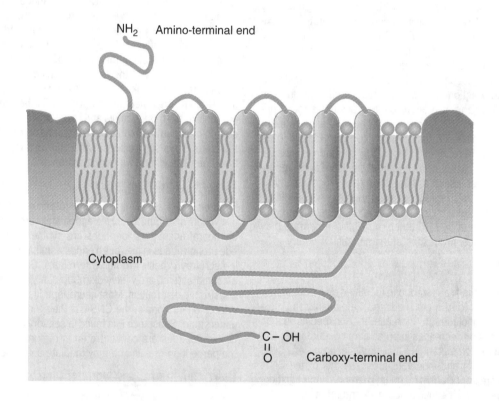

B Nicotinic receptor

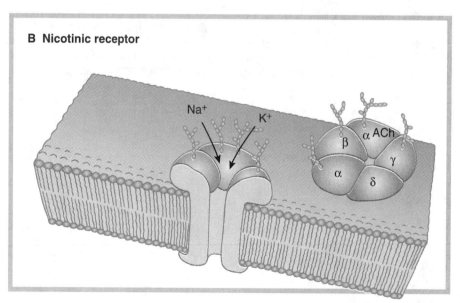

Nicotinic Receptors

The nicotinic receptor is present on skeletal muscle, at autonomic ganglia, and in the CNS. Nicotinic receptors consist of a rosette-like cluster structure of five protein subunits of varying types with a ligand-gated ion channel in its center. The receptor contains two α-subunits, and a β-, γ-, and δ-subunit. ACh binds to an α-subunit, but all subunits are necessary to bring about the appropriate protein conformation. By binding to recognition sites, ACh causes a spatial change to occur, opening the ion channel. Na^+ or K^+ pass through the excitable membrane, causing brief depolarization. Voltage-operated channels (VOR) open, resulting in spread of depolarization and muscle fiber contraction.

Subtypes. In the ANS, both sympathetic and parasympathetic ganglia receive impulses from preganglionic fibers through nicotinic receptors. They consist of five subunits but differ from nicotinic receptors at the neuromuscular junction in that they contain only two α- and three β-subunits.

Agonists and Antagonists. ACh activates all nicotinic receptors by binding to the α-subunit. Decamethonium, a potent antagonist at the neuromuscular junction (NMJ), has little effect at ganglia; in contrast, hexamethonium blocks ganglionic transmission with little effect at the NMJ. In the CNS, the alkaloids (−) nicotine and (−) epibatidine possess analgesic properties blocked by the centrally active mecamylamine but not by the autonomic ganglionic blocking drug, hexamethonium, and (−) lobeline, (−) nicotine, and (−) cytosine are reported to improve retention of learned tasks.

NICTOTINIC RECEPTOR AGONISTS AND ANTAGONISTS

Target	Agonists	Antagonists
Neuromuscular junction	Acetylcholine	Bungarotoxin
Autonomic ganglia	Anabasine	Decamethonium (C-12)
CNS	Cytosine	Dihydro-β-erythroidine
	Epibatidine	Hexamethonium (C-6)
	Lobeline	Mecamylamine
	Nicotine	*d*-Tubocurarine

Muscarinic Receptors

The response of tissues innervated by the parasympathetic nervous system to the alkaloid muscarine leads to the recognition of ACh-specific sites called *muscarinic receptors*. Three subtypes, the neural (M_1), cardiac (M_2), and glandular (M_3), are differentiated based on their pharmacologic function. Based on gene cloning, there are five forms of the receptor. The receptors are 7-TM GPCRs. The figure shows a muscarinic receptor residing in an excitable membrane. Each receptor has an amino-terminal end projecting away from membrane and a carboxy-terminal portion toward the cytoplasm. The site of interaction with ACh is believed to be somewhere in the second and third transmembrane domains. G proteins, consisting of α-, β-, and γ-subunits, can be either excitatory or inhibitory. Activation of muscarinic receptors activates guanylate cyclase and conversion of GTP to cyclic 3′,5′-GMP with second-messenger activity. Hydrolysis of GTP to GDP by the α-subunit of G protein is believed to result in inactivation of the G protein.

Subtypes. The M_1 receptors are found mainly in the peripheral nerve endings, on acid-secreting parietal cells, and in specific regions of the CNS. It is estimated that 95% of cholinergic receptors in the CNS are muscarinic. In contrast, the M_2 receptor is found in cardiac tissue in addition to other peripheral sites. Stimulation of the receptor causes increased K^+ conduction and decreased Ca^{2+} activity, slowing cardiac contraction. Glandular secretions from salivary, bronchial, and sweat glands, other secretions, and intestinal smooth muscle contractions result from activation of M_3 receptors.

Agonists and Antagonists. The muscarinic receptors have relatively few selective agonists. Atropine and scopolamine are relatively nonspecific antagonists, while pirenzepine is selective for the M_1 receptor. Gallamine, known to have curare-like actions at nicotinic receptors, is also a selective M_2 receptor antagonist.

MUSCARINIC RECEPTOR AGONISTS AND ANTAGONISTS

Target	Agonists	Antagonists
Peripheral system	Acetylcholine	Atropine
Eye	(Muscarine)	Benzotropine
iris	Bethanechol	Biperiden
ciliary body	Carbachol	lactate
trabecular membrane	Oxytremorine	Clinidium
canal of Schlemm	Pilocarpine	bromide
Heart		Dicyclomine
Intestine and sphincters		Eucatropine
gastric acid and		Homatropine
secretions		Ipotropium
GI motility		Methantheline
Exocrine gland secretions		bromide
salivary		Pirenzepine
lacrimal		Procyclidine
bronchial		Propantheline
sweat		Trihexiphenidyl
Bladder and ureters		
CNS		
Cortex		
Hippocampus		
Basal ganglia (neo-striatum and putamen)		

12 Anticholinesterases

John J. O'Neill, Ph.D.

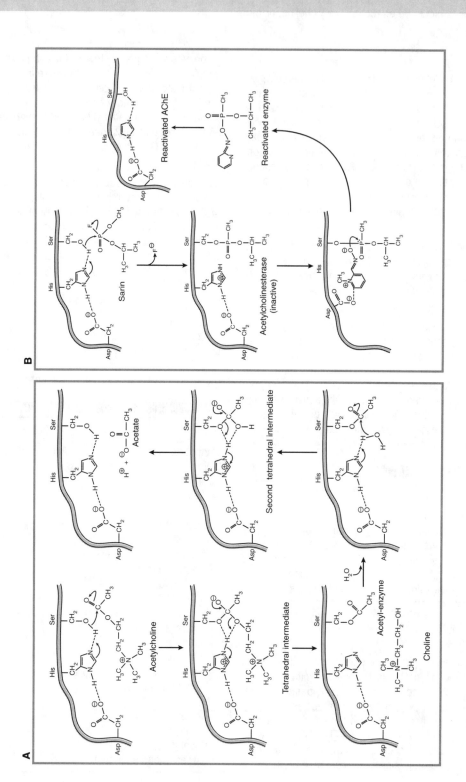

OVERVIEW

- The brief actions of ACh are terminated by hydrolysis, catalyzed by acetylcholinesterase (AChE) or by butyrylcholinesterase (BuChE).
- The cholinesterases are similar globular proteins bound through collagen tails to basement membranes of neurons (AChE) or to glia (BuChE) and cell stroma of RBCs.
- Soluble forms exist in plasma, referred to as plasma cholinesterase or pseudocholinesterase, and in spinal fluid (AChE).
- Neuronal AChE, or true cholinesterase, is specific for ACh, whereas BuChE has low specificity and reacts more readily with other aliphatic and aromatic esters of choline.

Pharmacology

Drugs that affect cholinesterase activity can be therapeutic in action. As shown in Fig. A, ACh first binds at the active center and interacts with the serine-histidine-aspartate triad. This results in acetylation of serine and removal of choline by hydrolysis. In a second step, acetylserine is hydrolyzed, releasing acetate ions. In an analogous manner, pyridostigmine and other carbamates react with cholinesterases by carbamylation. The carbamylated serine is more stable than the acetyl enzyme, leading to inhibition of cholinesterase activity, which is reversible with time. In contrast, organophosphorus compounds react to form stable serine bonds, which are only reversed by oximes such as 2-pyridine aldoxime methyl chloride (2-PAM), or pralidoxime. This drug in combination with atropine is an effective antidote for organophosphate poisoning.

The carbamates neostigmine and pyridostigmine, by inhibiting AChE at the neuromuscular junction, raise the concentration of ACh. They are among the most widely used drugs for the treatment of myasthenia gravis. Their actions are relatively short-lived (3–6 hours) but improve muscle performance by daily administration in myasthenic patients. Longer-acting organophosphate compounds like diisopropylphosphorofluoridate (DFP) are no longer used because of difficulty in controlling dosage proportional to patients' needs.

Toxicity

The adverse effects of all AChEs result from stimulation of muscarinic receptors. These effects include abdominal cramps, increased salivation, bronchial secretions, miosis, and bradycardia.

Intoxication from the more potent organophosphates, referred to as nerve gases, can be fatal unless treated. Treatment requires injection of atropine to block ACh at all muscarinic receptors and use of an oxime, such as pralidoxime, to reverse the inhibition of AChE (see Fig. A). Nerve agents can cause symptoms of acute toxicity, including profuse salivation and sweating, severe pulmonary edema, cardiac arrest, but also severe peripheral neuropathy and demyelination. This seems to result not from inhibition of cholinesterase but of neuropathy target esterase (NTE), specific to myelin.

Spontaneous hydrolysis of phosphorylated enzyme is extremely slow, which makes poisoning from the nerve agents Soman, Sarin, Tabun, and VX life threatening. When pralidoxime is brought in proximity to the phosphate bond at serine of the catalytic center, the oximate ion, a strong nucleophilic agent, causes transfer of the phosphorus compound from serine, leading to enzyme reactivation. With Soman, side-chain dealkylation leads to "aging" within minutes, a condition no longer activable by oximes. To prevent this from happening, pyridostigmine is administered prophylactically, thus carbamylating the enzyme. The enzyme is also inactivated, but the effect is reversible spontaneously. The mechanism of organophosphate inhibition and reactivation of AChE is shown in Fig. B. Shown also is the reactivation of inhibited enzyme by the nucleophilic attack of the oxime 2-PAM.

13 Cholinergic Antagonists

Peter H. Doukas, Ph.D.

A

Tissue response and pharmacologic effect

↑

Second-messenger events

↑

Muscarinic receptor

↕   ↕

ACh   Antagonist

B

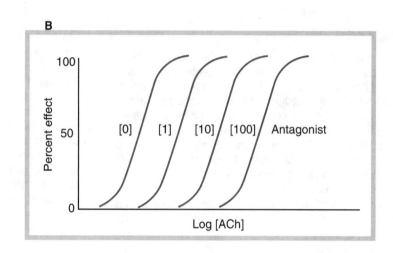

C

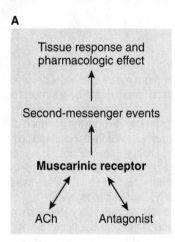

D

-H or -OH

Bulky groups → → X → N → 3⁰ or 4⁰ Terminal amine

Polar center (ester, ether, alcohol, amine)

E

F

G

Pharmacology

By competitively antagonizing the actions of the endogenous neurotransmitter ACh at muscarinic cholinergic receptors, antimuscarinics diminish or block the second-messenger–mediated events of ACh, such as IP_3 and DAG formation, or inhibition of cAMP production. Blockade of ACh in smooth muscle (other than vasculature) leads to muscle relaxation: in the GI tract there is a decrease in tone and motility and an increase in gastric emptying time; relaxation of the bladder and ureters reduces urinary voiding; bronchiolar relaxation leads to enhancement of the airway. Vagal blockade reverses vagally mediated bradycardia and leads to an increase in heart rate. Blockade of muscarinic receptors in the basal ganglia enhances dopaminergic activity and assists in diminishing the tremor associated with Parkinsonism or drug-induced extrapyramidal syndrome (EPS), such as that caused by potent dopamine-blocking antipsychotic agents. Antimuscarinic effects in the eye lead to pupillary dilation (mydriasis) and decreased contraction of the ciliary muscle (cycloplegia), which are used to facilitate ocular examinations. Centrally active antimuscarinics (especially atropine in large doses) are used to reverse the effects of excess cholinergic activity resulting from poisoning by cholinesterase inhibitors. Several subclasses of muscarinic receptors have been identified. Although currently there are no selective antagonists available for therapeutic application, several are under investigation (e.g., pirenzepine, an M_1 antagonist).

Medicinal Chemistry

The belladonna alkaloids atropine, hyoscine (scopolamine), and hyoscyamine are naturally occurring antimuscarinic agents. Atropine serves as the structural prototype for the pharmacologic class and is a tertiary aminoalcohol ester of an aromatic acid (Fig. C). As a tertiary amine, atropine is widely distributed and exerts important actions centrally. Its essential pharmacophore has been determined (Fig. D) and includes the presence of bulky groups adjacent to a polar center approximately three or four atomic units from a terminal amine. Although the most potent compounds contain an ester functionality, it is not essential for activity and may be replaced by other polar groups such as an ether, a hydroxyl, or an amino function. The terminal amino group can be either tertiary or quaternary, with the latter imparting a restricted physiologic distribution. Numerous synthetic congeners and analogs have been synthesized. The synthetic compounds differ primarily in their distribution characteristics. Tertiary amines possess central action, whereas quaternary amines are limited in their action to the periphery; thus compounds can be selected for therapeutic application on this basis. Examples include ipratropium (Fig. E), benztropine (Fig. F), and trihexyphenidyl (Fig. G).

Mechanism of Action

Antimuscarinics compete with ACh for association with the muscarinic cholinergic receptor (see Fig. A). These compounds possess affinity for the receptor but exhibit no intrinsic activity and inhibit the ability of ACh to bind to the site and elicit a stimulus. As reversible competitive antagonists, the antimuscarinics shift the dose–effect curve of ACh increasingly to the right (see Fig. B) with increasing concentrations of antagonist (the concentrations shown in the figure are arbitrary). The antagonism is surmountable with increasing concentrations of ACh.

Pharmacokinetics

Administration and Distribution. Antimuscarinics are usually administered orally; some are also used parenterally and via inhalation. Tertiary amines are widely distributed and enter the CNS. Quaternary amines are limited in their distribution to peripheral sites of action: GI tract, urinary tract, and lungs (e.g., ipratropium after inhalation).

Metabolism and Excretion. Compounds possessing an ester function can be hydrolyzed by liver and plasma esterases; aromatic, alicyclic, alkyl, and amino functions can be transformed by several hepatic oxidative pathways. Quaternary amino compounds are rapidly excreted via the urinary tract. The majority of antimuscarinics exhibit short half-lives, thus necessitating multiple daily doses at 4- or 6-hour intervals. Some are available in sustained-release forms that permit once or twice daily dosing.

Side Effects and Toxicity

Antimuscarinics can produce a cluster of side effects that are extensions of their primary pharmacologic actions and that are especially noticeable in elderly patients. These include: dry mouth, mydriasis and blurring of vision, increased intraocular pressure (these compounds are contraindicated in patients with glaucoma), urinary retention, and adynamic ileus. Centrally these compounds can cause sedation and, with excessive doses, can induce excitation, hallucinations, and coma. Antimuscarinics can suppress sweating and thus in large doses can induce elevated body temperature (children are especially sensitive to this effect).

SPECIFIC AGENTS

Tertiary Amines	Quaternary Amines
Atropine (generic) • Anticholinesterase poisoning Cyclopentolate (Cyclogyl) • Ocular refraction (eye drops) Oxybutynin (Ditropan) • Decrease bladder contractility, urinary urgency and frequency Benztropine (Cogentin) and trihexyphenidyl (Artane) • Antiparkinsonian, prevent EPS	Ipratropium (Atrovent) • Treat COPD via inhalation Glycopyrrolate (Robinul) • GI hypermotility and spasm

14 Neuromuscular Blocking Agents

Peter H. Doukas, Ph.D.

OVERVIEW

- Neuromuscular blocking agents are used to block cholinergic input at the junction between postganglionic cholinergic nerve fibers and skeletal muscle.
- Mechanism and sites of action: Most neuromuscular blockers are reversible, nondepolarizing, competitive antagonists of ACh at postsynaptic nicotinic receptors on the motor end plate of striated muscle fibers. One commonly used blocker, succinylcholine, exerts its effects via a prolonged depolarizing blockade.
- Therapeutic applications: to relax skeletal muscle so as to permit endotracheal intubation, general surgery, or mechanical ventilation.

Pharmacology

By antagonizing the action of the endogenous neurotransmitter ACh at the neuromuscular junction, these blockers hinder the intracellular accumulation of cations needed for contraction. *Nondepolarizing blockers* are competitive antagonists that bind to the receptors and prevent access to ACh. This leads to a flaccid paralysis of the muscle. Termination of the blockade depends on diffusion of the antagonist from the immediate site of action. Reversal of these blockers can be hastened by the intravenous administration of peripherally acting cholinesterase inhibitors, such as neostigmine, pyridostigmine, and edrophonium, which permit the accumulation of ACh and enhance its ability to displace the blocker at the receptor through the competitive mechanism. To limit the effects of the accumulated ACh to the nicotinic sites at the neuromuscular junction, the cholinesterase inhibitor is preceded by the intravenous administration of an antimuscarinic agent. The *depolarizing blocker* succinylcholine induces a prolonged depolarization, which prevents the normal cycle of Na^+ gating and repolarization and leads to a refractoriness of the muscle to further stimulation by ACh. This type of blockade is characterized initially by muscle fasciculations followed by flaccid paralysis. Since succinylcholine resists hydrolysis by acetylcholinesterase (it is hydrolyzed by plasma esterases), it persists longer than ACh in the synapse. Generally its effects are short-lived, and cholinesterase inhibitors *must not* be used to accelerate its reversal.

Medicinal Chemistry

The essential pharmacophore for neuromuscular blockers is based on the structure of D-tubocurarine curare (Fig. A), a naturally occurring nondepolarizing blocker (the term *curariform* is used to describe nondepolarizing blockade) used for centuries as a hunting poison in South America. Other than succinylcholine (Fig. B), which is a simple aliphatic diester, the commonly used agents belong to one of two classes whose major structural components provide a framework for maintaining the appropriate interatomic distance (about 10 atomic units) between the two positively charged nitrogens. They constitute two classes, the benzylisoquinolines (e.g., atracurium, shown in Fig. C) and the aminosteroids (e.g., pancuronium, shown in Fig. D); both groups are also known as *pachycurares*, based on their structural bulkiness (succinylcholine is known as a *leptocurare*, because of its streamlined structure). Structural variations account for differences in side effects and duration of action; the latter is used to categorize compounds as short-, intermediate-, or long-acting.

Pharmacokinetics

Administration and Distribution. Neuromuscular blockers are administered intravenously. Their distribution is limited to peripheral sites of action.

Metabolism and Excretion. The benzylisoquinolines and aminosteroids are primarily excreted unchanged, accompanied by varying degrees of hydrolysis by plasma esterases. Atracurium has been designed to undergo a spontaneous Hofmann elimination at plasma pH, which terminates its action (Fig. E). In Hofmann elimination, the mildly acidic hydrogens adjacent to the carbonyl groups are activated at plasma pH, thereby promoting the spontaneous breakdown of atracurium to yield the tertiary benzylisoquinoline laudanosine and the acrylate esters. Hydrolytic cleavage also occurs in patients with normal plasma esterase levels. Laudanosine is a tertiary amine capable of entering the CNS and potentially acting as a stimulant (the clinical importance of the latter is not clear). Succinylcholine is normally hydrolyzed by plasma esterases, first to succinyl monocholine and finally to succinic acid. Patients who have a deficiency of plasma esterase demonstrate prolonged apnea with succinylcholine and require an alternative blocker, such as atracurium, that is eliminated by a different mechanism.

Side Effects and Toxicity

Curare exhibits a number of side effects, such as vagal blockade, histamine release, and inhibition of norepinephrine uptake, that contribute to tachycardia and blood pressure changes. The newer synthetic derivatives are reported to be less prone to exhibit some, or all, of these effects. Certain patients may demonstrate an idiosyncratic life-threatening malignant hyperthermia in response to succinylcholine; treatment includes the administration of dantrium.

SPECIFIC AGENTS

Duration[a]		
Short-Acting [10–15 min]	Intermediate-Acting [20–30 min]	Long-Acting [45–60 min]
Succinylcholine	Atracurium	D-Tubocurarine
Mivacurium	Vecuronium	Dimethyl tubocurarine
	Rocuronium	Doxacurium
		Pancuronium

[a] Estimates of clinically effective blocking times after one ED95 dose.

15 Adrenergic Receptors

David B. Bylund, Ph.D.

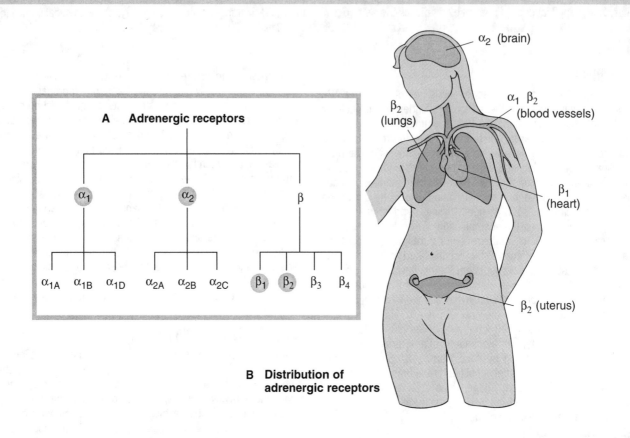

A **Adrenergic receptors**

α_1 α_2 β

α_{1A} α_{1B} α_{1D} α_{2A} α_{2B} α_{2C} β_1 β_2 β_3 β_4

α_2 (brain)

β_2 (lungs)

α_1 β_2 (blood vessels)

β_1 (heart)

β_2 (uterus)

B **Distribution of adrenergic receptors**

C **Mechanisms of action—adrenergic receptors**

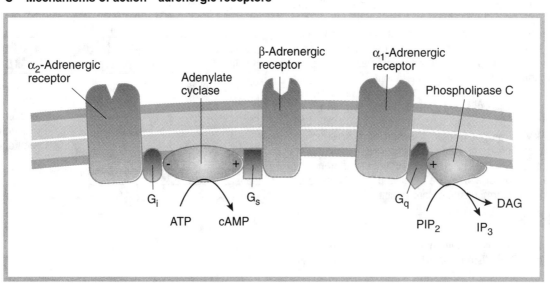

α_2-Adrenergic receptor

Adenylate cyclase

β-Adrenergic receptor

α_1-Adrenergic receptor

Phospholipase C

G_i G_s G_q

ATP cAMP PIP$_2$ IP$_3$ DAG

History and Classification

Epinephrine and norepinephrine are endogenous compounds that serve as hormones and neurotransmitters. The actions of these catecholamines are mediated by adrenergic receptors. In the 1940s, the adrenergic receptors were divided into two main types: α-adrenergic receptors and β-adrenergic receptors. As shown in Fig. A, it is now recognized that there are three major types of adrenergic receptors (α_1, α_2, and β), each of which can be further subdivided into three or four subtypes, making a total of ten adrenergic receptor subtypes. An understanding of these subtypes is important because a drug that is selective for a given subtype is likely to have fewer side effects than a drug that acts on several of the subtypes. Currently four of the adrenergic receptors are of particular clinical significance (α_1, α_2, β_1, and β_2). As better and more highly selective drugs are developed for the other subtypes, it is likely that they will become clinically significant.

Distribution and Effects of Adrenergic Receptors

Adrenergic receptors are widely distributed throughout the body, and thus drugs that act at these receptors can produce many different effects. The more important sites are indicated in Fig. B. Most blood vessels contain α_1-adrenergic receptors, which constrict the vessel when they are stimulated. The α_2-adrenergic receptors are distributed widely throughout the nervous system. Some α_2 receptors are located presynaptically and function to regulate the release of norepinephrine and other neurotransmitters. Most of the β-adrenergic receptors in the heart are of the β_1 subtype and regulate the force and rate of cardiac contractions. The lung, on the other hand, contains mostly the β_2 subtype, and stimulation of these receptors results in relaxation of bronchial smooth muscle. The blood vessels in skeletal muscle and the smooth muscle of the uterus also contain β_2-adrenergic receptors.

Prototypic Adrenergic Drugs

Epinephrine and norepinephrine are generally nonselective, as they have similar affinities at all ten subtypes, with the exception that norepinephrine is less potent at β_2-adrenergic receptors. An important feature of adrenergic drugs is their selectivity. Some adrenergic drugs, such as phenylephrine (α_1-selective) and isoproterenol (β-selective), are selective at the level of the three main types, whereas other drugs, such as metoprolol (β_1-selective) and terbutaline (β_2-selective), are selective at the subtype level. The selectivity of some of the more common adrenergic agonists and antagonists are listed in the following table.

SELECTIVITY OF ADRENERGIC DRUGS

Drug	Selectivity	Class
Phenylephrine	α_1	Agonist
Phentolamine	α_1, α_2	Antagonist
Prazosin	α_1	Antagonist
Clonidine	α_2	Agonist
Isoproterenol	β_1, β_2	Agonist
Propranolol	β_1, β_2	Antagonist
Timolol	β_1, β_2	Antagonist
Metoprolol	β_1	Antagonist
Atenolol	β_1	Antagonist
Terbutaline	β_2	Agonist
Ritodrine	β_2	Agonist

Therapeutic Uses of Drugs Acting at Adrenergic Receptors

The therapeutic uses of adrenergic drugs are consistent with the localization of the various subtypes and the selectivity of drugs for a particular type or subtype. For example, both α_1-adrenergic antagonists and α_2-adrenergic agonists reduce blood pressure and are thus useful in treating hypertension: α_1 antagonists cause vasodilatation by blocking the vasoconstricting effect of the endogenous catecholamines; α_2 agonists act postsynaptically in the brain to reduce sympathetic outflow, thus reducing the peripheral concentrations of the catecholamines (which act at α_1 and β_1 receptors to increase blood pressure). Additional examples of the therapeutic uses for drugs that act at various adrenergic receptors are listed below.

EFFECTS AND CLINICAL APPLICATIONS OF DRUGS ACTING AT ADRENERGIC RECEPTORS

Receptor	Class	Effect	Applications
α_1	Agonist	Vasoconstriction	Reduce bleeding; nasal decongestant; limit absorption of anesthetics
α_1	Antagonist	Vasodilatation	Hypertension, shock
α_2	Agonist	Sympathetic outflow decreased	Hypertension
β_1	Agonist	Cardiac stimulation	Bradycardia, heart failure
β, β_1	Antagonist	Several	Hypertension, angina, arrhythmias, glaucoma
β_2	Agonist	Smooth muscle relaxation	Asthma, premature labor

The side effects of adrenergic drugs are also consistent with the selectivity of the particular drug. For example, the use of propranolol (β_1 and β_2 antagonist) is contraindicated in a hypertensive patient who also has asthma; metoprolol and atenolol (β_1-selective antagonists) are expected to cause fewer bronchoconstrictive side effects.

Mechanisms of Adrenergic Receptor Action

The adrenergic receptors are members of the guanine nucleotide regulatory binding protein (G protein)–coupled superfamily of receptors. Each receptor is a single protein that is thought to transverse the membrane seven times. The binding of an agonist to the receptor causes it to associate with a G protein, permitting GDP, which was bound to the G protein, to be replaced by GTP. The GTP-bound G protein can then activate various effectors. As illustrated in Fig. C, β-adrenergic receptors are positively coupled to the effector enzyme adenylate cyclase through the stimulatory G_s protein (causing an increase in cAMP levels), whereas the α_2-adrenergic receptors are negatively coupled to adenylate cyclase through the inhibitory G_i protein (causing a decrease in cAMP levels). The α_1-adrenergic receptors, on the other hand, are coupled through a G_q protein to the stimulation of the enzyme phospholipase C, which breaks down a membrane PIP_2 to give DAG and IP_3. The products of these regulated reactions (cAMP, DAG, and IP_3) are called second messengers and are involved in regulating cellular processes, often through protein phosphorylation.

16 Adrenergic Receptor Agonists

David B. Bylund, Ph.D.

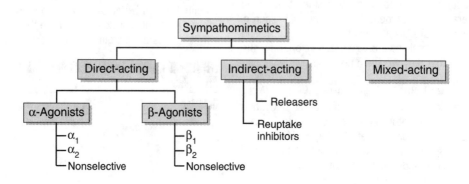

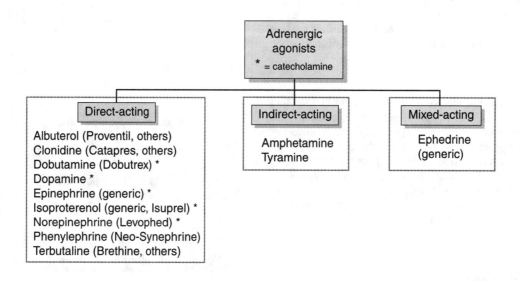

Adrenoreceptor-selective drugs			
α_1	α_2	β_1	β_2
Phenylephrine	Clonidine	Dobutamine	Albuterol and terbutaline

OVERVIEW

- Norepinephrine (noradrenaline) is the neurotransmitter at terminals of most postganglionic sympathetic neurons (exceptions include projections to sweat glands and some blood vessels in the neck and face).
- Epinephrine and some norepinephrine are released from the adrenal medulla during sympathetic activation (e.g., "fight or flight" response).
- Drugs that mimic or facilitate the actions of norepinephrine or epinephrine are termed *sympathomimetic* (=noradrenergic=adrenergic).
- Receptors that respond to norepinephrine or epinephrine are termed *adrenergic receptors* (adrenoceptors).

MEDIATION OF SYMPATHETIC EFFECTS

Sympathetic Effect	Adrenoceptor Type
Vasoconstriction; mydriasis	α
Increased heart rate, force of contraction	β_1
Bronchodilation (uterine relaxation; glycogen to glucose)	β_2
Lipolysis	β_3

Sympathomimetic Drugs

Sympathomimetics mimic the actions of norepinephrine and epinephrine. They can be direct-acting (directly activating adrenergic receptors), indirect-acting (increasing synthesis or release or by decreasing reuptake or metabolism), or mixed-acting (binding to adrenergic receptors and stimulating release of norepinephrine).

Catecholamines versus Noncatecholamines

The catecholamines (*3,4-dihydroxybenzamines*) norepinephrine, epinephrine, and dopamine are endogenous; others are synthetic. They are rapidly metabolized in gut wall by catechol *O*-methyltransferase (COMT) and in the liver and gut wall by monoamine oxidase (MAO). They are ineffective when given orally. Catecholamines are polar, that is, they do not readily (but do) penetrate the blood–brain barrier. Noncatecholamines (e.g., ephedrine) are poor substrates for MAO, hence they have greater oral activity and longer duration of action than catecholamines.

Direct-Acting Adrenoceptor Agonists

Epinephrine. β-receptor activation predominates at low concentration; α-receptor activation at high concentration. Epinephrine produces increases in blood pressure (systolic greater than diastolic) followed by overshoot before returning to baseline; it is used to treat bronchospasm, hypersensitivity reactions (anaphylactic shock), cardiac arrest, chronic open-angle glaucoma, and to prolong duration of infiltrative anesthesia. It can cause anxiety, headache, cerebral hemorrhage, cardiac arrhythmias, pulmonary hypertension, and pulmonary edema.

Norepinephrine. Norepinephrine acts on α- and β_1-adrenergic receptors more than β_2-adrenergic receptors. Norepinephrine produces increases in blood pressure (systolic and diastolic) followed by reflex tachycardia; it is used to treat hypotension during anesthesia when tissue perfusion is good. Adverse effects are similar to those of epinephrine.

Isoproterenol. Isoproterenol is a β-agonist. Unreliable for oral administration, it causes decreases in diastolic blood pressure, but cardiac output increases as a result of its positive inotropic and chronotropic effects. It is also used for relaxation of bronchioles, stimulation of insulin secretion, and as a cardiac stimulant or bronchodilator (tolerance can develop). Adverse effects are similar to those of norepinephrine and epinephrine (potentially fatal ventricular arrhythmias in overdose).

Dopamine. Dopamine is a β-agonist; its structure and pharmacokinetics are similar to norepinephrine and epinephrine. At low doses it increases systolic (but not diastolic) pressure. It is used in treatment of cardiogenic and septic shock and refractory congestive heart failure (CHF). Adverse sympathomimetic effects are similar to those of norepinephrine and epinephrine (usually short-lived because of rapid metabolism).

Phenylephrine. Acting on α_1-adrenergic receptors, phenylephrine is a vasoconstrictor (raises both systolic and diastolic blood pressure) and produces reflex bradycardia (no direct effect on heart). It is used in ophthalmic solutions for mydriasis and as a nasal decongestant. High doses cause hypertensive headache and cardiac irregularities.

Clonidine. Clonidine acts on α_2-adrenergic receptors. It is used in essential hypertension and to attenuate opiate-withdrawal symptoms.

Dobutamine. Dobutamine acts on β_1-adrenergic receptors and increases cardiac contractility with a minimal change in heart rate (does not significantly increase O_2 demand). It is used to increase cardiac output in CHF. It may have toxic effects on AV conduction.

Terbutaline and *Albuterol.* Affecting β_2-adrenergic receptors, terbutaline and albuterol are both bronchodilators. They also reduce uterine contractions during premature labor.

Indirect- and Mixed-Acting Adrenoceptor Agonists

Amphetamine. An agonist for α- and β-adrenergic receptors, amphetamine stimulates the release of norepinephrine and increases blood pressure (α-adrenergic receptors on the vasculature and β-adrenergic receptor stimulation of the heart). Abuse is related to its central stimulatory action.

Tyramine. An α- and β-adrenergic receptor agonist, tyramine is found in fermented foods (leads to drug interactions). It stimulates the release of norepinephrine and increases blood pressure (α-adrenergic receptor on the vasculature and β-adrenergic receptor stimulation of the heart).

17 Adrenergic Receptor Antagonists

J. Paul Hieble, Ph.D.

A Subclassification of α- and β-adrenoceptors

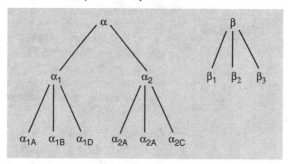

B Structural classes of molecules showing potent antagonist activity at α- and β-adrenoceptors

α-Adrenoceptor antagonists

R = Ar, Ar-O-,

β-Adrenoceptor antagonists

R = Ar, Ar-O-CH_2

R = -$C(CH_3)_3$, -$CH(CH_3)_2$

C Selectivity profiles of doxazosin (α_1-adrenoceptor antagonist), propranolol (β-adrenoceptor antagonist), metoprolol (β_1-adrenoceptor antagonist), and labetalol (α_1/β-adrenoceptor antagonist)*

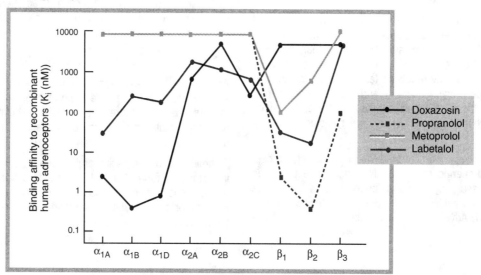

*As determined by radioligand binding assay using CHO cells expressing recombinant human receptors.

Pharmacology

Adrenergic receptor antagonists bind to the receptors normally activated by the catecholamine neurotransmitters norepinephrine and epinephrine. The presence of an antagonist on the receptor prevents its activation. Adrenergic receptors have been subdivided into α-adrenergic receptors, which primarily mediate smooth muscle contraction, and β-adrenergic receptors, which mediate cardiac stimulation and smooth muscle relaxation. Further subdivision of both α- and β-adrenergic receptors has led to drugs with improved therapeutic profiles, that is, adrenergic receptor antagonists that relax smooth muscle without stimulation of norepinephrine overflow and β_1-adrenergic receptor antagonists that block the cardiac stimulation but not the tracheobronchial relaxation induced by catecholamines. Both α_1- and α_2-adrenergic receptors have been further subdivided; selective α_{1A}-adrenergic receptor antagonists are being evaluated in benign prostatic hyperplasia. Specific agents are listed below.

Medicinal Chemistry

All potent β-adrenergic receptor antagonists are either 2-aryl-ethanol-1-amines or 3-aryloxy-propan-2-ol-1-amines (most common) with a bulky substituent on the amine nitrogen atom. β_1 versus β_2 selectivity is influenced by the nature and pattern of substituents on both the aromatic moiety and amine nitrogen. α-Adrenergic receptor antagonists are structurally diverse, containing an aromatic nucleus linked to an amine by an aliphatic chain. The amine nitrogen is often incorporated into a piperazine, piperidine, or imidazoline ring. The most widely used α_1-adrenergic receptor antagonists contain a quinazoline ring linked to a piperazine. Compounds blocking both α- and β-adrenergic receptors incorporate structural elements of both α- and β-adrenergic receptor antagonists in a single molecule.

Therapeutic Activity

α_1-Adrenergic receptor antagonists reduce blood pressure and relieve urethral obstruction induced by prostatic hyperplasia primarily via relaxation of vascular and prostatic smooth muscle, respectively, although a centrally mediated sympatholytic action may contribute. Although several therapeutic applications have been postulated for selective α_2-adrenergic receptor antagonists, the only marketed drug in this class is yohimbine, used occasionally for impotence.

β-adrenergic receptor antagonists, either nonselective or β_1-selective, are used as antihypertensives. The mechanism for this action is likely to involve interaction with β-adrenergic receptors at multiple sites, including heart, kidney, and CNS. Blockade of cardiac β-adrenergic receptors to attenuate the effects of excess sympathetic drive is useful in the therapy of angina pectoris, cardiac arrhythmia, following myocardial infarction, and for prevention of its recurrence. Therapeutic applications for selective β_2- or β_3-adrenergic receptor antagonists have not been identified.

Pharmacokinetics

Both α- and β-adrenergic receptor antagonists are well absorbed PO, and most agents are available in once-daily formulations, based either on a long half-life of the molecule or on sustained-release technology. Route of metabolism depends on the individual agent.

Toxicity

Side effects of α- and β-adrenergic receptor antagonists result from excessive pharmacologic activity or from blockade of receptors at an undesired site. For example, β-adrenergic receptor antagonists can produce bradycardia, bronchoconstriction, peripheral vasoconstriction, and asthenia. Bronchoconstriction is less common with selective β_1-antagonists. Cessation of β-adrenergic receptor antagonist therapy in patients with coronary artery disease can induce anginal symptoms, cardiac arrhythmias, and myocardial infarction. α_1-Adrenergic receptor antagonists are associated with tachycardia, orthostatic hypotension, dizziness, and asthenia. Cardiovascular effects are associated with initiation of dosing (first-dose phenomena); incidence can be reduced by dose titration.

SPECIFIC AGENTS

α-Adrenergic Receptor Antagonist	β-Adrenergic Receptor Antagonists	α-Adrenergic Receptor and β-Adrenergic Receptor Antagonists
Prazosin (generic, Minipress) • First selective α_1-adrenergic receptor antagonist • Extensive hepatic metabolism **Terazosin** (Hytrin) • Long duration of action **Doxazosin** (Cardura) • Long duration of action • Extensive hepatic metabolism **Tamsulosin** (Flomax, Omnic) • Marketed for benign prostatic hyperplasia • Selectivity for α_{1A}- and α_{1D}- versus α_{1B}-adrenergic receptor • Extensive hepatic metabolism	**Propranolol** (generic, Inderal) • First widely used β-antagonist • Nonselective for subtype **Atenolol** (Tenormin) • Selective for β_1 subtype • Relatively polar molecule **Metoprolol** (generic, Lopressor) • Selective for β_1 subtype • Relatively lipophilic	**Carvedilol** (Coreg, Kredex) • Market for congestive heart failure (United States, Europe) and hypertension (Europe) • Functional potency about tenfold greater at β- versus α_1-adrenergic receptors **Labetalol** (generic, Normodyne) • Market for hypotension • Functional potency about fivefold greater at β- versus α_1-adrenergic receptors

18 Prostaglandins and Related Compounds

Barrie Ashby, Ph.D.

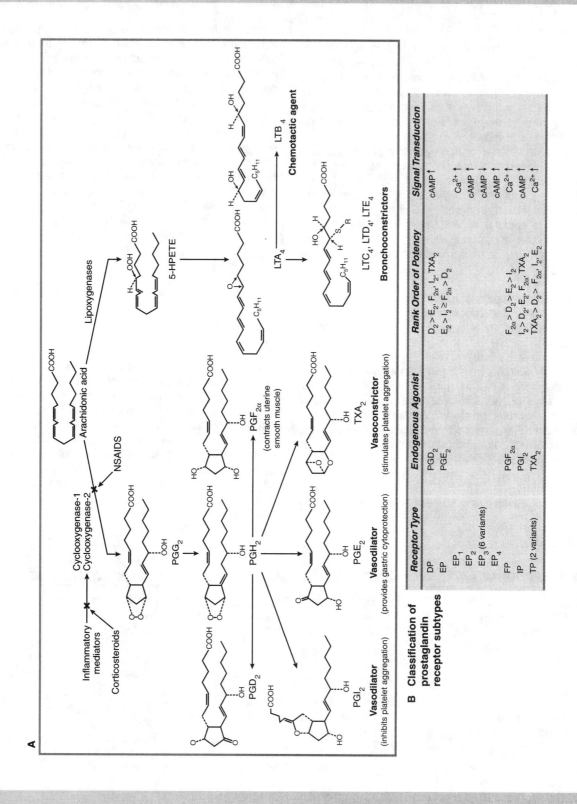

B Classification of prostaglandin receptor subtypes

Receptor Type	Endogenous Agonist	Rank Order of Potency	Signal Transduction
DP	PGD$_2$	D$_2$ > E$_2$, F$_{2\alpha}$, I$_2$, TXA$_2$	cAMP ↑
EP	PGE$_2$	E$_2$ > I$_2$ ≥ F$_{2\alpha}$ > D$_2$	
EP$_1$			Ca^{2+} ↑
EP$_2$			cAMP ↑
EP$_3$ (6 variants)			cAMP ↑
EP$_4$			cAMP ↑
FP	PGF$_{2\alpha}$	F$_{2\alpha}$ > D$_2$ > E$_2$ > I$_2$	Ca^{2+} ↑
IP	PGI$_2$	I$_2$ > D$_2$, E$_2$, F$_{2\alpha}$, TXA$_2$	cAMP ↑
TP (2 variants)	TXA$_2$	TXA$_2$ > D$_2$ > F$_{2\alpha}$, I$_2$, E$_2$	Ca^{2+} ↑

OVERVIEW

- Prostaglandins are oxygenated, unsaturated, 20-carbon fatty acids known as eicosanoids, that originate from arachidonic acid.
- Eicosanoids act on most cells and tissues and provide targets for pharmacologic intervention in several disease states.
- Prostaglandins are involved in pathologic processes such as inflammation and fever.
- Prostaglandin action can be prevented by blocking synthesis with NSAIDs, such as aspirin.

FIRST IDENTIFIED: von Euler, 1930

Synthesis of Prostaglandins and Other Eicosanoids

Arachidonic acid is formed from cell membrane phospholipids by the action of the enzyme phospholipase A_2. There are three pathways for enzymatic conversion of arachidonic acid: cyclooxygenases, lipoxygenases, and cytochrome P-450–dependent monooxygenases. Two distinct cyclooxygenases (COX-1, COX-2) have been identified. COX-2 is inducible during inflammation, and corticosteroids suppress induction of this form. Aspirin inhibits cyclooxygenases irreversibly by covalent acetylation of a serine residue; other NSAIDs are reversible cyclooxygenase inhibitors. The relatively stable prostaglandins, PGD_2, PGE_2, and $PGF_2\alpha$, originate from common intermediates, the cyclic endoperoxides PGG_2 and PGH_2. The endoperoxide PGH_2 is also metabolized into two unstable compounds that are highly active biologically: thromboxane A_2 (TXA_2) and prostacyclin (PGI_2). Lipoxygenases catalyze incorporation of oxygen into arachidonic acid to form hydroperoxyeicosatetraenoic acids (HPETEs), which give rise to the leukotrienes.

Metabolism of Prostaglandins

Prostaglandins are not stored but are synthesized in response to diverse stimuli and enter the extracellular space. They act as local hormones (autacoids), their biologic activities usually restricted to the cell or tissue where they are synthesized. Concentrations of PGE_2 and $PGF_2\alpha$ in arterial blood are very low because of pulmonary degradation, which removes more than 90% from the venous blood as it passes through the lungs.

Mechanisms of Action

Prostaglandins act through several G-protein–coupled receptor subtypes to cause stimulation or inhibition of adenylate cyclase or stimulation of phospholipase C. Prostaglandins induce vasodilation, bronchodilation, promotion of salt and water excretion, inhibition of lipolysis, glycogenolysis, and fatty acid oxidation.

Pharmacotherapeutics

Blood Flow Regulation. PGE_1, PGE_2, and PGI_2 are all potent vasodilators. TXA_2 is a potent vasoconstrictor. The peptide leukotrienes LTC_4 and LTD_4 also constrict coronary arteries and cause hypotension.

Platelet Aggregation. TXA_2 causes platelet aggregation, whereas PGI_2 inhibits it. Antithrombotic strategies attempt to maximize the effect of aspirin on platelet cyclooxygenase (blocking TXA_2 formation) while sparing the effect of cyclooxygenase on endothelial cells (allowing PGI_2 formation).

Ductus Arteriosus. The ductus arteriosus generally closes spontaneously at birth but in some cases it remains patent (open) so that 90% of cardiac output is shunted away from the lungs. The patency is probably due to high production of PGI_2 after delivery. Indomethacin inhibits prostaglandin production and closes the ductus. Conversely, neonates with certain congenital heart defects depend on an open ductus arteriosus for survival until corrective surgery can be performed. PGE_1 (alprostadil) is used therapeutically to dilate the ductus.

GI Tract. PGE_1 and PGE_2 inhibit gastric acid production and pepsin secretion, leading to the cytoprotective, antiulcer properties of prostaglandins. The methylester prodrug misoprostol, a 15-deoxy-16-hydroxy-16-methyl PGE, is useful in treatment of peptic ulcers.

Immune Responses. PGE_2 and its analogs influence inflammatory and immune responses.

Reproductive System. PGE_1 injected into the corpus cavernosum of the penis causes and maintains erection in impotent patients. Both PGE_2 and $PGF_2\alpha$ cause contraction of uterine smooth muscle and may modulate menstruation. Consequently, NSAIDs such as ibuprofen are prescribed for relieving menstrual cramps. Use of PGE_2 to induce labor is accompanied by uterine hypertonus and fetal bradycardia, so that the main use of prostaglandins in gynecologic practice has been as abortifacients.

Bronchoconstriction. The lungs produce PGE_2, PGI_2, PGD_2, $PGF_2\alpha$, TXA_2, LTC_4, and LTD_4. Mast cells lining the respiratory passages are the likely source of leukotrienes, and PGD_2 and overproduction of these substances lead to bronchoconstriction, so that they are potential mediators of asthma. $PGF_2\alpha$ and TXA_2 are also potent bronchoconstrictors, whereas PGE_1, PGE_2, and PGI_2 are potent vasodilators. However, inhaled prostaglandins irritate the airways and are not suitable as antiasthmatic drugs.

Nerve Transmission. There is evidence that eicosanoid-dependent mechanisms operate within the neuron of origin and externally at nerve endings to modulate autonomic transmission.

SPECIFIC AGENTS

Prostaglandins	NSAIDs
Alprostadil	Aspirin and other salicylates
Carboprost tromethamine	Ibuprofen
Dinoprostone	Indomethacin
Misoprostol	Meclofenamates
	Naproxen
	Others

Histamine and Histamine Antagonists
Robert B. Raffa, Ph.D.

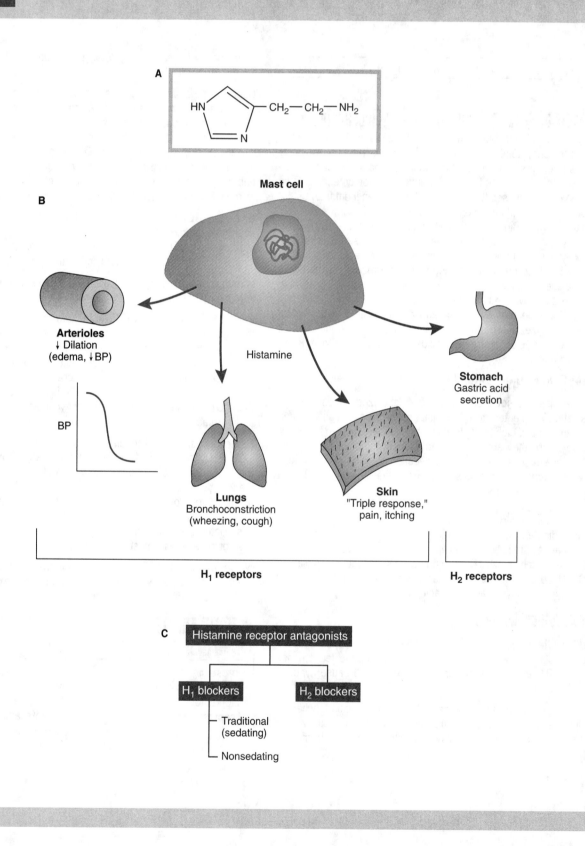

A

Mast cell

B

Arterioles
↓ Dilation
(edema, ↓BP)

BP

Histamine

Lungs
Bronchoconstriction
(wheezing, cough)

Skin
"Triple response,"
pain, itching

Stomach
Gastric acid
secretion

H_1 receptors

H_2 receptors

C Histamine receptor antagonists

H_1 blockers

H_2 blockers

— Traditional
(sedating)

— Nonsedating

OVERVIEW

- Histamine is ubiquitous in animals and plants and widely distributed within them.
- There is a species-dependent sensitivity to histamine-induced effects (e.g., humans, guinea pigs, cats, and dogs are more sensitive than mice and rats).
- Histamine is synthesized from the amino acid histidine (Fig. A).
- Most histamine in mammals is bound in granules of mast cells (or basophils). The bound form is inactive, but stimuli (or drugs such as morphine, codeine, succinylcholine, D-tubocurarine) release histamine into surrounding tissues, where it acts as a local hormone (autacoid).
- Histamine has roles in immediate allergic reaction, inflammation, gastric acid secretion, and as a neurotransmitter and neuromodulator.

Pharmacology

Sensitized mast cells degranulate when they are exposed to appropriate antigen (Fig. B); histamine, ATP, and other mediators are released, producing the "allergic reaction." Histamine causes local vasodilation, leakage of inflammatory mediators and inflammatory cells, producing inflammation. Histamine's mediating effects on the neuroendocrine cardiovascular and CNS are evidence of its function as neurotransmitter and neuro-modulator. All receptors identified to date are cell-surface 7-transmembrane G-protein–coupled receptors (7-TM GPCRs). H_1 receptors are located in smooth muscle (IP_3 and NO) and brain (IP_3); H_2 receptors are located in gastric mucosa, cardiac muscle, and brain (adenylate cyclase); H_3 are located in myenteric plexus and CNS (presynaptic autoreceptor negative feedback). All three receptor types are widely distributed in the CNS. H_1 and H_2 are mainly postsynaptic. H_3 is mainly presynaptic and serves as feedback inhibition of histamine release; it also inhibits the release of norepinephrine, 5-HT, ACh, and peptides. Release of histamine may be *cytolytic*, which involves damage to plasma membrane, is energy-independent, with Ca^{2+} not required, and results in leakage of cytoplasmic contents; or *noncytolytic*, with no damage and no leakage, requiring ATP and Ca^{2+}, and resulting in exocytosis.

Mechanism of Action

Histamine's predominant action is vasodilation resulting from relaxation of arteriolar smooth muscle and precapillary sphincters (leading to flushing, headache, edema, urticaria [hives] (H_1 and H_2 each can produce maximal effect); it produces a reflex decrease in systolic and diastolic blood pressure (requires H_1 and H_2 antagonists to block) and an increase in heart rate (direct and reflex), as well as bronchoconstriction (wheezing), particularly in sensitized individuals. Other effects are stimulation of sensory nerve endings (pain, itching) and of gastric acid secretion. Intradermal injection yields "triple response": reddening (vasodilation), wheal (edema), and red, irregular flare around wheal (axon reflex).

Histamine Antagonism

Inhibition of histamine release is produced by cromolyn (mechanism unknown); and β_2 adrenergic receptor agonists (increase cAMP). Physiologic inhibition is achieved with epinephrine, used for anaphylaxis and other massive release of histamine, such as allergy to insect stings. Pharmacologic antagonism utilizes reversible, competitive receptor antagonism (Fig. C).

H_1-Receptor Antagonists ("Antihistamines"). These are rapidly absorbed, widely distributed, and older ones readily pass the blood–brain barrier. They are extensively metabolized by hepatic microsomes. The newer agents have the advantages of less lipid solubility (less blood–brain barrier penetration), longer duration, and being more H_1-selective; examples are terfenadine (Seldane), astemizole (Hismanal), loratadine (Claritin), and others. Uses include: allergic reactions: drugs of choice in allergic rhinitis and urticaria, where hist-amine is the primary mediator (ineffective in bronchial asthma); motion sickness and vertigo; and uses related to other properties of nonselective agents.

H_2-Receptor Antagonists. These are reversible, competitive antagonists of histamine H_2 receptors. They inhibit gastric acid secretion. Uses include: reduction of gastric acid secretion; Zollinger-Ellison syndrome; gastroesophageal reflux disease (other drugs are generally more effective); and in combination with antibiotics to treat *Helicobacter pylori* associated peptic ulcer disease (the most common cause of ulcers not caused by NSAIDs).

Toxicity and Adverse Effects

H_1-Receptor Antagonists. Overdose of older agents resembles atropine overdose (treated similarly); newer agents can cause cardiac arrhythmias. Teratogenicity is possible with use of these agents.

H_2-Receptor Antagonists. Adverse effects are low (1%–2%). Cimetidine is an antiandrogen, producing inhibition of cytochrome P-450 enzymes, and ranitidine causes some inhibition of P-450 and inhibition of glucuronidation of acetaminophen.

H_1- AND H_2-RECEPTOR ANTAGONISTS

H_1 Blockers ("Antihistamines")

Astemizole (Hismanal)
Azatadine (Optimine)
Brompheniramine (Dimetane, Bromfed, others, generic)
Carbinoxamine (Clistin)
Cetirizine (Zyrtec)
Chlorpheniramine (Chlor-Trimeton, others, generic)
Clemastine (Tavist)
Cyclizine (Marezine)
Cyproheptadine (Penactin, generic)
Dexchlorpheniramine (Polamine, others, generic)
Dimenhydrinate (Dramamine, generic)
Diphenhydramine (Benadryl, generic)

Fexofenadine (Allegra)
Hydroxyzine (Atarax, Vistaril, generic)
Loratadine (Claritin)
Meclizine (Antivert, others, generic)
Methdilazine (Tacaryl)
Phenindamine (Nolahist)
Promethazine (Phenergan, others, generic)
Pyrilamine (generic)
Terfenadine (Seldane, generic)
Trimeprazine (Temaril)
Tripelenhamine (PBZ, generic)
Triprolidine (Actidil, generic)

H_2 Blockers

Cimetidine (Tagamet)
Famotidine (Pepcid)

Nizatidine (Axid)
Ranitidine (Zantac)

20 Drug-Induced Allergic Reactions

Sandra Knowles, B.Sc.Pharm., and Neal H. Shear, M.D.

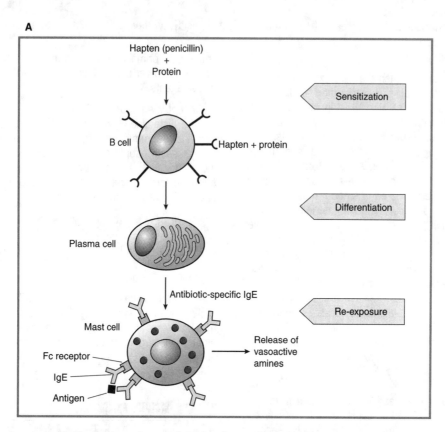

A

Hapten (penicillin)
+
Protein

Sensitization

B cell — Hapten + protein

Differentiation

Plasma cell

Antibiotic-specific IgE

Re-exposure

Mast cell

Fc receptor

IgE

Antigen

Release of vasoactive amines

B Mechanism of unpredictable adverse drug reactions

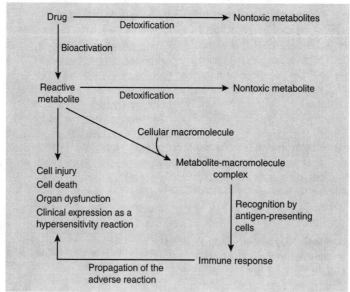

Drug — Detoxification → Nontoxic metabolites

Bioactivation

Reactive metabolite — Detoxification → Nontoxic metabolite

Cellular macromolecule

Metabolite-macromolecule complex

Cell injury
Cell death
Organ dysfunction
Clinical expression as a hypersensitivity reaction

Recognition by antigen-presenting cells

Immune response

Propagation of the adverse reaction

OVERVIEW

- Most adverse drug reactions do not have an allergic basis; allergic reactions account for only 6%–10% of all adverse reactions to drugs (Borda and Slone, 1968).
- Allergic reactions are caused by interaction of the drug or metabolites with effector cells of the immune system (i.e., are immunologically mediated).

Adverse Drug Reactions

Although patients and many clinicians may refer to an adverse event as an "allergic reaction," the mechanism of many of these events does not involve the immune system. A classification system has been described (Patterson, 1988), which groups adverse events into predictable and unpredictable reactions.

CLASSIFICATION SYSTEM FOR ADVERSE DRUG REACTIONS

Reaction	Definition
Predictable	Dose-dependent
Toxicity or overdose	Due to excess dose or impaired excretion of a medication
Side effects	Undesirable effects caused by pharmacologic effect of drug
Drug interaction	Action of one drug on toxicity or effectiveness of another
Unpredictable	Dose-independent
Intolerance	Lower threshold to normal pharmacologic action
Idiosyncratic	Genetically determined metabolic or enzyme deficiency; may involve the immune system
Allergy	Involves immunologic mechanisms
Pseudoallergic	Similar clinical manifestations to allergic reaction but not immunologically mediated
Psychogenic	Psychologic reaction

Classification of Allergic Reactions

Gell and Coombs (1975) defined four basic types of immunologic mechanisms for hypersensitivity reactions. There are a number of reactions that are partially immune mediated (e.g., serum sickness–like reaction, acute generalized exanthematous pustulosis, drug-induced lupus, hypersensitivity syndrome reactions [Fig. B]).

Antigenic Properties of Drugs

Large molecular size (e.g., insulin, chymopapain) and complexity is associated with an increased ability to elicit an immune response. However, most drugs are low-molecular-weight compounds. For these compounds to become immunogenic, a drug or the metabolite (the hapten) must bind to a macromolecular carrier (Fig. A). Only a small number of drugs, notably penicillin and sulfonamide antibiotics, have had the haptenic determinant identified.

Testing

Both in vivo and in vitro testing have been used to diagnose drug allergies (Weiss, 1992). In vitro testing involves exposing the cells of patients to drugs or drug metabolites and observing for changes in cell activities or other indices. In general, in vitro testing is not as sensitive as in vivo testing techniques. In vivo challenge reexposes the patient to the drug in question. It is used in cases where the history of drug allergy is vague and the drug is considered essential. Oral challenges should not be confused with desensitization—the administration of minute quantities of drug to patients in whom drug allergy has been clearly established. Skin tests are the most useful and most sensitive method of determining IgE-mediated events (type I reactions). They have been used for high-molecular-weight proteins such as insulin and chymopapain and for major and minor determinants of penicillin. Skin tests are not useful for low-molecular-weight compounds unless the hapten has been identified (penicillin). Patch testing can be used for determination of delayed-type immune reactions, especially contact dermatitis.

Management

A systematic and rational approach to diagnosing an allergic drug reaction has been suggested: clinical diagnosis of the reaction, analysis of drug exposure, differential diagnosis, literature search regarding the adverse event and the drug, confirmation using in vivo or in vitro testing, advice to patient and his or her health care providers (i.e., which drugs to avoid in the future), and reporting to the licensing authorities or manufacturer (Recchia and Shear, 1994). During an acute reaction, withdrawal of the offending agent is recommended, especially for severe reactions such as anaphylaxis, hepatitis, and toxic epidermal necrolysis. Supportive care includes administration of antihistamines, systemic or topical corticosteroids, and other specific therapy (e.g., epinephrine for anaphylactic reaction).

Selection of medications for drug-allergic patients is based on three principles: (1) use of a drug with similar therapeutic efficacy but no cross-reactivity (macrolides in patients with β-lactam allergies), (2) use of suppressive medication (e.g., antihistamines and systemic corticosteroids prior to radiocontrast media administration), and (3) acute desensitization (e.g., gradually increasing doses of the drug over a period of hours to days).

FOUR CLASSIC ALLERGIC REACTION TYPES

Description	Primary Effector Mechanism	Clinical Reaction
Anaphylactic	IgE antibodies	Urticaria, hypotension, angioedema, bronchospasm, anaphylaxis
Cytotoxic IgG or IgM	Hemolytic anemia	
Immune complex reaction	Soluble immune complexes	Leukocytoclastic vasculitis
Delayed or cell-mediated hypersensitivity	Sensitized T lymphocytes	Contact dermatitis, fixed drug eruptions, exanthematous eruptions

PART II: QUESTIONS

Directions: For each of the following questions, choose the **one best** answer.

1. Which of the following descriptions of succinylcholine's mechanism of neuromuscular block is true?

(A) It is a competitive antagonist of muscarinic ACh receptors.

(B) It is a competitive antagonist of nicotinic ACh receptors.

(C) It is an irreversible antagonist of nicotinic ACh receptors.

(D) It is a depolarization block.

(E) It is highly susceptible to acetylcholinesterase.

2. Parkinson's disease is characterized by progressive degeneration of neurons containing the neurotransmitter

(A) GABA

(B) acetylcholine

(C) serotonin

(D) dopamine

(E) somatostatin

3. Which one of the following statements about prostaglandins is true?

(A) Prostaglandin synthesis is inhibited by aspirin.

(B) Prostaglandins play an important role in inflammation.

(C) Prostaglandins are products of cyclooxygenase activity.

(D) Prostaglandins act exclusively to stimulate adenylate cyclase.

(E) Prostaglandin E_2 can induce labor.

4. Which of the following statements about adrenergic receptors is true?

(A) Most blood vessels contain only α_1-adrenergic receptors.

(B) α_2-Adrenergic receptors are located only in the nervous system.

(C) Most of the β-adrenergic receptors in the heart are of the β_2 type.

(D) Most of the β-adrenergic receptors in the lung are of the β_2 type.

5. Allergic reactions to drugs are best described by which of the following statements?

(A) They account for the majority of adverse drug reactions.

(B) They involve effector cells of the immune system.

(C) They cannot be caused by metabolites.

(D) Large size and complexity of a drug molecule are associated with decreased risk of allergic reaction.

6. What structural features are common to all clinically useful β-adrenergic receptor antagonists?

(A) Aromatic ring system, aliphatic hydroxyl group, amine nitrogen

(B) Heterocyclic ring system, amine nitrogen

(C) Adjacent ring hydroxyl groups, amine nitrogen

(D) Aromatic and aliphatic portions linked by oxygen atom

7. Monoaminergic neurons are best differentiated from amino acid–containing neurons in that they

(A) always have an inhibitory function in the CNS

(B) are relatively few in number but extensively innervate most areas of the CNS

(C) synthesize neurotransmitters in the cell body and transport them to synaptic terminals

(D) do not coexist with other neurotransmitters in a single neuron

(E) mediate their effects by altering Cl^- conductance

8. Clinical indications for eicosanoids or their inhibitors include all of the following EXCEPT

(A) transposition of the great arteries

(B) hypertension

(C) patent ductus arteriosus

(D) abortion

(E) treatment of peptic ulcers

9. A typical adverse effect of cholinesterase inhibitors is

(A) abdominal cramps

(B) decreased salivation

(C) bronchial drying

(D) mioisis

(E) tachycardia

10. Which of the following agents is a muscarinic cholinergic receptor (mAChR) agonist?

(A) Atropine

(B) Carbachol

(C) Pirenzepine

(D) Scopolamine

11. What is an advantage of the newer antihistamines?

(A) They are more lipid soluble.

(B) They have a shorter duration of action.

(C) They are more selective for H_2 receptor subtypes.

(D) They produce fewer CNS effects.

12. A poor strategy for selection of medications for drug-allergic patients would be

(A) acute desensitization

(B) acute high-dose challenge, then tapering

(C) to choose a drug from a different chemical class

(D) to use suppressive medication

13. Antihypertensive therapeutic efficacy is improved for phentolamine-like drugs by subtype selectivity at which one of the following pharmacologic classes of adrenergic receptors?

(A) α-Adrenergic

(B) β-Adrenergic

(C) α_2-Adrenergic

(D) α_1-Adrenergic

14. Which of the following agents is a nicotinic cholinergic receptor (nAChR) agonist?

(A) Decamethonium

(B) Hexamethonium

(C) Nicotine

(D) Tubocurarine

15. Which of the following agents is the most selective for α-adrenergic receptors?

(A) Epinephrine

(B) Isoproterenol

(C) Norepinephrine

(D) Phenylephrine

(E) Terbutaline

16. Prolonged apnea in a patient who is administered succinylcholine is most likely due to a deficiency of

(A) acetylcholinesterase

(B) plasma cholinesterase

(C) tyrosine hydroxylase

(D) cytochrome P-450

17. All of the following statements are true EXCEPT

(A) leukotrienes are products of lipoxygenases

(B) prostaglandins act through G-protein–linked receptors

(C) thromboxane A_2 is a stable metabolite of arachidonic acid

(D) prostaglandin synthesis can be inhibited by corticosteroids

(E) prostaglandins act primarily as local hormones (autacoids)

18. Which of the following cholinesterases is more specific?

(A) Acetylcholinesterase (AChE)

(B) Butyrylcholinesterase (BuChE)

19. All of the following antimuscarinics enter the CNS EXCEPT

(A) atropine

(B) ipratropium

(C) benztropine

(D) trihexyphenidyl

20. Systemic administration of isoproterenol would produce

(A) increased diastolic blood pressure

(B) decreased heart rate

(C) decreased insulin secretion

(D) inotropic effect

21. All of the following responses are characteristic of muscarinic blockade EXCEPT

(A) mydriasis

(B) excessive salivation

(C) urinary retention

(D) adynamic ileus

22. Typical adverse effects of conventional H_1 antihistamines include all of the following EXCEPT

(A) diarrhea

(B) blurred vision

(C) orthostatic hypotension

(D) sleepiness

23. Carvedilol reduces morbidity and mortality in congestive heart failure. Based on the pharmacology of this agent, this can be explained by its ability to

(A) block both α_1- and β-adrenergic receptors

(B) increase sympathetic outflow to heart and blood vessels

(C) produce an intrinsic sympathomimetic effect

(D) selectively block cardiac β-adrenergic receptors

24. All of the following statements about eicosanoids are true EXCEPT

(A) eicosanoids are unsaturated fatty acids

(B) eicosanoids all contain a pentane ring

(C) eicosanoids originate primarily from arachidonic acid

(D) eicosanoids may act through several second messengers

(E) eicoisanoid synthesis results from activation of phospholipase A_2

25. Which of the following agents is the most selective β_2 agonist?

(A) Atenolol

(B) Isoproterenol

(C) Phenylephrine

(D) Prazosin

(E) Terbutaline

1. The answer is D.

Succinylcholine does not produce nondepolarizing antagonism of either muscarinic or nicotinic ACh receptors. By producing depolarization block, succinylcholine prevents the normal cycle of Na^+ gating and repolarization and leads to a refractoriness of the muscle to further stimulation by the neurotransmitter at neuromuscular junctions (ACh). Succinylcholine resists hydrolysis by acetylcholinesterase and persists longer in the neuromuscular synapse than does ACh.

2. The answer is D.

Parkinson's disease is characterized by a progressive degeneration of dopamine neurons located primarily in the substantia nigra. Loss of dopamine function results in motor dysfunction, which includes tremor, muscular weakness and rigidity, and akinesia. Treatment includes dopamine agonists and large doses of the dopamine precursor L-dopa, which are intended to help restore a more normal dopaminergic tone.

3. The answer is D.

Prostaglandins act through a variety of second-messenger systems to stimulate adenylate cyclase exclusively.

4. The answer is D.

Most of the β-adrenergic receptors in the lung are of the β_2 type. This difference allows for selective drug therapy in heart (mostly β_1-adrenergic receptors) or lung tissue. Most blood vessels do contain more than just the α_1 type of adrenergic receptors, and α_2-adrenergic receptors are distributed widely in the periphery as well as throughout the nervous system.

5. The answer is B.

Allergic reactions, which can be mild or serious, have been estimated to account for 6%–10% of all adverse reactions to drugs. Either the drug or one or more of its metabolites can elicit an allergic reaction involving effector cells of the immune system. Most drugs are small, low-molecular-weight compounds that require attachment to a much larger molecule before they can elicit an allergic reaction.

6. The answer is A.

Unlike α-adrenergic receptor antagonists, which show a high degree of structural diversity, all β-adrenergic receptor antagonists have an aromatic ring system, an alphatic hydroxyl group, and amine nitrogen, which are also found in the catecholamine neurotransmitters.

7. The answer is B.

Monoamine neurons comprise neurons containing dopamine, norepinephrine, histamine, and serotonin. Their cell bodies are relatively few in number and are located in discrete brainstem nuclei. However, each neuronal axon arborizes extensively so that virtually all areas of the CNS receive a significant monoaminergic input. In this manner a few neurons can extensively regulate neuronal activity throughout the brain. Cell bodies of amino acid–containing neurons are numerous and found throughout the CNS.

8. The answer is B.

None of the vasodilator eicosanoids has a long enough duration of action to be useful in hypertension.

9. The answer is A.

The adverse effects of anticholinesterases result from stimulation of muscarinic cholinergic receptors and hence produce parasympathomimetic side effects such as abdominal cramps. Increased salivation, bronchial secretions, mydriasis, and bradycardia are parasympathetic effects that result from stimulation of muscarinic receptors secondary to increased synaptic levels of ACh brought about by cholinesterase inhibition.

10. The answer is B.

Carbachol is an agonist at muscarinic cholinergic receptors and mimics the action of ACh at these sites. Atropine and scopolamine are relatively nonselective muscarinic cholinergic receptor antagonists, whereas pirenzepine is a relatively selective antagonist of the M_1 subtype of muscarinic receptor.

11. The answer is D.

Compared to the older agents, the newer antihistamines are less lipid soluble and, hence, penetrate the blood–brain barrier less readily than the older agents and produce less sedation. They have a longer duration of action (increased convenience). H_2 selectivity is of no advantage.

12. The answer is B.

Exposure of the patient to a high dose of the allergenic drug could result in greater harm. Acute densensitization might be achieved by gradually increasing the dose of the drug over a period of hours to days. A drug from a different chemical class (different structure) might not act as a hapten. The use of suppressive medication (e.g., antihistamines or corticosteroids) might be sufficient for mild, anticipated reactions (e.g., prior to administration of radiocontrast agents).

13. The answer is A.

The first α-adrenergic receptor antagonists such as phenoxybenzamine and phentolamine, which block both α_1- and α_2-adrenergic receptors, were not effective in the treatment of hypertension. The development of highly selective α_1-adrenergic receptor antagonists led to a group of clinically useful antihypertensive drugs.

14. The answer is C.

Nicotine is an agonist at nicotinic cholinergic receptors (hence the name of this subtype), and it mimics the action of ACh at these sites. Decamethonium potently acts at the neuromuscular junction and has little effect at ganglia, whereas the reverse is true for hexamethonium. Curare, long used for poison darts, is now commonly used in surgical procedures to produce skeletal muscle relaxation.

15. The answer is D.

Epinephrine and norepinephrine are not highly adrenergic receptor subtype selective. Isoproterenol and terbutaline are β-selective drugs.

16. The answer is B.

In most patients, succinylcholine normally is hydrolyzed by plasma esterases. Patients who have a deficiency of plasma esterase can demonstrate prolonged apnea with succinylcholine and require an alternative drug that can be eliminated by a different mechanism. Succinylcholine resists hydrolysis by acetylcholinesterase and is not affected by tyrosine hydroxylase. Cytochrome P-450 levels are not critical in patients who have sufficient plasma cholinesterase activity.

17. The answer is C.

Thromboxane is a highly unstable metabolite with a half-life on the order of seconds.

18. The answer is A.

Neuronal AChE, or "true" cholinesterase, is specific for ACh, whereas BuChE has low specificity and reacts more readily with other aliphatic and aromatic esters of choline.

19. The answer is B.

Ipratropium is a derivative of atropine with a permanent positive charge resulting from a quaternary nitrogen. As such it is unable to cross the blood–brain barrier in pharmacologically meaningful amounts, and its distribution is limited to the periphery. It is available in an aerosolized dosage form for direct application to the bronchioles. Atropine, benzotropine, and trihexyphenidyl are all tertiary amines and are thus lipophilic and readily enter the CNS; this distributive characteristic permits benzotropine and trihexyphenidyl to be used in the treatment of Parkinson's disease and drug-induced extrapyramidal syndrome.

20. The answer is D.

Isoproterenol is a relatively selective β-adrenergic receptor agonist. Systemic administration normally decreases diastolic blood pressure, but cardiac output increases due to its positive inotropic and chronotropic effects. Isoproterenol stimulates insulin secretion, which is another β-adrenergic receptor–mediated effect.

21. The answer is B.

Antimuscarinics exhibit strong antisecretory effects and thus are used preoperatively to reduce salivary secretions; an important side effect of these drugs is dry mouth. Mydriasis, urinary retention, and adynamic ileus are all typical responses to the decreased tone of smooth muscle effected by the antimuscarinics as competitive antagonists of ACh.

22. The answer is A.

In most patients, adverse effects of conventional antihistamines include a combination of antihistamine and anticholinergic actions (particularly for the less selective compounds). Therefore, blurred vision, orthostatic hypotension and sleepiness are encountered. Constipation, not diarrhea, is the more common GI effect.

23. The answer is A.

The β-adrenergic receptor antagonist activity of carvedilol reduces the cardiac effects of excess sympathetic drive associated with heart failure. Its α_1-adrenergic receptor antagonist activity produces vasodilation, reducing cardiac afterload. The combination of these two actions produces a synergistic improvement in cardiac function, resulting in symptomatic benefit.

24. The answer is B.

Not all eicosanoids contain a pentane ring. Thromboxane contains a six-membered oxane ring.

25. The answer is E.

Terbutaline is more selective for β_2-adrenergic receptors than are any of the other agents listed. As such, it is useful in producing smooth muscle contraction for treating asthma or premature labor. Atenolol is a selective antagonist of β_1-adrenergic receptors, and isoproterenol is a nonselective β antagonist. Both phenylephrine and prazosin are α-adrenergic receptor selective.

PART III
Peripheral Systems Pharmacology

21 Antiarrhythmic Agents

J. Andrew Wasserstrom, Ph.D.

A   Phases of cardiac action potential and underlying ionic currents

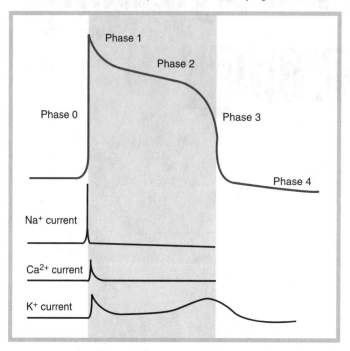

B   Antiarrhythmic drug binding to different states of cardiac Na⁺ channels

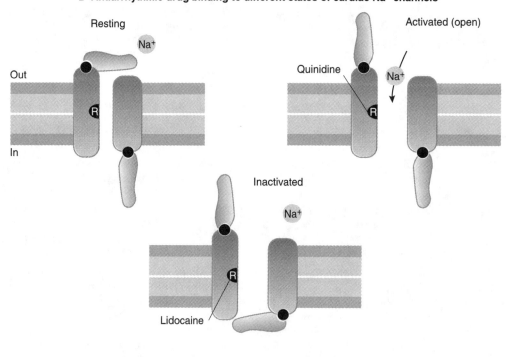

54

OVERVIEW

- There are four classifications of antiarrhythmic drugs that are loosely based on cellular mechanisms of action: local anesthetic block of cardiac sodium (Na^+) channels, β-adrenoceptor blockade, prolongation of action potential duration, and calcium (Ca^{2+}) channel antagonism.
- Channel blocking agents demonstrate use-dependent actions that improve their efficacy with more rapid arrhythmias.
- Most agents are taken orally and have the potential for numerous cardiac and CNS secondary actions.

General Strategies for Antiarrhythmic Drug Therapy

There are several ways in which antiarrhythmic drugs can slow or eliminate rapid excitation of the ventricle. One strategy is to reduce the excitation rate of a pacemaker site that is driving the heart at an abnormally high rate; reduction of pacemaker rate will restore the normal SA node rhythm. Another strategy is to reduce the number of action potentials that can conduct into the ventricular myocardium. If a rapid arrhythmia is the result of repetitive ventricular excitations (as in most ventricular tachycardias), ventricular rate can be reduced by (1) action potential prolongation so that fewer impulses can be activated or by (2) reducing excitability of the cell membrane so that it becomes more difficult to generate an action potential. In some cases (e.g., atrial tachycardias, flutter, and fibrillation), simply slowing AV nodal conduction slows ventricular rate even though atrial rate will be unaltered.

Drug Classifications

Class I—Na$^+$-Channel Blocking Agents. As shown in Fig. A, inward Na^+ current is activated at the onset of membrane depolarization and is responsible for the upstroke (phase 0) of the cardiac action potential. Activation of Na^+ channels is followed within 1–2 msec by channel closure during maintained depolarization to a state known as inactivation, from which channels cannot reopen. Only following repolarization to the resting potential are Na^+ channels available once again to be reactivated. Drugs that block Na^+ channels alter the excitability of the cardiac cell membrane; with reduction of excitability, the likelihood of rapid reexcitation is reduced, thus slowing or abolishing arrhythmias. Different agents bind to the various states of the channel (Fig. B). For example, lidocaine preferentially binds to the inactivated channel, slowing its recovery even at normal resting potential. Quinidine binds to the open channel, again slowing its recovery rate and maintaining a reduced level of excitability well after full repolarization. Na^+-channel blocking activity also produces a use-dependent effect; the extent of block is cumulative between action potentials so that block increases with successive depolarization, making the drug more effective with more rapid tachycardias. Finally, most of these agents directly reduce the rate of secondary pacemakers.

There are three subcategories of Na^+-channel blocking agents: class IA agents (e.g., quinidine and procainamide) reduce excitability and prolong action potential duration; class IB agents (e.g., lidocaine and mexiletine) have modest effects on excitability but shorten action potential duration; and class IC agents (e.g., flecainide and propafenone) reduce excitability but have little effect on repolarization. Most antiarrhythmic agents can be taken orally with the exception of lidocaine, which must be administered acutely intravenously. See Appendix, A, for specific agents and their properties.

Class II—Sympatholytic (β-Adrenergic) Blocking Agents. The prototype of these agents is propranolol, although sotalol is currently in wide use. These agents are effective in instances where premature ventricular contractions (PVCs), AV junctional arrhythmias, or atrial or ventricular tachycardias are generated as the result of excessive adrenergic tone.

Class III—Agents That Prolong Action Potential Duration. By prolonging action potential duration, ventricular rate must necessarily be slowed because the ventricle takes much longer to repolarize, therefore delaying recovery of Na^+ channels and cell excitability. Amiodarone is the most widely used of these agents, although bretylium is also effective. Amiodarone blocks both Na^+ and Ca^{2+} channels but also blocks several types of K^+ channels; as shown in Fig. A, the activation of K^+ channels is primarily responsible for cell repolarization both at the beginning (phase 1) and at the end of the plateau (phase 3). Effects of these agents to reduce delayed activation of K^+ channels is thought to underlie their ability to prolong action potential duration and to abolish rapid ventricular tachyarrhythmias.

Class IV—Ca^{2+}-Channel Antagonists. Voltage-dependent Ca^{2+} channels are activated early in depolarization during the beginning of the action potential plateau (phases 1 and 2) and allow Ca^{2+} influx across the sarcolemma, which is critical to activate contraction. These drugs produce state-dependent ion channel interactions similar to those described for class I agents with the Na^+ channel. These agents (e.g., verapamil) reduce conduction through the AV node, where cell activation is primarily dependent on Ca^{2+} channels, thus, they are effective in arrhythmias where atrial rate is very high and the goal of therapy is to reduce ventricular rate.

Efficacy of Agents with Multiple Actions. It is very likely that it is this combination of cellular actions that makes these agents so effective, rather than an interaction with a single ion channel target. Quinidine blocks both Na^+ and K^+ channels, which is responsible for both class I and class III characteristics. Amiodarone, currently the most effective and widely used antiarrhythmic agent for ventricular tachyarrhythmias, displays characteristics of classes I, II, and III.

Toxicity

Secondary actions of antiarrhythmic drugs are extensive: CNS toxicity such as convulsions with lidocaine, arrhythmias such as torsade de pointes with action potential–prolonging agents (class IA), and alterations in autonomic tone (e.g., quinidine block of vagal tone). Amiodarone can cause pulmonary fibrosis, corneal drug deposits, and skin discoloration.

22 Antianginal Agents

Jan M. Kitzen, R.Ph., Ph.D.

A Sites of action in the heart and circulation

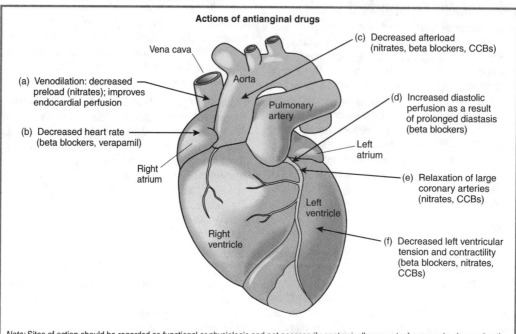

Actions of antianginal drugs

(a) Venodilation: decreased preload (nitrates); improves endocardial perfusion

(b) Decreased heart rate (beta blockers, verapamil)

Vena cava

Aorta

Pulmonary artery

Right atrium

Left ventricle

Right ventricle

(c) Decreased afterload (nitrates, beta blockers, CCBs)

(d) Increased diastolic perfusion as a result of prolonged diastasis (beta blockers)

Left atrium

(e) Relaxation of large coronary arteries (nitrates, CCBs)

(f) Decreased left ventricular tension and contractility (beta blockers, nitrates, CCBs)

Note: Sites of action should be regarded as functional or physiologic and not necessarily anatomically accurate; for example, decreasing the afterload does not actually refer to action on the aorta but to a decrease in arterial blood pressure that results from peripheral vasodilation.

B Mechanisms of action for nitrates and CCBs

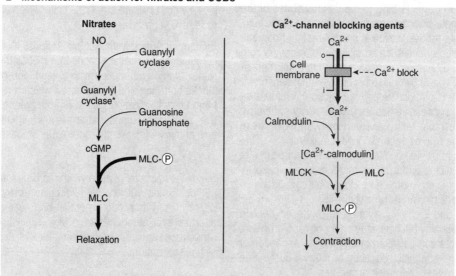

Nitrates

NO

Guanylyl cyclase

Guanylyl cyclase*

Guanosine triphosphate

cGMP   MLC-P

MLC

Relaxation

Ca^{2+}-channel blocking agents

Ca^{2+}

Cell membrane $\leftarrow$ - - -Ca^{2+} block

Ca^{2+}

Calmodulin

[Ca^{2+}-calmodulin]

MLCK   MLC

MLC-P

Contraction

Note: Heavy arrows = critical steps for causing relaxation; MLC = myosin light chain; MLCK = myosin light chain kinase; NO = nitric oxide; o = outside; i = inside; P = phosphate. *Activated guanylyl cyclase

Background, Definition, and Classification

A temporary imbalance in the myocardial supply and demand for oxygen can lead to an anginal attack, defined as precordial chest pain lasting approximately 3–5 minutes. The pain may radiate to the neck, jaw, and arm.

Angina is classified into three general categories:

- Chronic stable angina: Caused by an atherosclerotic obstruction of the coronary arteries. Physical exertion leads to increases in myocardial demand for oxygen that cannot be supplied by flow through the partially obstructed artery, resulting in chest pain.
- Unstable angina: Characterized by frequent episodes of chest pain occurring at rest. Ischemia is due to thrombotic occlusion consequent to plaque fissuring and platelet aggregation.
- Vasospastic or variant angina (also Prinzmetal's angina): Active vasospasm of larger coronary arteries. This can occur at rest or on exercise, is unpredictable, and may occur in normal vessels.

Medicinal Chemistry

There are three types of agents used in the treatment of angina: the nitrates, the Ca^{2+}-channel blockers, and beta-blocking agents. These may be used individually or as combination therapy.

Nitrates. Sublingual nitroglycerin (nitrate) is the mainstay of treatment. The organic nitrates are polyol esters of nitric acid. The organic nitrates and several other compounds that are capable of denitration to release NO are collectively referred to as *nitrovasodilators*.

Ca^{2+}-Channel Blockers. The nine compounds approved for clinical use in the United States are derived from four chemical classes: phenylalkylamines (verapamil), dihydropyridines (nifedipine), benzothiazepines (diltiazem), and a diarylaminopropylamine (bepridil). Newer compounds are primarily dihydropyridine derivatives with improvements in pharmacokinetic profile, greater vascular selectivity, and fewer direct negative inotropic effects.

Beta-blockers. Most of the effective beta-blocking agents may be thought of chemically as derivatives of the beta-agonist isoproterenol.

Clinical and Pharmacologic Effects

Nitrates. Several effects of the nitrates contribute to their clinical efficacy in relieving anginal pain (Fig. A). By causing dilation of the systemic veins, the preload of the heart is reduced (site a), which improves endocardial perfusion and also decreases myocardial wall tension (site f) and oxygen demand. Nitrates also cause vasodilation of large and medium-sized coronary arteries (site e). This improves the oxygen delivery and perfusion of the subendocardial region of the heart. Nitrates actively promote relaxation by releasing NO, which then activates guanylyl cyclase (Fig. B). Cyclic GMP (cGMP) then leads to the dephosphorylation of myosin light chain (MLC), resulting in a decreased interaction with actin. Nitrates also inhibit platelet aggregation, a beneficial effect in unstable angina.

Ca^{2+}-Channel Blockers. These agents selectively inhibit the influx of Ca^{2+} into vascular and myocardial cells (Fig. B). They are generally considered to do this by blocking the L type of Ca^{2+} channel (gray-hatched area in Fig. B). Relaxation of arterial smooth muscle leads to decreased peripheral resistance and a reduction in cardiac afterload (Fig. A, site c). Verapamil is effective in reducing heart rate (site b).

Beta-blockers. Reduce the oxygen demand of the heart by decreasing the double product (heart rate × blood pressure; Fig. A, sites b and c) and by depressing contractility (site f). By prolonging the period of relaxation (diastasis), coronary perfusion is facilitated (site d).

Pharmacokinetics

Because of the ability of the liver to remove nitrate groups, the organic nitrates have low bioavailability. Nitroglycerin (NTG) is absorbed from the skin and oral mucosa, and less readily from the gut. Sublingual NTG leads to an onset of clinical effects within 1–2 minutes and can last up to 1 hour. Isosorbide dinitrate (ISDN) is also absorbed from the oral mucosa and gut, with a somewhat slower onset and longer duration of action. Nitrates are primarily excreted renally as the glucuronide conjugate of the denitrated metabolite. Ca^{2+}-channel blockers are well absorbed; however, as with the other antianginal agents, significant first-pass metabolism reduces bioavailability. Dosages should be reduced in patients with hepatic cirrhosis.

Toxicity, Side Effects, and Drug Interactions

Nitrates. Headache is the most common side effect and can be severe. It usually decreases after a few days and can be controlled by decreasing the dose and treatment with a mild analgesic. Other untoward reactions include dizziness, weakness, and other manifestations of postural hypotension. Continued exposure can lead to development of tolerance in just a few hours. For this reason, combination therapy with a beta-blocker or Ca^{2+}-channel blocker is frequently employed. Sildenafil (Viagra), recently introduced for the treatment of male erectile dysfunction, interacts with nitrates to produce profound hypotension with an associated risk of myocardial infarction resulting from coronary hypoperfusion.

Beta-blockers. The major risk is cardiac depression as a result of excessive beta-blockade. Since the nonselective beta-blockers can cause increases in airway resistance, they are contraindicated in patients with asthma.

Ca^{2+}-Channel Blockers. Side effects are primarily due to excess vasodilation and are manifested as headaches, flushing, dizziness, and pedal edema. The Ca^{2+}-channel blockers all have the potential to cause myocardial depression; however, with proper use this is not usually a problem. Constipation has been associated with verapamil, especially in elderly subjects.

23 Agents for the Treatment of Congestive Heart Failure

Tai Akera, M.D., Ph.D.

A Action of digoxin and dobutamine

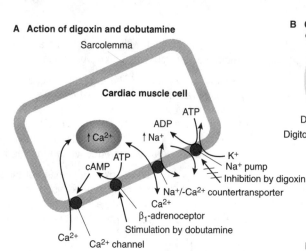

Sarcolemma

Cardiac muscle cell

↑ indicates drug-induced increase

B Chemical structure of digoxin

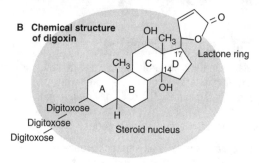

Lactone ring

Digitoxose

Digitoxose

Digitoxose

Steroid nucleus

C Na⁺ pump inhibition and effects of digoxin

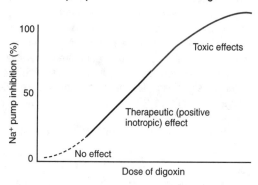

Toxic effects

Therapeutic (positive inotropic) effect

No effect

Dose of digoxin

D Accumulation and plasma concentration of digitoxin during repeated administration

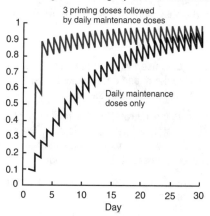

3 priming doses followed by daily maintenance doses

Daily maintenance doses only

Day

E Imbalance between cardiac force of contraction and work load*

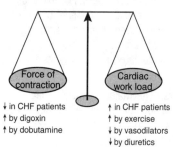

Force of contraction	Cardiac work load
↓ in CHF patients	↑ in CHF patients
↑ by digoxin	↑ by exercise
↑ by dobutamine	↓ by vasodilators
	↓ by diuretics

* Resulting from body's attempts to maintain blood pressure by activation of sympathetic, renin-angiotensin, and endothelin systems and by ↑ circulating plasma volume in patients with CHF.

F Three-month mortality in SOLVD treatment, exercise studies, and ELITE

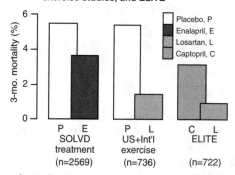

- Placebo, P
- Enalapril, E
- Losartan, L
- Captopril, C

P E SOLVD treatment (n=2569)

P L US+Int'l exercise (n=736)

C L ELITE (n=722)

Source: Reprinted with permission from Pitt et al: Randomized trial of losartan versus captopril in patients over 65 with heart failure (Evaluation of Losartan in the Elderly study, ELITE). *Lancet* 349:747, 1997.

Treatment of Congestive Heart Failure

CHF is a condition wherein the ability of the heart to pump blood is compromised and the heart cannot meet the demand when motor activity is increased. This imbalance can be corrected by either increasing the force of heart contraction (cardiotonic drugs) or decreasing the work load (vasodilators and diuretics). All these treatments are palliative, because no drug can restore damaged heart muscle.

The effects of another class of vasodilator, calcium-channel blockers, are controversial. Short-acting calcium-channel blockers have problems of substantial and fluctuating inhibition of cardiac contractions; however, modern long-acting calcium-channel blockers, such as amlodipine, appear to provide beneficial effects.

Losartan has been reported to be more effective than angiotensin-converting enzyme (ACE) inhibitors in reducing sudden death and cardiac events. The mechanism for the difference is unknown, however.

Pharmacology

Digitalis glycosides and allied drugs inhibit the sodium pump of the cell membrane. A slight increase in intracellular Na^+ increases cellular Ca^{2+} via sarcolemmal Na^+-Ca^{2+} countertransporter. Dobutamine increases cAMP by stimulating β_1-adrenergic receptors and amrinone and milrinone by inhibiting phosphodiesterase subtype III. An increase in cAMP enhances Ca^{2+} influx via calcium channels. These drugs enhance the force of myocardial contraction and improve hemodynamics. (For vasodilators and diuretics, see other chapters.)

Medicinal Chemistry

Digitalis glycosides have a steroid structure. These steroids, however, have a trans-C-D fusion, unlike the corticosteroids, which have a cis-C-D fusion. An unsaturated lactone ring is essential, whereas sugar moieties contribute to high receptor affinity.

Pharmacokinetics

Administration and Distribution. Digitalis glycosides, vasodilators, and diuretics are usually administered orally. Absorption of digoxin could be variable (45%–85%), depending on tablet preparations. Absorption of digitoxin is above 90%. Because of the narrow margin of safety of digitalis glycosides, variable absorption of digoxin may result in toxicity or lack of efficacy. Dobutamine, amrinone, and milrinone require intravenous administration and, therefore, are not suitable for long-term treatment.

Metabolism and Excretion. Renal excretion is the major route of elimination for digoxin. Digitoxin is metabolized by the liver. Because of a large apparent volume of distribution, digoxin (1.7 days) and digitoxin (7 days) have a long half-life.

Drug Interactions

Quinidine increases digoxin (but not digitoxin) concentration in plasma and may trigger digitalis toxicity. Diuretics reduce K^+ concentration in plasma and enhance toxic actions of digoxin or digitoxin.

Toxicity

Overdose of digitalis glycosides causes arrhythmia by inhibiting AV conduction, primarily through parasympathetic activation, and by directly enhancing excitability of cells in the conduction system and ventricular muscle proper. Digitalis toxicity results from excessive sodium pump inhibition and excessive cellular Ca^{2+} overloading. Low plasma K^+ concentration enhances digitalis toxicity. Dobutamine, amrinone, and milrinone may cause mild chronotropic, hypertensive, and arrhythmogenic effects. Clinical studies show that long-term treatment with amrinone or milrinone may increase mortality in heart failure patients. (For other classes of drugs, see respective chapters.)

SPECIFIC AGENTS

Digitalis glycosides
Digoxin (generic, Lanoxin)
- Narrow margin of safety

Digitoxin (generic, Crystodigin)
- Slow onset of action; digitalization needed
- Narrow margin of safety

Angiotensin II receptor antagonist
Losartan (Cozaar)
- Marked reduction of cardiovascular events in patients with advanced CHF
- Very few side effects

Diuretics
- Enhances digitalis toxicity by plasma K^+ depletion

β_1-Adrenergic receptor agonist
- IV use only for short-term support. Note that β-adrenergic receptor antagonists may also be used for the treatment of CHF.

Phosphodiesterase (type III) inhibitors
Amrinone (Inocor) and milrinone (Primacor)
- For short-term support only. These drugs are shown to increase mortality over long-term use.

ACE inhibitors
Captopril (Capoten
- 1st ACE inhibitor (1977)

Enalapril (Vasotec)
- Metabolite (enalapriate) is the active form.

24 Antihypertensive Agents

Robert B. Raffa, Ph.D.

A

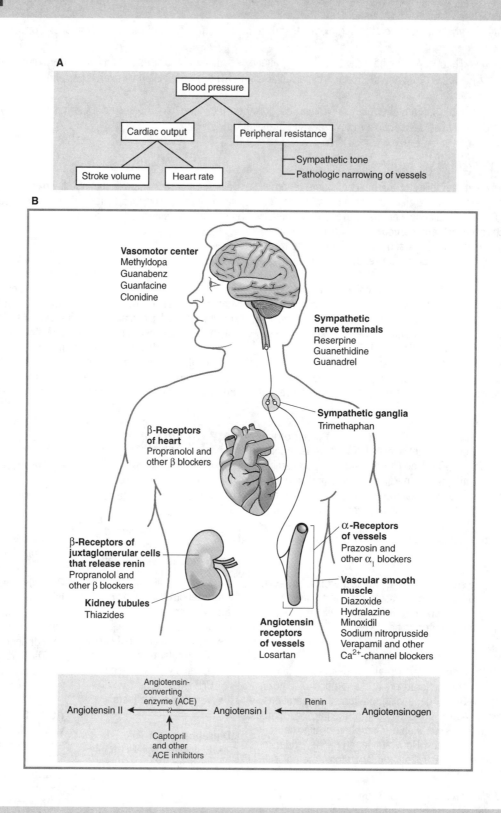

Blood pressure
— Cardiac output
— Stroke volume
— Heart rate
— Peripheral resistance
— Sympathetic tone
— Pathologic narrowing of vessels

B

Vasomotor center
Methyldopa
Guanabenz
Guanfacine
Clonidine

Sympathetic nerve terminals
Reserpine
Guanethidine
Guanadrel

Sympathetic ganglia
Trimethaphan

β-Receptors of heart
Propranolol and other β blockers

β-Receptors of juxtaglomerular cells that release renin
Propranolol and other β blockers

Kidney tubules
Thiazides

α-Receptors of vessels
Prazosin and other α_1 blockers

Vascular smooth muscle
Diazoxide
Hydralazine
Minoxidil
Sodium nitroprusside
Verapamil and other Ca^{2+}-channel blockers

Angiotensin receptors of vessels
Losartan

Angiotensin II ← Angiotensin-converting enzyme (ACE) ← Angiotensin I ← Renin ← Angiotensinogen

Captopril and other ACE inhibitors

OVERVIEW

- Antihypertensive agents counteract the rise in blood pressure that accompanies pathologic changes in cardiac function or blood vessel diameter (e.g., atherosclerosis). These changes have been associated with increased risk of morbidity and mortality.
- Choice of agent is based on precipitating factor (if known) or degree of hypertension; degree of end-organ damage; comorbidity; patient compliance with drug, exercise, or dietary regimens; and mechanism and toxicity profile of the drug or combination of drugs.
- Mechanisms of action: reduction of cardiac output, peripheral resistance, or CNS influence.
- Sites of action: CNS, heart, smooth muscle of blood vessels (mainly arterioles), kidney, and angiotensin.

Diuretics

These lower blood pressure by decreasing blood volume and thus cardiac output (early in therapy) and by decreasing peripheral resistance (after 6–8 weeks). The latter may result from decreased Na^+, subsequent decreased Na^+-Ca^{2+} exchange, and hence decreased intracellular Ca^{2+} within smooth muscle of blood vessels. Generally are effective for mild or moderate hypertension in patients with normal renal and cardiac function and are used in combination with other antihypertensives for more severe hypertension. Thiazide diuretics can produce hypokalemia and its sequelae, can precipitate gout, and can result in drug-drug interactions (e.g., with digitalis). "Potassium-sparing" and "loop" diuretics have lesser and greater ion-depleting actions, respectively. (For specific drugs, see Chap. 27.)

Sympathetic Nervous System Modifiers

α_1-*Adrenoceptor Antagonists.* Decrease sympathetic tone by pharmacologic antagonism of the vasoconstricting action of NE or epinephrine on smooth muscle of the vasculature. Because sympathetic tone normally predominates, α_1 antagonism results in vasodilation if the vessel is not already maximally dilated.

- Doxazosin (Cardura); prazosin (Minipress); terazosin (Hytrin)

α_2-*Adrenoceptor Agonists.* Decrease sympathetic tone by activation of (presynaptic) negative feedback on release of NE from sympathetic innervation of smooth muscle of the vasculature. These agents have central and peripheral actions. Dry mouth, sedation, and mental depression are possible adverse effects. As with most antihypertensive therapy, withdrawal should be gradual.

- Clonidine (generic, Catapres); guanabenz (Wytensin); guanfacine (Tenex); methyldopa (generic, Aldomet)

β-*Adrenoceptor Antagonists.* Decrease sympathetic tone by pharmacologic antagonism of the chronotropic and inotropic actions of NE or epinephrine on the heart. The more β_1-selective agents have less adverse effect on lung (e.g., in asthma) or other functions involving β_2 adrenoceptors.

- Acebutolol (Sectral); atenolol (generic, Tenormin); betaxolol (Kerlone); bisoprolol; carteolol (Cartrol); labetalol (Normodyne, Trandate); metoprolol (Lopressor); nadolol (Corgard); penbutolol (Levatol); pindolol (generic, Visken); propranolol (generic, Inderal); timolol (generic, Blocadren)

Ganglionic Blockers. Decrease sympathetic tone by pharmacologic antagonism of the action of ACh on nicotinic receptors (N_N-AChR) located on the ganglia of the autonomic nervous system. Adverse effects generally are extensions of N_N-AChR block, such as orthostatic hypotension, sexual dysfunction, constipation, blurred vision, and dry mouth.

- Mecamylamine (Inversine)

Indirect-Acting Drugs. Decrease sympathetic tone by inhibiting the synthesis, storage, or release of NE from nerve terminals.

- Guanadrel (Hylorel); guanethidine (generic, Ismelin); reserpine (generic, Serpasil)

Vascular Agents

Direct Vasodilators. These act by a variety of mechanisms (e.g., enhanced action of nitric oxide, cAMP, cGMP). Sympathetic reflexes remain intact; hence orthostatic hypotension or sexual dysfunction are not common adverse effects.

- Diazoxide (generic, Hyperstat I.V.); hydralazine (generic, Apresoline); minoxidil (generic, Loniten); sodium nitroprusside (generic, Nipride)

Ca^{2+} -*Channel Blockers.* Inhibit Ca^{2+} influx into smooth muscle cells. Several Ca^{2+} channels are known; most present drugs inhibit the L type.

- Amlodipine (Norvasc); diltiazem (generic, Cardizem); felodipine (Plendil); isradipine (DynaCirc); nicardipine (Cardene); nisoldipine (Sular); nifedipine (generic, Adalat, Procardia); verapamil (generic, Calan, Isoptin)

Adverse Effects. Common adverse effect include headache and, in the case of the direct vasodilators, excess hypotension. Each agent can have serious adverse effects or drug-drug interactions; thus more detailed accounts of agents should be consulted.

Angiotensin-Directed Agents

ACE Inhibitors. Decrease peripheral vascular resistance, generally without reflex tachycardia. Angiotensinogen is converted (by renin) to angiotensin I and then the potent vasoconstricting angiotensin II (by ACE). Converting enzyme (kininase II) also mediates the breakdown of bradykinin. Adverse effects include severe hypotension, acute renal failure, hyperkalemia (possible interaction with K^+ supplements or K^+-sparing diuretics), and dry cough. NSAIDs can impair ACE inhibitor efficacy by blocking bradykinin-induced vasodilation (which involves prostaglandins).

- Benazepril (Lotensin); captopril (Capoten); enalapril (Vasotec); fosinopril (Monopril); lisinopril (Prinivil, Zestril); moexipril (Univasc); perindopril (Aceon); quinapril (Accupril); ramipril (Altace)

Angiotensin-Receptor Antagonists. These agents block the action of angiotensin. Adverse effects are similar to the ACE inhibitors with the notable exception of cough and other bradykinin-mediated effects.

- Losartan (Cozaar); valsartan (Diovan)

25 Antianemia Agents

Robert B. Raffa, Ph.D.

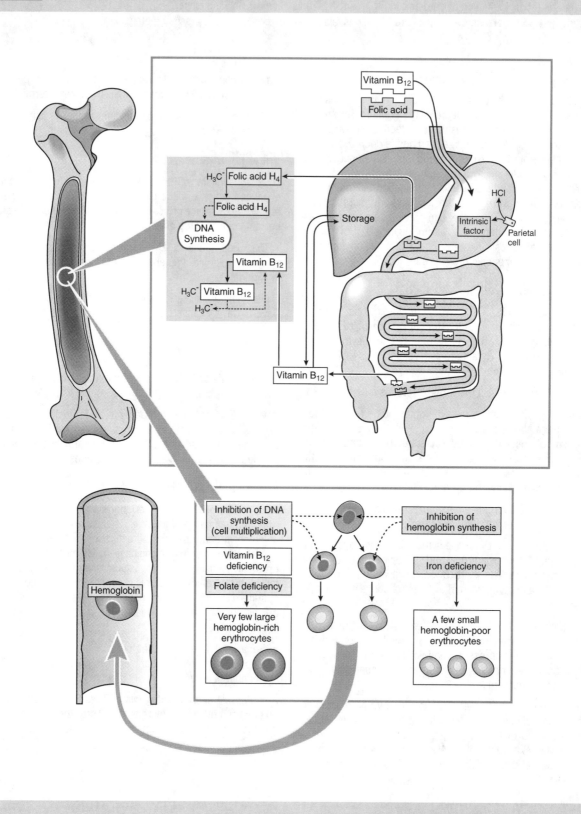

OVERVIEW

- Antianemia agents reestablish the hemoglobin function of the blood to levels that are necessary to satisfy the oxygen demands of the body. The choice of agent is based on the type (cause) of the anemia.
- Mechanisms of action: replenishment of deficient nutrients and vitamins or stimulation of red blood cell production.
- Sites of action: diet (replacement therapy) or bone marrow (RBC colony-stimulating factors).
- Therapeutic uses: treatment of specific anemia disorder (e.g., aplastic, autoimmune, congenital, Cooley's, megaloblastic, microcytic, pernicious, sickle cell, etc.) or anemia secondary to other disorders or therapies (e.g., radiation or cancer chemotherapy).
- Overuse of iron supplements can lead to iron toxicity. Overly aggressive use of colony-stimulating growth factors can lead to a too rapid rise in hemoglobin or hematocrit.

Pharmacology

The iron in hemoglobin reversibly binds oxygen. Iron supplements release iron that is absorbed (following oral or parenteral administration) and is incorporated into hemoglobin. Vitamin B_{12} and folic acid are essential for DNA synthesis, and deficiency leads to impaired DNA synthesis and hence to abnormal cell production or function—particularly of rapidly dividing cells like RBCs. Replacement therapy reverses the impaired hematopoiesis. Hematopoietic growth factors stimulate the proliferation and differentiation of hematopoietic progenitor cells in the bone marrow.

Medicinal Chemistry

Hemoglobin in RBCs reversibly binds oxygen and is the major carrier for oxygen transport from lungs to tissues. Hemoglobin consists of an iron-porphyrin ring (heme) and associated globin chains. Iron is a critical component of the oxygen-binding region of heme. Therapeutic iron supplements contain elemental iron in the form of iron salts or as complexes of iron with inorganic substances (e.g., dextran).

Folates are required as cofactors for several enzymes necessary for DNA synthesis, specifically in reactions leading to thymidylic acid and the purine heterocycle. Vitamin B_{12} contains a prophyrin-like ring with a cobalt atom. Vitamin B_{12} catalytically converts 5-CH_3-H_4 folate and homocysteine to H_4 folate and methionine. Without folic acid or vitamin B_{12} these reactions cannot occur and the necessary continuous production of RBCs is interrupted.

Human erythropoietin is produced by recombinant DNA technology (r-HuEPO) as a heavily glycosylated 165–amino acid peptide (MW = 30,400).

Direct and Indirect Anemias

Anemia results when the blood is unable to meet the normal oxygen demands of the body. This situation can be brought about by:

- Blood loss
- Reduced number (production) of circulating RBCs
- Reduced concentration of RBCs in blood
- Reduced amount of hemoglobin
- Reduced oxygen-binding capacity of hemoglobin

These conditions can arise as the result of injury, genetic defects, and as symptoms of illness and disease. The treatment can be symptomatic or directed at the underlying cause.

Pharmacokinetics

Administration and Distribution. Iron (commonly administered orally as ferrous salts) is rapidly absorbed under normal conditions, mostly in the duodenum and proximal jejunum. Different preparations contain different percentages of elemental iron (typically 12%–33%). Oral therapy might be recommended for several (3–6) months to replenish the iron stores that were depleted during the body's early attempt to compensate for the iron loss. Folic acid is usually well absorbed even in patients with malabsorption problems. In contrast, vitamin B_{12} usually must be injected, because most causes of its deficiency are related to malabsorption of the vitamin from the GI tract. r-HuEPO usually is administered intravenously or subcutaneously (it is broken down in the GI tract).

Metabolism and Excretion. As replacement therapy, these substances are metabolized and excreted in the same manner as the endogenous material. There is no efficient method for excretion of excess iron.

Adverse Effects or Toxicity

Iron. Injection of iron can cause local discomfort, discoloration, and possible malignant skin changes. By any route, headache, fever, arthralgias, and lymphadenopathy can occur, and anaphylactic reactions (rare) can be fatal. Iron toxicity in adults is rare, but young children are much more susceptible. Acute oral iron overdose can cause necrotizing gastroenteritis and serious sequelae. Chronic iron toxicity can lead to organ failure and death.

Folic Acid and Vitamin B_{12}. Large doses of folic acid and vitamin B_{12} are promptly eliminated (urine and stool); hence neither is associated with significant toxicity.

Erythropoietin. The most common adverse experiences with erythropoietin derive from too-rapid administration and thus can be minimized. Allergic reactions or overt toxicity are rare.

SPECIFIC AGENTS

Iron	Folic Acid	Vitamin B_{12}	Erythropoietin (epoetin alfa, Epo, r-HuEPO)
Ferrous sulfate, hydrated Ferrous sulfate, dessicated Ferrous gluconate Ferrous fumarate Iron dextran (INFeD) [parenteral only]	Folacin, pteroylglutamic acid (generic) [oral or parenteral]	Cyanocobalamin or hydroxocobalamin (generic)	Recombinant erythropoietin epoetin alfa, r-HuEPO (Epogen, Procrit)

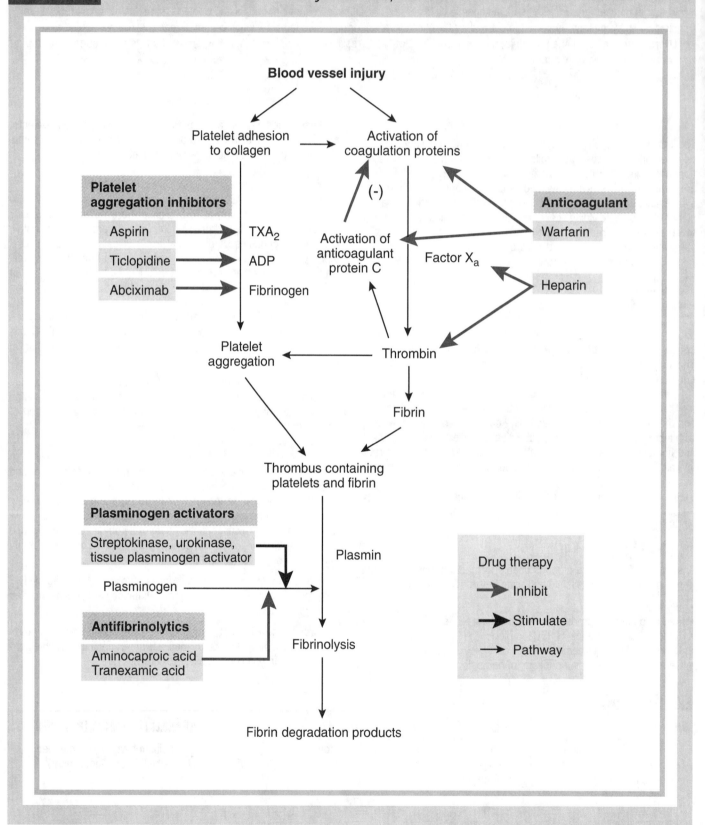

OVERVIEW

- Disorders of coagulation factors, platelets, or the vessel wall, often as a consequence of trauma, surgery, or cardiovascular disease, can lead to thrombosis in the arterial and venous circulation.
- Major antiplatelet drugs to reduce arterial thrombosis and stroke are aspirin, ticlopidine, and abciximab.
- Major anticoagulants to prevent arterial and venous thromboembolism are warfarin, heparin, and enoxaparin.
- Major fibrinolytics to remove unwanted thrombi are streptokinase, urokinase, and tissue plasminogen activator.
- Drugs used to decrease bleeding (often caused by anticoagulants or fibrinolytics) include vitamin K, protamine sulfate, aminocaproic acid, and tranexamic acid.

Antiplatelet Agents

Aspirin. Irreversibly inhibits constitutive cyclooxygenase (COX-1) in platelets by acetylating a serine residue near the active site, preventing formation of thromboxane A_2 (TXA_2) from arachidonic acid released from platelet membrane phospholipids. TXA_2 augments the aggregation process that occurs after platelets adhere to collagen.

Ticlopidine. Inhibits ADP-induced binding of fibrinogen to platelet integrin $\alpha_{IIb}\beta_3$, which is necessary for platelet aggregation. ADP is released from platelet granules when platelets adhere to collagen or are exposed to thrombin.

Abciximab. The Fab fragment of a chimeric human-murine monoclonal antibody to the $\alpha_{IIb}\beta_3$. It competes with fibrinogen for binding sites. In contrast to aspirin and ticlopidine, abciximab inhibits aggregation induced by all agents, including thrombin.

Anticoagulants

Warfarin. Coumarin derivative that resembles vitamin K. It prevents the formation of active molecules of several coagulation proteins by blocking regeneration of vitamin K. It also prevents formation of naturally occurring anticoagulant proteins C and S.

Heparin. Mixture of highly acidic mucopolysaccharides, heparin is abundant in liver and lungs. By binding to a lysine-rich site in plasma antithrombin III (AT-III), it accelerates inactivation of coagulation factors Xa and thrombin.

Enoxaparin. Low-molecular-weight fraction of heparin. Causes more effective neutralization of factor Xa than thrombin, as compared to unfractionated heparin, and has a longer biologic half-life.

Fibrinolytics

Streptokinase. Bacterial product that forms a complex with plasminogen to activate other plasminogen molecules to the enzyme plasmin. Plasmin degrades fibrin clots.

Urokinase (u-PA). Proteolytic enzyme produced by the kidney and found in the urine; urokinase cleaves plasminogen to plasmin.

Tissue Plasminogen Activator (t-PA). t-PA cleaves a susceptible bond in plasminogen to generate plasmin.

Agents for Controlling Blood Loss

Vitamin K. Fat-soluble vitamin whose presence is partly dependent on its synthesis by intestinal bacteria that is required for the synthesis of several coagulation proteins and the anticoagulant proteins C and S. It is given prophylactically as phytonadione to prevent hemorrhage in newborns and is used to treat warfarin overdosage.

Protamine Sulfate. Electropositive, low-molecular-weight protein that binds to heparin and forms an inert complex. It is used to treat heparin overdosage.

Aminocaproic Acid. Antifibrinolytic drug useful in fibrinolytic bleeding complications such as those following heart surgery. It acts principally by inhibition of plasminogen activators.

Tranexamic Acid. Acts like aminocaproic acid.

Pharmacokinetics

Aspirin. Effect on platelets is rapid and persists longer than one day, as recovery of the ability to synthesize TXA_2 requires the entry of new platelets into the circulation. It is maximally effective as an antithrombotic at 160–320 mg/d.

Ticlopidine. Requires about 10 days of oral ingestion to achieve full effect. It is well absorbed, binds to plasma proteins, and is metabolized by the liver.

Abciximab. Platelet function generally recovers over 48 hours, although the drug remains in the circulation for up to 10 days in a platelet-bound state.

Warfarin. Administered orally; full effect is not observed until all coagulation factors in blood are catabolized. Heparin treatment is used for the first 5 days. More than 95% of circulating warfarin is bound by plasma albumin. It is the free drug that inhibits vitamin K regeneration; displacement of bound warfarin by other drugs may result in bleeding. Warfarin is hydroxylated in the liver; its metabolites are excreted via bile.

Heparin. IV administration results in immediate anticoagulant effect with a half-life of about 1 hour. It is not bound by plasma proteins. Its action is terminated by uptake by the reticuloendothelial system and liver and by renal excretion of unchanged drug and metabolites.

Enoxaparin. Has approximately twice the half-life of heparin. Neither is absorbed orally.

Fibrinolytics. Streptokinase, u-PA, and t-PA are given IV, are rapidly metabolized, and have half-lives of less than 20 minutes. Recombinants ru-PA and rt-PA may have some benefit over streptokinase by virtue of selective binding to the fibrin clot and less extensive fibrinogen degradation, but bleeding occurs with similar incidence.

Protamine Sulfate. Used IV to rapidly control bleeding resulting from excessive heparin.

Vitamin K (Phytonadione). Readily absorbed following IM administration, but acute bleeding resulting from warfarin overdosage can be treated only by transfusion of plasma containing normal clotting proteins.

Aminocaproic Acid and Tranexamic Acid. Both used as bolus IV injections to reduce fibrinolytic bleeding. In life-threatening situations, transfusions of fresh whole blood or fibrinogen may be required.

27 Diuretics

Edwin K. Jackson, Ph.D.

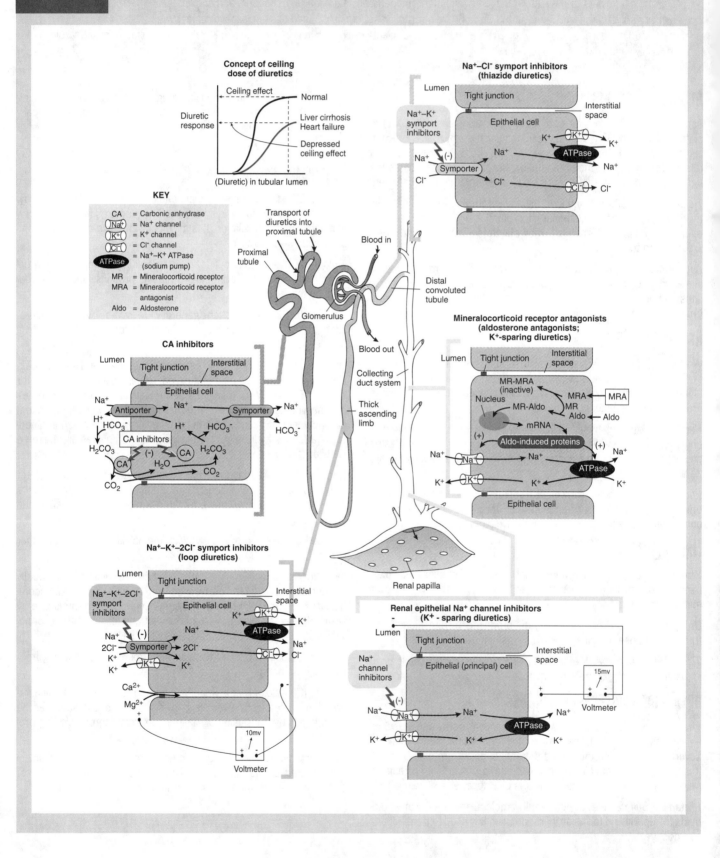

OVERVIEW

- Definition of diuretics: agents that increase urine flow (diuresis) and sodium excretion (natriuresis).
- Mechanism of action: carbonic anhydrase (CA) inhibition; $Na^+-K^+-2Cl^-$ symport inhibition; Na^+-Cl^- symport inhibition; Na^+-channel blockade; mineralocorticoid receptor (MR) antagonism; osmotic effect.
- Site of action: epithelial cells in nephrons; specific drugs are selective for specific nephron segments.
- Major therapeutic uses: to decrease edema in heart, kidney, and liver disease; to lower arterial blood pressure in hypertension.
- Ceiling dose: an important concept for the rational use of diuretics.

Medicinal Chemistry

Inhibitors of CA, $Na^+-K^+-2Cl^-$ symport, and Na^+-Cl^- symport are organic acids and (except for ethacrynic acid) are sulfonamides. The Na^+-channel inhibitors are organic bases, and the MR antagonists are steroids. Osmotic diuretics are a diverse group of relatively inert, but osmotically active, compounds. See Appendix, B, for specific agents.

Basic Pharmacology

Mechanisms and Sites of Action. CA inhibitors block CA in the luminal membrane and intracellular compartment of the proximal tubule epithelial cell (Fig. A). Inhibitors of $Na^+-K^+-2Cl^-$ symport and Na^+-Cl^- symport (commonly called *loop diuretics* and *thiazide diuretics*, respectively) inhibit these ion cotransporters in the luminal membrane of epithelial cells in the thick ascending limb (Fig. B) and distal convoluted tubule (Fig. C), respectively. Renal epithelial Na^+-channel inhibitors and MR antagonists (both commonly called *potassium-sparing diuretics*) block luminal membrane Na^+ channels (Fig. D) and intracellular MRs (Fig. E), respectively, in the collecting duct system epithelial cell. Osmotic diuretics decrease water and Na^+ reabsorption in the proximal tubule and loop of Henle (primary site of action) in part by limiting the osmosis of water out of the tubular lumen.

Effects on Urinary Excretion. Diuretic efficacy (maximum attainable excretion of Na^+ expressed as a percentage of filtered load of Na^+) is 25%, 5%, and 2% for $Na^+-K^+-2Cl^-$ symport, Na^+-Cl^- symport, and Na^+-channel inhibitors, respectively. Diuretic efficacy for MR antagonists depends on the prevailing levels of aldosterone, and diuretic efficacy of CA inhibitors is reduced by "downstream" absorption of the proximal rejectate and is self-limiting as a result of metabolic acidosis. The major anion that accompanies Na^+ is Cl^-, with the exception of CA inhibitors, where HCO_3^- is the major anion. CA, $Na^+-K^+-2Cl^-$ symport, and Na^+-Cl^- symport inhibitors increase K^+ excretion by increasing distal delivery of Na^+. $Na^+-K^+-2Cl^-$ symport inhibitors increase Ca^{2+} and Mg^{2+} excretion, and Na^+-channel inhibitors and MR antagonists decrease K^+ excretion in part by abolishing transepithelial potential differences at their respective sites of action (Figs. B and D).

Other Actions. CA inhibitors reduce intraocular pressure. $Na^+-K^+-2Cl^-$ symport inhibitors, particularly furosemide, increase venous capacitance. Osmotic diuretics reduce intracranial and intraocular pressures.

Clinical Pharmacology

Pharmacokinetics. No broad generalizations regarding oral bioavailability, half-lives, or routes of elimination are possible for this chemically diverse group of drugs. Glomerular filtration of $Na^+-K^+-2Cl^-$, Na^+-Cl^- symport, and Na^+-channel inhibitors is limited by binding to plasma proteins; thus these drugs reach their sites of action in the tubular lumen primarily via the organic acid (symport inhibitors) or organic base (channel inhibitors) secretory mechanisms in the proximal tubule.

Drug Interactions. NSAIDs may attenuate diuretic efficacy. Aminoglycosides may increase ototoxicity of $Na^+-K^+-2Cl^-$ symport inhibitors. Diuretic-induced K^+ depletion may increase digitalis-induced arrhythmias. The combination of potassium-sparing diuretics with other drugs that diminish K^+ excretion (e.g., ACE inhibitors, NSAIDs, other potassium-sparing diuretics) or with K^+ supplements may cause life-threatening hyperkalemia.

Pharmacotherapeutics

Indications. Major indications are for edema resulting from acute and chronic heart failure, liver cirrhosis (particularly MR antagonists), chronic renal failure, nephrotic syndrome, and for treatment of hypertension (particularly Na^+-Cl^- symport inhibitors). Other indications include:

- CA inhibitors—Glaucoma, epilepsy, acute mountain sickness, familial periodic paralysis
- $Na^+-K^+-2Cl^-$ symport inhibitors—Acute renal failure, hypercalcemia, hyponatremia
- Na^+-Cl^- symport inhibitors—Nephrogenic diabetes insipidus
- Na^+-channel inhibitors—Liddle's syndrome, lithium nephrotoxicity
- Osmotic diuretics—Acute renal failure, cerebral edema, intraocular hypertension, dialysis disequilibrium syndrome.

Diuretic Resistance (Edema Refractory to a Given Diuretic). Solutions include: confirming compliance, restricting Na^+ intake, increasing dose of diuretic to ceiling dose (see Fig. F; pointless and possibly harmful to exceed ceiling dose), switching to more efficacious diuretic, administering diuretic more frequently, and employing sequential blockade (e.g., giving two or more diuretics that act at different sites in the tubule).

Toxicity and Adverse Effects

- All diuretics—Extracellular fluid volume (ECFV) depletion leading to hypotension and reduced organ perfusion
- CA inhibitors—Metabolic acidosis
- $Na^+-K^+-2Cl^-$ and Na^+-Cl^- symport inhibitors—Hyponatremia, hypochloremia, hypokalemia, metabolic alkalosis, hypomagnesemia, hyperuricemia, hyperglycemia, sexual dysfunction (Na^+-Cl^- symport inhibitors only), ototoxicity ($Na^+-K^+-2Cl^-$ symport inhibitors only)
- Na^+-channel inhibitors and MR antagonists—Hyperkalemia, metabolic acidosis
- Osmotic diuretics—Shift of water from intracellular to extracellular compartments causing ECFV expansion and hyponatremia.

28 Ocular Pharmacology

Sayoko E. Moroi, M.D., Ph.D.

Some targets of ocular pharmacology

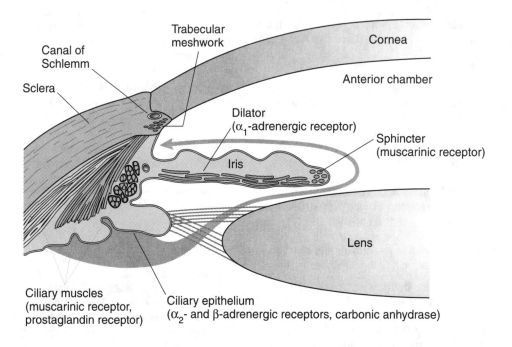

Aqueous humor is secreted by the ciliary epithelium of the ciliary body, flows in the anterior chamber, and exits primarily by the trabecular meshwork. Some receptors and carbonic anhydrase are indicated as pharmacologic targets for glaucoma therapies and for diagnostic purposes.

- The eye is a complex sensory organ with unique opportunities and challenges for drug design and delivery.
- Ocular medical therapeutic areas: infectious and inflammatory diseases, glaucoma, diagnostic purposes, and agents for surgical applications.

Pharmacokinetics

Drug Delivery. Since the eye is relatively isolated from systemic circulation, most drugs are administered topically. Other routes include injections to regions surrounding and within the eye, implantable devices, collagen shields, and oral or IV administration.

Absorption, Distribution, Metabolism, and Elimination. Most diseases of the conjunctiva and cornea are treated by medications introduced into the tear film. For glaucoma and uveitis, drugs must be absorbed by penetrating barriers, such as the cornea, conjunctiva, and sclera, to reach sufficient therapeutic intraocular drug concentrations. Once absorbed, a drug distributes to the iris, lens, ciliary body, retina, and other structures. Enzymes in the cornea metabolize prodrugs used in glaucoma treatment (e.g., latanoprost, a prodrug of 17-phenyl substituted prostaglandin $F_2\alpha$). Undesired systemic absorption occurs via the nasolacrimal system, where tears drain from the ocular surface and onto the nasal mucosa.

Pharmacology

Iris. Pupil size is determined by two opposing smooth muscle systems in the iris, the circular smooth muscle and the radial dilator muscle. Innervated by parasympathetic nerve fibers containing ACh, the iris circular smooth muscle contracts by stimulation of muscarinic cholinergic receptors by ACh or cholinergic agonists. This contraction causes the pupil to become smaller (miosis). Cholinergic antagonists block the action of ACh; hence, these drugs allow the radial dilator muscle to dominate, which leads to pupil dilation (mydriasis). The iris radial dilator muscle is innervated by sympathetic nerve fibers containing NE. On stimulation of $\alpha1$-adrenergic receptors by NE or adrenergic agonists, this muscle contracts, which leads to pupil dilation. Antagonists block endogenous NE, allowing the circular smooth muscle to dominate, so the pupil constricts.

Ciliary Body. The ciliary body epithelium contains adrenergic receptors that, in part, regulate the secretion of aqueous humor. α_2- and β_2-adrenergic receptors are therapeutic targets for glaucoma.

The ciliary body smooth muscle is innervated by the parasympathetic system. Contraction of this muscle causes two effects: (1) relaxation of the zonules supporting the lens, which leads to a change in lens shape, resulting in a stronger refractive power (accommodation), which facilitates reading; and (2) "stretching open" the trabecular meshwork in the drainage angle of the eye, thus enhancing aqueous humor outflow. Conversely, cholinergic muscarinic antagonists interfere with accommodation (cycloplegia) and may elevate intraocular pressure in susceptible persons.

Pharmacotherapeutics

Infectious Disease and Inflammatory Disease. Antimicrobial agents are prescribed empirically from the clinical appearance and then adjusted based on culture and drug sensitivity test. When ocular inflammation is associated with systemic disease, treatment is directed toward the underlying etiology. Uveitis (intraocular inflammation) and postoperative inflammation are typically treated with topical corticosteroids. Allergic conjunctivitis, cystoid macular edema, and postoperative inflammation may be treated with NSAID drops.

Glaucoma Pharmacology. With the premise that elevated intraocular pressure causes a characteristic pattern of optic nerve damage, current glaucoma therapy is directed toward lowering intraocular pressure. The main determinants of intraocular pressure are the production of aqueous humor by the ciliary body, or "inflow," and the egress of this fluid from the eye, or "outflow," primarily via the trabecular meshwork. Most patients are treated with several medications that either decrease aqueous humor production or enhance outflow. In addition to the cholinergic and adrenergic agents, two other drug classes are prescribed—prostaglandins to enhance outflow and carbonic anhydrase inhibitors to decrease secretion.

Cholinergic and Adrenergic Drugs. These drugs and their ophthalmic indications are summarized in Appendix, C.

Other Drugs

Topical Anesthetics. These drugs provide short-term anesthesia for minor procedures on the cornea and conjunctiva (e.g., measuring eye pressure, removing foreign bodies, performing laser surgery). The most frequently used are proparacaine and tetracaine (for mechanism of action, see Chap. 47).

Diagnostic Dyes. Rose bengal stains devitalized epithelial surfaces on either the conjunctiva or cornea. Fluoroscein stains epithelial defects and is also used intravenously to assess the retina, retinal pigment epithelium, and choroid.

Agents for Ocular Surgery. Viscoelastic substances are used to protect the cornea and to maintain anatomic stability during anterior segment surgery, (e.g., cataract removal and intraocular lens placement). Intraocular gases and silicone oil are used to reposition detached retinas.

Tear Replacement Agents. Adequate ocular surface coverage with tears requires a balance of mucous, aqueous, and lipid components. Disturbance of any component can potentially lead to severe corneal problems. Current tear replacement agents substitute for the aqueous component.

Toxicity

Any topical eye medication can potentially cause a periocular allergic reaction from either the preservative or drug. Other ocular side effects include: deposits within the cornea from ciprofloxacin and the conjunctiva from epinephrine, and accelerated cataract growth and secondary glaucoma from corticosteroids.

Systemic side effects may occur from drug absorption via the nasolacrimal system into the systemic circulation. For instance, the β-adrenergic receptor antagonists can cause bradycardia, asthma, or depression. Oral carbonic anhydrase inhibitors commonly cause paresthesias, fatigue, nephrolithiasis (less frequently), and hematologic disorders (rarely).

29 Agents for the Treatment of Asthma

Robert B. Raffa, Ph.D.

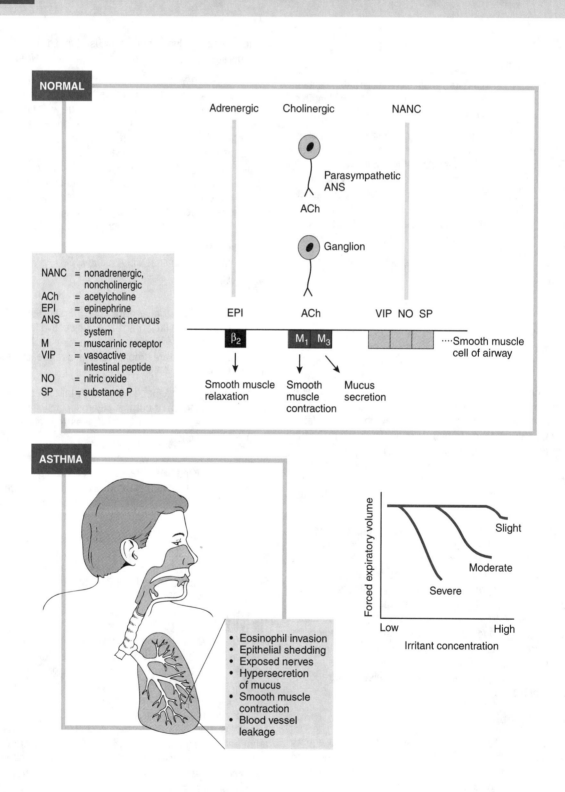

NORMAL

Adrenergic   Cholinergic   NANC

Parasympathetic ANS

ACh

Ganglion

EPI   ACh   VIP NO SP

β₂   M₁ M₃   ····Smooth muscle cell of airway

Smooth muscle relaxation   Smooth muscle contraction   Mucus secretion

NANC = nonadrenergic, noncholinergic
ACh = acetylcholine
EPI = epinephrine
ANS = autonomic nervous system
M = muscarinic receptor
VIP = vasoactive intestinal peptide
NO = nitric oxide
SP = substance P

ASTHMA

- Eosinophil invasion
- Epithelial shedding
- Exposed nerves
- Hypersecretion of mucus
- Smooth muscle contraction
- Blood vessel leakage

Forced expiratory volume

Slight
Moderate
Severe

Low   High
Irritant concentration

Asthma

Characteristics. Asthma is characterized by reversible narrowing of trachea and bronchi; recurrent episodic coughing, shortness of breath, chest tightness, and wheezing; fall in forced expiratory volume in 1 second (FEV_1); correlated with inflammation of the bronchi (damage to epithelium and eosinophil infiltration); hypersensitivity to stimuli (allergens, cold air, exercise, fumes); contraction of bronchial smooth muscle, and increased mucus secretion and viscosity. It is often associated with an increase in ACh activity or sensitivity.

Phases. Phases are distinguished as immediate (0–2 hours)—mainly the result of spasm of bronchial smooth muscle—and late (4–8 hours)—inflammatory reaction (cytokine-releasing T cells, eosinophils) initiated during the immediate phase (damage to epithelia). How inflammation increases airway sensitivity is unknown, but eosinophils and neutrophils have been implicated. Other cell products also lead to hyperreactivity (macrophages, mast cells, sensory neurons, epithelial cells), suggesting that bronchospasm in asthma results from a combination of release of mediators and exaggerated response to their effects. Hence, treatment with combinations of drugs having different modes of action might be most effective (or required).

Pharmacotherapy

The contraction of smooth muscle (early phase) is most easily reversed by therapy; edema and cell infiltration (late phase) requires sustained treatment with anti-inflammatory agents. General strategies consist of administering drugs that reverse bronchoconstriction (e.g., β-adrenergic receptor agonists and, more precisely, selective β_2-adrenergic receptor agonists, xanthines, anticholinergics), and those with anti-inflammatory effects (e.g., cromolyn sodium, steroids). Antihistamines are relatively ineffective (probably because other mediators, such as leukotrienes, are the primary bronchoconstrictors in asthma in humans) and traditional Ca^{2+}-channel blockers are relatively ineffective, probably because of a different Ca^{2+}-channel type on mast cells from those on cardiac or other tissues. See Appendix, D, for specific agents.

Bronchodilators

β-Adrenergic Receptor Agonists. β-Adrenergic receptor agonists increase cAMP, relax smooth muscle, and increase mucociliary transport (increase ciliary activity and affect the composition of mucus). They have a relatively rapid (minutes) onset and are long lasting (hours). They are effective by inhalation and are used for mild, intermittent attacks. Adverse effects include tachycardia, hypertension, and muscle tremor.

Methylxanthines. Methylxanthines are used for acute asthma and to decrease symptoms of chronic disease. The mechanism of action is uncertain, but methylxanthines inhibit cAMP breakdown by phosphodiesterase (PDE) enzymes and are adenosine receptor antagonists. Theophylline clearance is influenced by diet, cigarette smoking, physiologic factors, and drug–drug interactions (e.g., via induction of hepatic enzymes). There is a narrow range of safe therapeutic doses (frequent serum-level tests advisable). An overdose can result in seizures and arrhythmias, without any warning symptoms.

Anticholinergics. Anticholinergic receptor antagonists inhibit that portion of the response mediated by mAChRs (varies among asthmatics). Ipratropium bromide, a quaternary-nitrogen derivative of atropine, is poorly absorbed, hence produces few systemic effects.

Anti-Inflammatory Agents

Cromolyn Sodium (Disodium Cromoglycate) and Nedocromil. Cromolyn sodium has no bronchodilator activity; thus, it is not good for acute attacks. It is used as a prophylactic agent. It inhibits immediate and delayed reactions to inhalation of antigen and blocks exercise- and aspirin-induced bronchoconstriction. It inhibits histamine and other mediator release to stabilize membrane, and it may also inhibit PDE (increases cAMP). Cromolyn sodium can be used with β_2 antagonists to prevent exercise-induced asthma. It should be inhaled as it is poorly absorbed orally. There is a delayed onset (weeks), and it is rapidly metabolized. There are few systemic adverse effects.

Corticosteroids. Corticosteroids are for prophylactic, not acute use. They decrease inflammation, edema, and capillary permeability. They inhibit arachidonic acid release (aspirin can provoke symptoms in some asthmatics), phospholipase A, and gene transcription of cytokines. Chronic use reduces bronchial hyperreactivity (unlike beta agonists or theophylline), but maximum effect might require 9–12 months. Chronic use of oral steroids leads to thinning of skin, osteoporosis, GI and CNS disturbances, decreased adrenal function; abrupt withdrawal can precipitate adrenal crisis. With inhaled steroids, the major side effect is yeast in oral cavity.

Other Agents

Leukotriene antagonists block leukotriene receptors. Zafirlukast (Accolate) is modestly effective for maintenance therapy and is particularly good for aspirin-induced asthma. Montelukast (Singulair) has been approved for once-daily dosing in children younger than 12. Lipoxygenase inhibitors (e.g., zileutin [Zyflo]) block the synthesis of leukotriene receptors.

30 Antidiarrheal Agents

Thomas F. Burks, Ph.D.

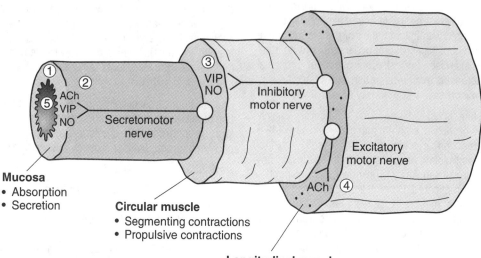

Wall of intestine

① ②
⑤ ACh
VIP
NO Secretomotor nerve

③ VIP NO Inhibitory motor nerve

Excitatory motor nerve

ACh ④

Mucosa
• Absorption
• Secretion

Circular muscle
• Segmenting contractions
• Propulsive contractions

Longitudinal muscle
• Propulsive contractions

Condition or drug	① Fluid absorption	② Fluid secretion	③ Segmenting contractions	④ Propulsive contractions	⑤ Luminal secretogogues
Diarrhea	0	↑	↓	↑	↑
Opioids	↑	↓	↑	↓	
Clonidine		↓			
Atropine		↓	↓	↓	
Octreotide		↓			
Bismuth subsalicylate					↓
Cholestyramine					↓
Note: 0 = normal; ↑ = increase; ↓ = decrease					

OVERVIEW

- Drugs produce antidiarrheal effects by 1 or more of 5 mechanisms: (1) increasing fluid absorption from lumen, (2) decreasing fluid secretion into lumen, (3) increasing segmenting contractions, (4) decreasing propulsive contractions, and (5) binding secretogogues in the lumen.
- Opiates are most often used in nonspecific therapy of diarrhea.
- Opiates may act in the brain, spinal cord, and at enteric nerves to produce antidiarrheal effects.
- Optimal treatment of diarrhea is to remove the cause.
- The most severe health threat from diarrhea is dehydration.

FIRST:	**OPIUM** (antiquity)
FIRST SYNTHETIC:	**DIPHENOXYLATE**
MOST WIDELY USED:	**LOPERAMIDE**

Pharmacology

The main objectives of antidiarrheal therapy are to reduce net accumulation of fluid in the lumen of the small intestine and colon, reduce propulsive contractions, and retard flow by increasing segmenting contractions. Drugs can act by different mechanisms to achieve these objectives.

Sites and Mechanisms of Action

Opiates such as diphenoxylate and loperamide, which do not effectively cross the blood–brain barrier, act at secretomotor neurons to diminish release of neurotransmitters, such as ACh, VIP, and NO, that stimulate secretion by epithelial cells in crypts. Opiates also increase absorption by villus cells. Opiates decrease release of VIP and NO from nerves that inhibit circular smooth muscle, thereby increasing segmenting contractions. They also inhibit release of excitatory neurotransmitters, such as ACh, in longitudinal smooth muscle, thereby decreasing propulsive contractions. α-Adrenergic agonists (clonidine), somatostatin agonists (octreotide), and muscarinic antagonists (atropine) also decrease secretion by reducing effects of secretomotor neurons on crypt cells. Bismuth subsalicylate binds bacterial toxins and prevents formation of secretogogues in the bowel lumen. Cholestyramine binds and inactivates bile acids, which are secretogogues.

Pharmacokinetics

Opiates, clonidine, atropine, and octreotide act systemically and are inactivated by hepatic biotransformation. Bismuth subsalicylate and cholestyramine act in the bowel lumen and are excreted in the feces.

Toxicity

Adverse effects of opiates, α_2 agonists, muscarinic antagonists, and somatostatin agonists are caused largely by extension of their pharmacologic effects. Opiates most often used as antidiarrheals do not cross the blood–brain barrier and rarely cause respiratory depression or abuse; they often induce constipation. α_2-Adrenergic agonists produce hypotension, which limits their use. Muscarinic antagonists produce dry mouth, visual disturbances, urinary hesitancy, and constipation. Somatostatin agonists must be administered parenterally.

SPECIFIC AGENTS

Opiates	α_2 Agonists	Antimuscarinics	Somatostatin Agonists
Morphine (generic) • Effective • Crosses blood–brain barrier Codeine (generic) • Effective • Crosses blood–brain barrier Diphenoxylate (+ atropine = Lomotil) • Crosses blood–brain barrier poorly • Atropine in Lomotil to prevent abuse Loperamide (Immodium) • Very little crosses blood–brain barrier • Low abuse liability	Clonidine (Catapres) • Not often used • Lowers blood pressure	Atropine (generic) • Causes intolerable side effects	Octreotide (Sandostatin) • Effective in AIDS diarrhea • Requires parenteral injection Bismuth subsalicylate (Pepto-Bismol) • Useful in prevention and treatment of traveler's diarrhea Cholestyramine (Questran) • Binds bile acids • Useful in treating bile acid catharsis

31 Laxatives

Thomas F. Burks, Ph.D.

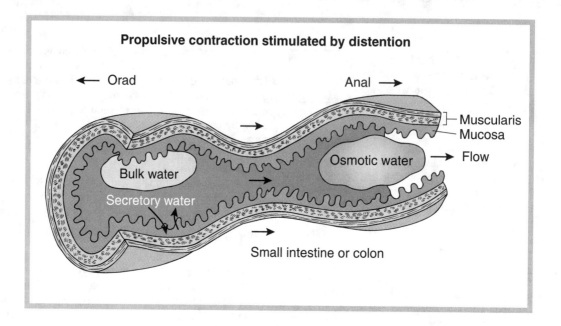

Propulsive contraction stimulated by distention

← Orad Anal →

Muscularis
Mucosa

Osmotic water → Flow

Bulk water

Secretory water

Small intestine or colon

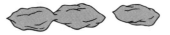

Laxatives:

Increase volume ⎤ Increased flow ⎤ Increased
Decrease viscosity ⎦ Increased propulsive ⎦ defecation
contractions

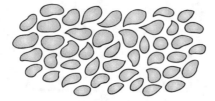

Condition inside colonic lumen

Constipation

Compact, dessicated content

Laxative

Bulky, fluid content

Natural and plant-derived chemicals have been used as laxatives since antiquity.

Pharmacology

Laxatives increase the amount of water in the lumen of the colon. Water increases fluidity of colonic contents, increases bulk, distends the colon to increase propulsive contractions and initiate the defecation reflex, and facilitates passage of stool.

Mechanisms of Action

Osmotic laxatives capture and retain water in the lumen by osmotic forces. These agents include poorly absorbed inorganic salts and non-absorbed sugars. Secretory laxatives act at the intestinal or colonic mucosa, at least in part through formation of nitric oxide, to stimulate secretion of water and electrolytes into the lumen. Bulk laxatives consist of nonabsorbed vegetable fiber that takes up water to form a hydrophilic mass. Softening agents are surfactants or lubricants that decrease viscosity of colonic contents.

All laxatives can decrease transit time (enhance propulsion) through the GI tract. Bulk laxatives have the least overall effect and osmotic laxatives the most dramatic effects. Time to first defecation after oral administration is somewhat dose-dependent. Osmotic agents take effect within 1–3 hours; secretory agents, within 6–8 hours; and bulk laxatives and stool softeners, within 24–72 hours.

Pharmacokinetics

Laxatives act from the intestinal and colonic lumen. They are usually given orally, but some may be administered via the rectum. For the most part they are poorly absorbed and are eventually excreted in the feces. Some undergo modest biotransformation, such as hydrolysis of glycosides or acetyl groups, by pancreatic or microbial enzymes.

Toxicity

Most adverse effects occur by extension of laxative pharmacologic actions: explosive, watery stools; abdominal pain; borborygmi; flatulence. Bulk laxatives usually produce the fewest adverse effects. Danthron and phenolphthalein have recently been removed from the market because of concerns about hepatotoxicity and carcinogenic potential. Dependence on laxatives for bowel movements has been reported with all agents. Laxatives must not be administered in the presence of appendicitis-like symptoms or in cases of mechanical obstruction of the bowel.

Uses

Laxatives can stimulate bowel movements in patients with occasional or drug-induced constipation. Elderly patients and patients with chronic idiopathic constipation often benefit from bulking agents. Osmotic agents may be used to cleanse the bowel before examination or surgery.

SPECIFIC AGENTS

Bulking Agents	Osmotic Agents	Secretory Agents	Softening Agents
• Bran (generic) • Psyllium husk fiber (Metamucil) • Methylcellulose (Citrucel) • Polycarbophil (Mitrolan)	Saline • Magnesium hydroxide (Milk of Magnesia, generic) • Sodium phosphate (Fleet Phospho-Soda) Other • Polyethylene glycol (GoLYTELY, NuLYTELY) • Lactulose (Cephulac, Chronulac)	• Bisacodyl (Dulcolax) • Castor oil (generic, Neoloid) • Phenolphthalein (Ex-Lax, Modane) • Sennosides (Perdiem, Senokot) • Cascara (Peri-Colace) • Aloes	• Mineral oil • Glycerin suppositories • Dioctyl sodium sulfosuccinate (Docusate)

32 Agents for the Treatment of Peptic Ulcers

Henry I. Jacoby, Ph.D.

Gastrointestinal tract and regulation of HCl secretion by the gastric parietal cell

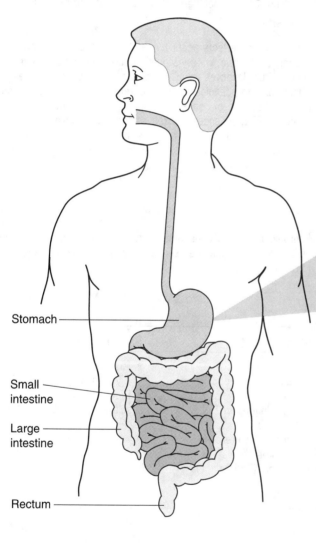

Stomach

Small intestine

Large intestine

Rectum

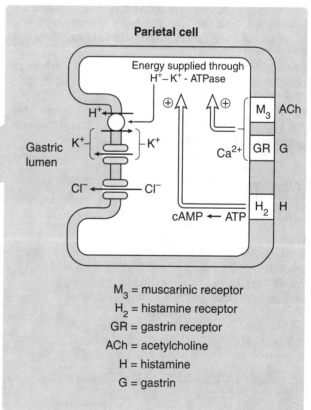

Parietal cell

Energy supplied through
$H^+ - K^+ - ATPase$

Gastric lumen

H^+

K^+ — K^+

Cl^- ← Cl^-

Ca^{2+}

cAMP ← ATP

M_3 ACh

GR G

H_2 H

M_3 = muscarinic receptor
H_2 = histamine receptor
GR = gastrin receptor
ACh = acetylcholine
H = histamine
G = gastrin

OVERVIEW

- A peptic ulcer is a lesion of the luminal surface of the GI tract in areas exposed to gastric acid and pepsin. They may occur in the lower esophagus, stomach, or duodenum.
- Etiology: The lesions are due to an imbalance between mucosal defense mechanisms and erosive activity of acid and pepsin.
- When activated by low pH, pepsin can damage mucosa and produce lesions and ulceration.
- The colonization of the stomach by *Helicobacter pylori* has recently been found to be associated with 90% of duodenal ulcers and 65%–70% of gastric ulcers.
- One of the few organisms that can live in the acid conditions of the stomach, *H. pylori* produces ammonia, using the enzyme urease, which can buffer the acid in the immediate vicinity of the bacteria. The high localized concentration of ammonia produced by the bacteria is thought to cause the mucosal damage. There is also evidence that colonization with *H. pylori* is a risk factor in the development of gastric malignant tumors.
- Another factor in the production of ulcerations is chronic dosing with NSAIDs. This class of agent inhibits the formation of prostaglandins, which are crucial for protection of the gastric and duodenal mucosa.

Pharmacology

Receptors in the parietal cell membrane for ACh, histamine, and gastrin interact when activated by antagonists to increase the availability of Ca^{2+} and stimulate H^+-K^+-ATPase of the luminal membrane (see Fig.). Acid secretion is decreased by blockade of ACh muscarinic (M_3) receptors, histaminic H_2 receptors, intracellular adenylate cyclase, or H^+-K^+-ATPase.

Pharmacotherapeutics

If the presence of *H. pylori* has been established by endoscopy or non-invasive diagnostic test, the goal of therapy is to eradicate colonization. If tests are negative, treatment is with antisecretory or gastroprotective agents. If the peptic ulcers are due to NSAIDs, either treatment consists of either stopping medication or giving a prostaglandin substitute.

Proton Pump Inhibitors. These strongly inhibit acid production; used for peptic ulcers and gastroesophageal reflux disease (GERD); only available on prescription.

Histamine H_2 Inhibitors. These moderately inhibit acid secretion; useful for mild peptic ulcer and GERD; available OTC for self-medication of GERD.

Anticholinergics. These inhibit stimulation of acid production resulting from M3 stimulation; can be effective but usually produce a significant degree of adverse effect related to blockade of M3 receptors.

Gastrin Antagonists. These block stimulation of acid as a result of gastrin released from antrum; also related to cholecystokinin.

Antacids. These neutralize acid in the stomach or esophagus and raise pH above level for pepsin activation.

Prostaglandins. These replace natural prostaglandins and restore mucosal integrity.

Prostaglandin Synthesis Inducers. These induce mucosa to produce protective levels of prostaglandins.

Antibiotics and Bismuth Salts. These kill *H. pylori* colonizing gastric mucosa; sometimes used with proton pump inhibitors.

SPECIFIC AGENTS

Class	Drug	Comments
Proton pump inhibitors	Omeprazole	Enteric-coated; onset 1 hour; duration > 24 hours; many drug interactions; few adverse effects
	Lansoprazole	Delayed-release dosage; few adverse effects; interaction with fewer compounds than omeprazole
Histamine H_2 antagonists	Cimetidine	Once or twice a day administration; many drug interactions; adverse effects rare (headaches and confusion, agitation may occur; weak antiandrogenic activity); available prescription and OTC
	Famotidine	Administration once or twice a day; interactions only with ketoconazole and theophylline; adverse effects rare (headaches and confusion); available prescription and OTC
	Nizatidine	Administration once or twice a day; interactions with antacids, ketoconazole, and salicylates; adverse effects rare; available prescription and OTC
	Ranitidine	Administration once or twice a day; drug interactions with antacids, cefuroxime, ketoconazole, nifedipine, theophylline; adverse effects rare; available prescription and OTC
Prostaglandins	Misoprostol	Synthetic, orally effective prostaglandin E_1 analog; used mainly for NSAID-induced gastric and duodenal lesions; inhibits acid production as well as provides mucosal protective effect; administration four times a day required; can produce abortion (contraindicated in pregnant women); often produces diarrhea (contraindicated in patients with inflammatory bowel disease); interactions with antacids, cyclosporine

33 Agents for Altering Uterine Motility

Mercedes Perusquía, Ph.D.

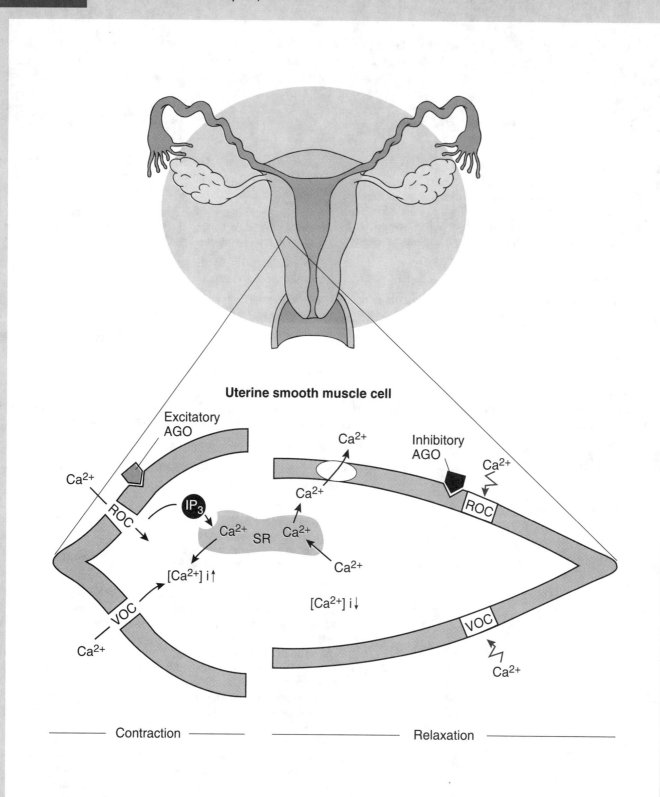

Uterine smooth muscle cell

Contraction — Relaxation

- The uterus of mammals is a complex organ with contractile activity under myogenic, neuronal, and hormonal control.
- Uterine smooth muscle is characterized by numerous excitatory, inhibitory, and modulatory inputs via neurotransmitters, hormones, and paracrine substances. The most relevant modulating agents of uterine contractility are summarized in the accompanying table.

Pharmacology

Drugs may elicit changes in cytoplasmic calcium concentration ($[Ca^{2+}]i$) of the uterine smooth muscle cell by promoting or inhibiting Ca^{2+} influx or efflux (see Fig.). Agonist binding to a receptor may initiate: (1) a contraction by increasing $[Ca^{2+}]i$ by activation of voltage (VOC)- or receptor (ROC)-operated Ca^{2+} channels and Ca^{2+} release from the sarcoplasmic reticulum (SR) by inositol 1,4,5-triphosphate (IP_3); or (2) a relaxation by lowering $[Ca^{2+}]i$ by inactivation of VOC or ROC, intracellular Ca^{2+} sequestration, or increased Ca^{2+} efflux from the cytoplasm.

Pharmacotherapeutics

The uterus is mainly innervated by adrenergic and cholinergic nerves. All subtypes of adrenoceptors have been identified in myometrial tissues. The generalization can be made that the uterine relaxant effects of catecholamines are exerted primarily through β_2 adrenoceptors, whereas the uterine contractile effects are mediated via α_1 adrenoceptors. Cholinergic agents stimulating the muscarinic receptors induce uterine contraction.

Hormones. The primary endocrine factors involved in uterine contractility are the sex steroid hormones secreted by the ovary (during pregnancy, the placenta). The number of α and β adrenoceptors and $5-HT_2$ receptors in the myometrium can be altered by changes in estrogen concentrations. The myometrium-stimulating effect of estrogens and the inactivating effect of progesterone have been known for more than 50 years. The withdrawal of progestational hormones is a necessary prerequisite for the conversion of the relaxed pregnant uterus to an active, contracting organ. Uterus-activating agents are also responsible for the conversion of the pregnant uterus to the contracting parturient uterus. Oxytocin and prostaglandins (PGs) are powerful uterotonics by their interaction with their myometrial-specific receptors. Oxytocin is also known to stimulate the production of $PGF_2\alpha$ by the decidua. Oxytocin may thus serve a dual function in initiating labor by its action on both the decidua and the myometrium. The failure of oxytocin to interrupt gestation in women is considered evidence against an important role for oxytocin in parturition. Vasopressin, another neurohypophyseal hormone, is a more potent myometrial stimulant than oxytocin in nonpregnant women and during the first trimester of pregnancy.

Eicosanoids. The eicosanoids, particularly PGE_2 and $PGF_2\alpha$, play a central role in labor initiation; at midgestation PGs are much more effective than oxytocin for the induction of uterine contractions. It has been reported that the isolated rat uterus is highly sensitive to serotonin (5-HT), interacting with $5-HT_2$ receptors present in the plasma uterine membrane to induce contraction. In addition, histamine induces uterine contraction in numerous mammals by interacting with H_1 receptors.

Peptides. Vasoactive intestinal peptide (VIP) inhibits myometrial activity in both nonpregnant women and in early pregnancy, and substance P has been reported to produce uterine contraction.

Ca^{2+}-Entry Blockers. A diverse group of compounds have the ability to alter Ca^{2+} movement across the cell membrane. These agents are referred to as *Ca^{2+}-entry blockers*. Conversely, the dihydropiridine-Ca^{2+}-channel activator, Bay K 8644, is capable of inducing uterine contraction.

FACTORS AFFECTING UTERINE SMOOTH MUSCLE ACTIVITY

Factor	Excitation	Inhibition
Receptors		
Cholinergic	Muscarinic	
Adrenergic	α_1	β_2
Hormones		
Female sex	Estrogens	Progestins
Neurohypophyseal	Oxytocin	
Autacoids	Vasopressin	
Histamine	H_1	H_2 (rat/mouse)
5-Hydroxytryptamine	$5-HT_2$	
Prostaglandins		
Nonpregnant human	$F_{2\alpha}$	E_2
Pregnant human	$E_2, F_{2\alpha}$	I_2
Peptides	VIP (nonpregnant and early pregnancy)	Substance P
Ion channels	Ca^{2+}-channel activators	Ca^{2+}-entry blockers

Mechanisms of Action

Smooth muscle contractile agents such as ACh, oxytocin, and PGs raise the intracellular Ca^{2+} concentration. In addition, PGE_2, $PGF_2\alpha$, or oxytocin decrease ATP-dependent Ca^{2+} uptake; interestingly, PGE_2 can also release Ca^{2+}. A vast array of agents, such as Ca^{2+}-entry blockers or steroid hormones, have the ability to block Ca^{2+} influx. It is generally assumed that the increase of the second messenger cAMP is the mediator of relaxing effects of a variety of agents such as β-adrenoceptor agonists.

Clinical Applications

The relaxing effect of progestins shifts the regulatory balance that maintains the quiescent uterus in midpregnancy. Thus progesterone has been used to prevent abortions. Labor at term can be induced either by giving exogenous oxytocin or by stimulating endogenous oxytocin release. To treat obstetric hemorrhage caused by postpartum uterine atony, PGE_2, $PGF_2\alpha$, or ergonovine are used. PG synthetase inhibitors and β_2 adrenoceptors have been most widely used in the treatment of preterm labor to induce uterine relaxation; at present, ritodrine is the only drug approved by the FDA for this use. $PGF_2\alpha$ is used as an abortifacient, either alone or in combination with the progesterone antagonist RU 486 (mifepristone).

34 Dermatologic Agents

Robert B. Raffa, Ph.D.

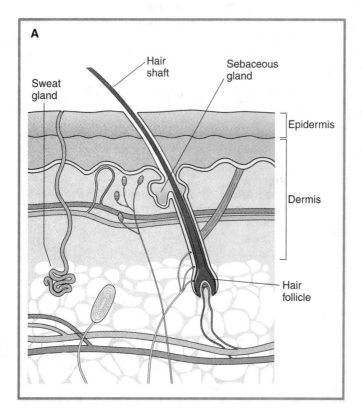

A

- Sweat gland
- Hair shaft
- Sebaceous gland
- Epidermis
- Dermis
- Hair follicle

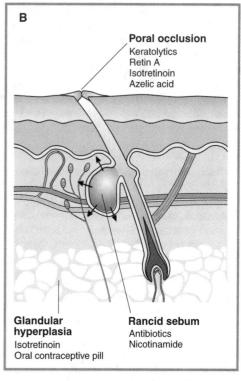

B

Poral occlusion
Keratolytics
Retin A
Isotretinoin
Azelic acid

Glandular hyperplasia
Isotretinoin
Oral contraceptive pill

Rancid sebum
Antibiotics
Nicotinamide

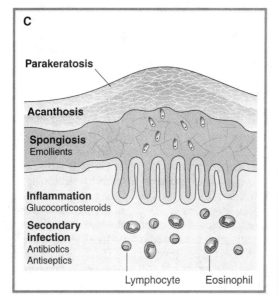

C

Parakeratosis

Acanthosis

Spongiosis
Emollients

Inflammation
Glucocorticosteroids

Secondary infection
Antibiotics
Antiseptics

Lymphocyte   Eosinophil

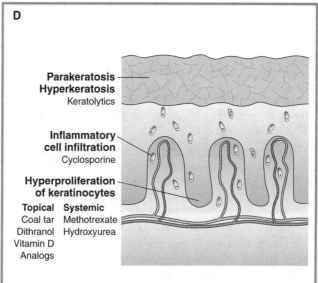

D

Parakeratosis
Hyperkeratosis
Keratolytics

Inflammatory cell infiltration
Cyclosporine

Hyperproliferation of keratinocytes

Topical	Systemic
Coal tar	Methotrexate
Dithranol	Hydroxyurea
Vitamin D	
Analogs	

OVERVIEW

- Drugs used to treat dermatologic disorders can be administered either directly to the skin or systemically, depending on the nature of the disorder, the drug, and the condition of the skin. An advantage of topical application is the administration of the drug at the highest concentration at its site of action. A disadvantage can be local irritation or allergic contact dermatitis.
- Topical anti-inflammatory agents include corticosteroids and coal-tar preparations. As with all dermatologic agents, topical or systemic adverse reactions can occur.
- Topical antibiotic preparations are available for the prevention and treatment of gram-positive and gram-negative bacteria infection of wounds, axillary deodorization, and the treatment of acne vulgaris (*Propionibacterium acnes*). Some preparations also contain corticosteroids or multiple antibiotics.
- Superficial fungal infections can be treated with topical or oral antifungal agents. Allergic contact dermatitis occurs only rarely, but co-administration of the oral azole derivatives with certain other drugs is absolutely contraindicated.
- Topical antiviral agents are available. As with the other drugs cited above, the indiscriminate use of these preparations can result in drug resistance.
- Dermatologic agents are also available to treat hyper- or hypopigmentation of skin, acne, warts, psoriasis, pruritus, seborrhea, parasites, and hair loss.

Pharmacology

Hyperpigmentation of skin is treated by the reversible inhibition of an enzyme (tyrosinase) involved in the biosynthesis of melanin or by a toxic action on melanocytes (permanent depigmentation). Vitiligo (lack of pigmentation) is treated with psoralens activated by long-wave UV light.

Acne is treated by drugs that are antimicrobial to *P. acnes* (e.g., benzoyl peroxide and azelaic acid), have peeling and comedolytic effects (e.g., benzoyl peroxide), inhibit sebaceous gland size and function (e.g., isotretinoin), or disrupt epidermal cell cohesion and enhance epidermal cell turnover (retinoic acid).

Anti-inflammatory agents are described in Chap. 46; antibiotic agents are described in Chap. 51; antifungal agents are described in Chap. 56; antiviral agents are described in Chap. 58.

Medicinal Chemistry

Hydrocortisone is an endogenous adrenal cortex glucocorticosteroid. Prednisolone and methylprednisolone are as active topically. Triamcinolone and fluocinolone are acetonide derivatives of the fluorinated steroids.

Coal tar is a mixture of about 10,000 compounds, arising as the principal by-product of bituminous coal distillation. Among the compounds are naphthalene, phenanthrene, fluoranthrene, benzene, xylene, toluene, creosols and other aromatic compounds, pyridine bases, ammonia, and peroxides.

Retinoic acid (tretinoin; all-*trans*-retinoic acid) is the acid form of vitamin A; isotretinoin is a synthetic retinoid; and etretinate is an aromatic retinoid. Azelaic acid is a straight-chain saturated dicarboxylic acid.

Toxicity

All of the topical agents have the potential to cause local irritation, allergic responses, skin alterations, and systemic toxicity if absorbed (particularly likely in damaged skin). Each agent has its own toxicity profile. The full toxicologic profile (along with advice about the clinical use of these agents) is available from other sources.

REPRESENTATIVE SPECIFIC AGENTS

Class	Drug
Acne preparations	Adapalene (Differin), azelaic acid (Azelex), benzoyl peroxide (generic), isotretinoin (Accutane), tretinoin (Retin-A)
Antibacterials	Bacitracin (in Neosporin, others), mupirocin (Bactroban), polymyxin B sulfate (in Betadine, Neosporin, others), neomycin (in Neosporin, others), clindamycin (Cleocin, others), erythromycin (several), metronidazole (MetroCream, others), tetracycline (Topicycline), and meclocycline (Meclan)
Antifungals	Imidazoles: e.g., clotrimazole (Lotrimin, Mycelex), econazole (Spectazole), ketoconazole (Nizoral), miconazole Monistat, MicaTin), oxiconazole (Oxistat), sulconazole (Exelderm). Others: e.g., ciclopirox olamine (Loprox), naftifine Naftin), terbinafine (Lamisil), tolnaftate (Aftate, Tinactin), nystatin (several), amphotericin B (Fungizone). Oral: fluconazole (Diflucan), griseofulvin (several), itraconazole (Sporanox), ketoconazole (Nizoral)
Antivirals	Acyclovir (Zovirax), famciclovir (Famvir), penciclovir (Denavir), valacyclovir (Valtrex)
Corticosteroids	Hydrocortisone
Keratolytics	Cantharidin, fluorouracil (Efudex), podofilox (Condylox) and podophyllum resin, propylene glycol, salicyclic acid, urea
Parasiticides	Crotamiton (Eurax), ivermectin (Mectizan), lindane (Kwell), malathion (Prioderm, Ovide), permethrin (Nix, Elimite), piperonyl butoxide (Rid, several), sulfur
Pigmentation or depigmentation	Hydroquinone (several), monobenzone (Benoquin), methoxsalen (Oxsoralen), and trioxsalen (Trisoralen)
Pruritus preparations	Doxepin (Zonalon), Pramoxine (several)
Psoriasis preparations	Calcipotriene (Dovonex), etretinate (Tegison)

Directions: For each of the following questions, choose the **one best** answer.

1. Which of the following drugs is most likely to cause hyperkalemia?

(A) Acetazolamide

(B) Furosemide

(C) Hydrochlorthiazide

(D) Spironolactone

2. Which drug is most likely to produce skin discoloration as a toxic action?

(A) Amiodarone

(B) Lidocaine oral

(C) Lidocaine IV

(D) Quinidine

3. For a patient who is newly diagnosed with glaucoma and has asthma that is treated with bronchodilators, which of the following agents would be an appropriate medication to prescribe?

(A) Atropine

(B) Timolol

(C) Brimonidine

(D) Gentamicin

(E) Tropicamide

4. Acne is unlikely to respond to which of the following agents?

(A) Azelaic acid

(B) Benzoyl peroxide

(C) Clotrimazole

(D) Isotretinoin

(E) Retinoic acid

5. Which of the following drugs is a proton pump inhibitor?

(A) Omeprazole

(B) Cimetidine

(C) Nizatidine

(D) Ranitidine

(E) Misoprostol

6. Which one of the following is an agonist at somatostatin receptors?

(A) Clonidine

(B) Octreotide

(C) Loperamide

(D) Cholestyramine

7. Which of the following drugs is most useful in anemia caused by bone marrow suppression?

(A) Cyanocobalamin

(B) Erythropoietin

(C) Ferrous sulfate

(D) Folic acid

8. Laxatives act primarily in which of the following ways?

(A) After systemic absorption

(B) In the brain to increase parasympathetic outflow

(C) In the liver to increase production of bile acids

(D) From the lumen of the intestine and colon

9. All of the following statements regarding asthma therapy are true EXCEPT

(A) β-receptor down-regulation is not a major problem with the use of β-agonist inhalers

(B) theophylline has a relatively narrow range of safe therapeutic doses

(C) ipratropium is a quaternary nitrogen derivative of atropine

(D) the major pharmacologic action of zafirlukast is inhibition of lipoxygenase

(E) cromolyn sodium is not a bronchodilator; therefore, it is not very useful in acute asthma attack

10. The major mechanism of action of the nitrates responsible for their ability to relieve chest pain in chronic stable angina is thought to be which of the following?

(A) Dilation of the coronary vasculature distal to the ischemic region

(B) Redistribution of flow within the ischemic region

(C) Reducing the myocardial oxygen demands and improving the supply of oxygen to the heart

(D) Reducing the preload of the heart

(E) Inhibition of platelet aggregation

11. Laxatives increase defecation because they

(A) increase absorption of water from the colon

(B) increase content of water within the colon

(C) act in the enteric nervous system to stimulate segmenting contractions

(D) produce sustained relaxation of the external anal sphincter

12. Characteristics of warfarin include which of the following?

(A) It must be given by intravenous injection.

(B) It acts rapidly to destroy clotting factors.

(C) It is potentiated by barbiturates.

(D) It affects the synthesis of clotting factors in the liver.

(E) It is an antagonist of the fat-soluble vitamin E.

13. Which drug is used primarily in cases of severe iron deficiency and iron malabsorption syndromes?

(A) Cyanocobalamin

(B) Ferrous sulfate

(C) Folic acid

(D) Iron dextran

14. Systemic toxicity from topically applied medications is a result of which of the following?

(A) Corneal absorption

(B) Intravenous administration

(C) Scleral absorption

(D) Accelerated cataract formation

(E) Mucosal absorption

15. Which type of drug modifies pepsin activity by altering pH?

(A) Anticholinergics

(B) H_1 antagonists

(C) Gastrin antagonists

(D) Antacids

(E) Prostaglandin synthesis inducers

16. The rationale for combination therapy of angina is based on which of the following?

(A) Combination therapy enhances bioavailability of nitrates.

(B) Combination therapy minimizes tolerance to nitrates, improves hemodynamic status, and establishes a longer duration of protection against precipitation of angina.

(C) Combination therapy reduces the incidence of side effects.

(D) Combination therapy increases patient compliance.

(E) Combination therapy enhances efficacy of nitrates as a result of the improvement in hemodynamic status.

17. Preoperative cleansing of the bowel can best be achieved by administration of

(A) psyllium

(B) docusate

(C) methylcellulose

(D) polyethylene glycol

18. Which of the following would produce uterine contractions?

(A) Muscarine

(B) Nitrendipine

(C) Propranolol

(D) Verapamil

19. Propulsive small intestinal and colonic contractions induced by laxatives result primarily from

(A) direct drug actions at excitatory nerve pathways

(B) direct drug actions that block inhibitory nerve pathways

(C) peristaltic reflexes activated by luminal distention

(D) biotransformation of laxatives into prokinetic agents

20. A physician told a patient that he was prescribing a presynaptic α_2-adrenergic receptor agonist, which produces negative feedback on norepinephrine release. The drug that was mostly likely prescribed is

(A) phenoxybenzamine (Dibenzyline)

(B) hydralazine (Apresoline)

(C) reserpine (Serpasil)

(D) losartan (Cozaar)

(E) clonidine (Catapres)

21. Effective antidiarrheals have which of the following actions?

(A) They block GI contractions.

(B) They form viscous residue in the bowel lumen.

(C) They decrease secretion of fluid into the lumen.

(D) They stimulate propulsive contractions.

22. A 55-year-old man has a sudden increase in blood pressure that requires immediate reduction using a direct vasodilator. All of the following drugs would be appropriate therapy EXCEPT

(A) hydralazine (Apresoline)

(B) diazoxide (Hyperstat I.V.)

(C) minoxidil (Loniten)

(D) reserpine (Serpasil)

23. An example of an antidiarrheal drug that acts at μ opioid receptors is

(A) clonidine

(B) loperamide

(C) atropine

(D) cholestyramine

24. The risk of bleeding in patients taking heparin is

(A) increased in patients with protein C deficiency

(B) reduced when the patients take aspirin

(C) increased when the patients take warfarin

(D) reduced in patients with thrombocytopenia

(E) increased when the drug is used orally

25. VIP and NO are examples of neurotransmitters that

(A) increase secretion into the lumen

(B) decrease secretion into the lumen

(C) stimulate contractions of circular smooth muscle

(D) stimulate contractions of longitudinal smooth muscle

26. What ion do the drugs ACh, oxytocin, PGE_2, and $PGF_{2\alpha}$ have in common in their uterine actions?

(A) Ca^{2+}

(B) Cl^-

(C) K^+

(D) Na^+

27. The laxative of choice for extended use in elderly patients is

(A) a bulk laxative, such as bran

(B) a secretory laxative, such as senna

(C) an osmotic laxative, such as magnesium hydroxide

(D) a stool softener, such as mineral oil

28. Which of the following drugs is an osmotic diuretic?

(A) Acetazolamide

(B) Furosemide

(C) Triamterene

(D) Mannitol

29. All of the following agents are effective for treating acute attacks of bronchial asthma EXCEPT

(A) antimuscarinics

(B) β_2-adrenergic receptor agonists

(C) methylxanthines

(D) steroids

30. Cholestyramine has which of the following actions?

(A) It inhibits release of VIP.

(B) It inhibits release of ACh.

(C) It stimulates absorptive activity of villus cells.

(D) It binds and inactivates bile acids.

31. Which of the following antiarrhythmics reduces action potential duration?

(A) Amiodarone

(B) Bretylium

(C) Lidocaine

(D) Quinidine

PART III: ANSWERS AND EXPLANATIONS

1. The answer is D.

Unlike the other diuretics listed, potassium-sparers such as spironolactone can cause mild to life-threatening hyperkalemia. The same is true for potassium-sparers that work by a different mechanism than spironolactone, such as triamterene and amiloride. All three drugs increase N^+clearance and decrease K^+-H^+ exchange. These drugs should not be administered together with potassium supplements or with high-potassium diets.

2. The answer is A.

Amiodarone can cause pulmonary fibrosis, corneal drug deposits, and skin discoloration. Lidocaine, which must be given intravenously, can pass the blood–brain barrier and cause convulsions. Quinidine is a class IA agent with the potential to produce torsades de pointes.

3. The answer is C.

Brimonidine is an α_2-adrenergic receptor agonist that decreases intraocular pressure by presumably decreasing humor secretion. Atropine, a muscarinic receptor antagonist, is a mydriatic and cycloplegic agent and could possibly elevate intraocular pressure in susceptible individuals. Though used for lowering intraocular pressure, timolol is a β-adrenergic receptor antagonist and may exacerbate this patient's asthma by causing bronchospasm, specifically by competing with the bronchodilator drug and the endogenous catecholamine hormone/neurotransmitter. Gentamicin is an antibiotic. Tropicamide is also a muscarinic receptor antagonist.

4. The answer is C.

Acne is unlikely to respond to an antifungal agent such as clotrimazole. Acne is treated by drugs that are antimicrobial to *Propionibac-*

terium acnes (e.g., benzoyl peroxide and azelaic acid) and have peeling and comedolytic effects (e.g., benzoyl peroxide), inhibit sebaceous gland size and function (e.g., isotretinoin), or disrupt epidermal cell cohesion and enhancement of epidermal cell turnover (retinoic acid).

5. The answer is A.

Omeprazole inhibits the proton pump of parietal cells. Cimetidine, nizatidine, and ranitidine are H_2-receptor antagonists. Misoprostol is a synthetic prostaglandin.

6. The answer is B.

Octreotide is an octapeptide that acts as an agonist at somatostatin receptors. Clonidine acts at α_2-adrenergic receptors and loperamide at μ opioid receptors. Cholestyramine is an ion exchange resin and does not act at receptors.

7. The answer is B.

Erythropoietin is one of the growth hormones involved in the regulation of differentiation and maturation of stem cells within the bone marrow. Cyanocobalamin and folic acid are used as supplement therapy in vitamin B_{12} and folic acid deficiencies, respectively. Ferrous sulfate is used for iron-replacement therapy.

8. The answer is D.

All presently available laxatives act from the lumen, primarily by increasing the amount of water in the lumen of the colon. Systemic or brain actions would be undesirable. Excessive production of bile acids can induce diarrhea (bile acid catharsis) but is not used as a mechanism for laxatives.

9. The answer is D.

The major pharmacologic action of zafirlukast is not the inhibition of lipoxygenase enzyme; it is the antagonism of leukotriene receptors. Theophylline has a relatively narrow range of safe therapeutic doses and frequent checks of plasma levels are advisable. Ipratropium is a quaternary nitrogen derivative of atropine, and hence, blood–brain barrier passage (CNS adverse effects) is limited. Cromolyn sodium is more useful as a prophylactic agent. Inhalation of β-adrenergic receptor agonists does not lead to clinically significant receptor downregulation.

10. The answer is C.

The nitrates have several sites of action both within the heart and in the peripheral circulation. By relaxation of the capacitance veins, the preload of the heart is reduced. Relaxation of the arterial vasculature leads to a decrease in blood pressure, which decreases the afterload of the heart. This leads to a decrease in left ventricular wall tension, resulting in a decrease in the demand for oxygen. Dilation of the coronary vasculature increases blood flow to the heart, thus improving the delivery of oxygen to myocardial cells. The overall effect of these pharmacologic actions of nitrates at these sites of action is to cause a decrease in myocardial demand for oxygen and to increase the arterial supply of oxygen to the heart. All of these nitrate-induced changes are responsible for the relief of anginal pain. Although nitrates are known to inhibit platelet aggregation, it is not a major effect of these drugs.

11. The answer is B.

Laxatives act in the small intestine and colon to increase content of water in the colonic lumen. Segmenting contractions retard flow through the bowel and tend to reverse laxation. Relaxation of the anal sphincter would lead to incontinence.

12. The answer is D.

Warfarin, which can be taken orally, acts by inhibiting vitamin K regeneration, thus preventing the posttranslational modification of clotting factors in the liver. Warfarin metabolism is accelerated by barbiturates and other drugs that stimulate the activity of cytochrome P-450, thereby reducing its pharmacologic activity.

13. The answer is D.

Parenteral therapy is usually reserved for patients with iron deficiency coupled with oral intolerance or malabsorption. Iron dextran is a stable complex of ferric hydroxide and low-molecular-weight dextran that can be given intramuscularly or intravenously. Cyanocobalamin and folic acid are used as supplement therapy for vitamin B_{12} and folic acid deficiencies, respectively. Ferrous sulfate is not appropriate therapy when malabsorption syndrome is present.

14. The answer is E.

Corneal absorption and scleral absorption are important considerations for drug design to effect therapeutic intraocular drug levels. Intravenous administration is a different route of drug delivery. Accelerated cataract formation is a local side effect from either topical or systemic corticosteroid.

15. The answer is D.

Antacids neutralize stomach or esophageal acid and raise pH above the level needed for pepsin activation. Anticholinergics inhibit the stimulation of acid production via M_3-cholinergic receptors. H_1-receptor antagonists (antihistamines), unlike H_2 blockers, typically do not have antiulcer action. Gastrin antagonists block stimulation of acid due to gastrin released from the antrum, and prostaglandin synthesis inducers cause mucosa to produce protective quantities of prostaglandins.

16. The answer is B.

Monotherapy with nitrates alone presents a pharmacologic challenge to provide round-the-clock protection against angina because tolerance develops. Optimal therapy with nitrates includes an 8–12-hour nitrate-free interval. It is desirable to supplement therapy with other agents such as the Ca^{2+}-channel blockers or beta-blockers, since these agents can provide additional actions to improve the supply–demand relationship for oxygen. Option C is not true since multitherapy would be expected to increase the incidence of side effects. Although combination therapy decreases the development of tolerance to nitrates as the result of decreased exposure, it does not enhance the efficacy of the nitrates.

17. The answer is D.

Psyllium, docusate, and methylcellulose do not act rapidly or completely enough to empty the bowel lumen. Polyethylene glycol combined with isotonic salts is effective in cleansing the bowel without dehydration of the patient.

18. The answer is A.

The mammalian uterus is innervated by the autonomic nervous system (adrenergic and cholinergic nerves) along with numerous other inputs. In general, muscarinic cholinergic receptor agonists such as muscarine induce uterine contractions. Uterine relaxant effects are exerted primarily through β_2-adrenergic receptors and would be blocked by propranolol. Uterine contraction/relaxation is a function of intracellular Ca^{2+} concentration. Hence, Ca^{2+}-channel blockers, such as nitrendipine and verapamil, would inhibit uterine smooth muscle activity.

19. The answer is C.

Cannon's law of the bowel applies. Luminal distention activates propulsive contractions that move contents toward the rectum. Laxatives in current use do not act at enteric nerves. Most laxatives remain in the lumen, and biotransformation is limited.

20. The answer is E.

Phenoxybenzamine is an α-adrenergic receptor antagonist; hydralazine is a direct vasodilator; reserpine is an indirect-acting sympathomimetic that disrupts the vesicular storage of norepinephrine in presynaptic nerve terminals; and losartan is an angiotensin-receptor antagonist.

21. The answer is C.

Net accumulation of excess fluid in the lumen is the cause of diarrhea. The goal of therapy is to reduce net fluid accumulation. The most effective antidiarrheal drugs decrease propulsive contractions and increase segmenting, nonpropulsive contractions. Formation of a viscous gel in the lumen would not improve fluid dynamics.

22. The answer is D.

Hydralazine, diazoxide, and minoxidil are all direct vasodilators. Reserpine is an indirect-acting sympathomimetic that disrupts vesicular storage of norepinephrine in presynaptic nerve terminals.

23. The answer is B.

Loperamide is an agonist at μ opioid receptors. Clonidine acts at α_2-adrenergic receptors and atropine (as an antagonist) at muscarinic cholinergic receptors. Cholestyramine is an ion exchange resin and does not act at receptors.

24. The answer is C.

In contrast to warfarin, heparin must be given by injection, has a short half-life, and may cause platelet aggregation and thrombocytopenia. It acts by binding to antithrombin III, thereby increasing the activity of this serine protease inhibitor against activated coagulation factors. Its effects on bleeding are increased by aspirin, which inhibits platelet aggregation, by warfarin, which inhibits the synthesis of coagulation factors, and by thrombocytopenia (low levels of platelets).

25. The answer is A.

Secretomotor neurons that innervate the mucosal epithelial cells release VIP, NO, and other secretory neurotransmitters to promote secretion of fluid into the lumen of the bowel. Both VIP and NO generally cause relaxation, not contraction, of smooth muscle.

26. The answer is A.

An increase in the intracellular Ca^{2+} concentration enhances uterine contractions and a decrease in intracellular Ca^{2+} concentration inhibits them. Smooth muscle contractile agents such as ACh, oxytocin, and prostaglandins raise the intracellular Ca^{2+} concentration. In addition, PGE_2, $PGF_{2\alpha}$, and oxytocin decrease ATP-dependent Ca^{2+} uptake.

27. The answer is A.

Bulk laxatives produce the fewest side effects and are safest for chronic use. Secretory and osmotic laxatives, which increase formation of NO, can damage the mucosa. Mineral oil can interfere with absorption of fat-soluble vitamins and may leak past the anal sphincter.

28. The answer is D.

Mannitol decreases water and Na^+ reabsorption in the proximal tubule and loop of Henle in part by limiting the osmosis of water out of the tubular lumen. Acetazolamide inhibits carbonic anhydrase activity within the luminal membrane and the intracellular compartment of epithelial cells along the proximal tubule of the nephron. Furosemide inhibits Na^+–K^+–$2Cl^-$ and Na^+–Cl^--cotransportor activity in the luminal membrane of epithelial cells of the thick ascending limb of the loop of Henle. Triamterene blocks luminal membrane Na^+ channels in the collecting duct system epithelial cell.

29. The answer is D.

In the usual clinical situation, β_2-adrenergic receptor agonists, antimuscarinics, and methylxanthines are much more effective in treating acute attacks of asthma than are steroids.

30. The answer is D.

Cholestyramine is a basic anion exchange resin that binds bile acids to promote their excretion in the feces. It is useful when diarrhea is caused by excessive production of bile acids. It is also used to reduce body content of cholesterol.

31. The answer is C.

Drugs such as lidocaine block Na^+ channels and alter cardiac cell excitability, thus reducing the likelihood of rapid reexcitation. Class III agents *prolong* action potential duration (and necessarily slow ventricular rate). Amiodarone, bretylium, and quinidine have class III characteristics.

PART IV
Central Nervous System Pharmacology

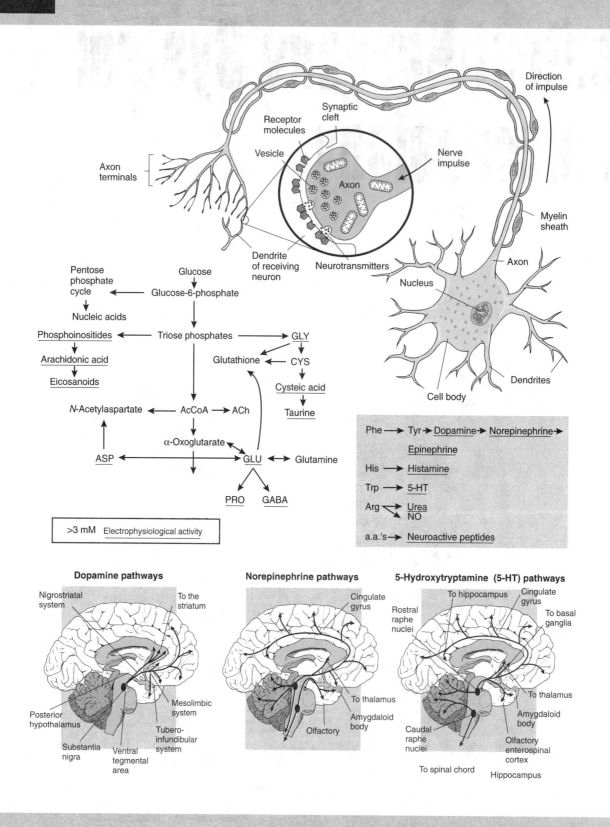

Direction of impulse

Receptor molecules

Synaptic cleft

Vesicle

Axon terminals

Nerve impulse

Axon

Myelin sheath

Axon

Nucleus

Dendrite of receiving neuron

Neurotransmitters

Dendrites

Cell body

Pentose phosphate cycle

Glucose

Glucose-6-phosphate

Nucleic acids

Phosphoinositides ← Triose phosphates → GLY

Arachidonic acid

Glutathione ← CYS

Eicosanoids

Cysteic acid

N-Acetylaspartate ← AcCoA → ACh

Taurine

α-Oxoglutarate

ASP ↔ GLU ↔ Glutamine

PRO   GABA

>3 mM Electrophysiological activity

Phe → Tyr → Dopamine → Norepinephrine →

Epinephrine

His → Histamine

Trp → 5-HT

Arg → Urea / NO

a.a.'s → Neuroactive peptides

Dopamine pathways

Nigrostriatal system

To the striatum

Posterior hypothalamus

Mesolimbic system

Substantia nigra

Ventral tegmental area

Tubero-infundibular system

Norepinephrine pathways

Cingulate gyrus

To thalamus

Amygdaloid body

Olfactory

5-Hydroxytryptamine (5-HT) pathways

To hippocampus

Cingulate gyrus

Rostral raphe nuclei

To basal ganglia

To thalamus

Amygdaloid body

Caudal raphe nuclei

Olfactory enterospinal cortex

To spinal chord

Hippocampus

OVERVIEW

- Virtually all drugs that act on the CNS produce their effects by modifying some aspect of synaptic transmission.
- Many features of central neurotransmission are similar to those of neurotransmission in the periphery.
- The peripheral neurotransmitters, such as ACh, norepinephrine, and dopamine, also are central neurotransmitters.
- The metabolic enzymes and pathways are qualitatively similar in nervous and nonnervous tissue, but the relative importance of certain paths differs.
- The neurotransmitters in highest concentration in the CNS derive from glucose metabolism, which is the major energy source for the Na^+-K^+ pump, which is required to maintain the neuronal membrane potential difference.

Some notable distinguishing features of central neurotransmission in contrast to peripheral neurotransmission include:

- Greater number of neurotransmitters (more than 40)
- Greater variety of neurotransmitters, such as peptides, nonpeptides, NO
- Cotransmitters commonly occurring within the same neuron
- Nondirected synapses in which the neurotransmitter can affect more than one postsynaptic site
- Inhibitory neurotransmitters (e.g., GABA)
- More complicated neuronal connections
- More complicated neural networks (e.g., hierarchical or diffuse)

Membrane Potential

The nerve membrane is electrically polarized (i.e., intracellular is more negative than extracellular) as a result of the relative distribution of ions (more Na^+, Ca^{2+}, and Cl^- outside, K^+ and protein inside). Neurotransmitters that enhance the flow of minus ions to the inside make the neuron more negative (hyperpolarized) and less likely to fire. Drugs that enhance the influx of plus ions into the neuron make it less negative (depolarization) and closer to its firing threshold. Neurotransmitters produce excitatory or inhibitory postsynaptic potentials (EPSPs and IPSPs) that are summed (at the axon hillock) and determine the neuron's general excitability. It should be noted that the relative state of excitation (or inhibition) of a particular neuron does not necessarily translate into behavioral excitation (or inhibition), because of the complex arrangements of the neurons. For example, inhibition of an inhibitory pathway results in behavioral excitation (termed *disinhibition*).

Axonal Transport

Owing to the greater reliance of central neurotransmission on peptide transmitters or cotransmitters, axonal transport is a significant factor in central neurotransmission (because peptide synthesis, unlike synthesis of nonpeptides, occurs in the cell body). Drugs that affect axonal transport can modulate transmitter action to a greater extent centrally than in the periphery.

Receptor Regulation

Chronic administration of CNS-active drugs typically (if not invariably) leads to a compensatory response, which results in a change in receptor number or transduction. An increase in receptor number is termed *up-regulation*. A decrease in receptor number is termed *down-regulation*. Up-regulation (usually in response to an antagonist) and down-regulation (usually in response to an agonist) play critical roles in the actions of CNS-active drugs.

Inverse Agonists

Drugs that produce effects opposite to those of the endogenous neurotransmitter are termed *inverse agonists*. Perhaps the most common examples of such drugs involve the $GABA_A$ receptor complex.

Sites of Drug Action in the CNS

Common sites of drug action in the CNS include: axonal transport; membrane potential difference; organelles for synthesis, storage, and release of neurotransmitter; enzymes for catabolizing neurotransmitter after release; postsynaptic receptor; second messengers (transduction); transcription, translation, and posttranslational processing; modifiable processes (plasticity, learning, memory); membrane potential difference; impulse propagation; presynaptic inhibition; autoreceptors (negative feedback); and postsynaptic catabolism.

SOME CENTRAL NEUROTRANSMITTERS

Acetylcholine and norepinephrine

Amino acids
- High concentration in CNS
- Inhibitory: glycine (Gly, G)
- Excitatory: glutamate (Glu, E), aspartate (Asp, D)

Amino acid derivatives
- Tryptophan (Trp, W) → 5-HT (serotonin)
- Phenylalanine (Phe, F) → catecholamines (DA, NE, EPI)
- Glycine → taurine
- Glutamate → GABA
- Histidine (His, H) → histamine

Peptides
- Opioid (e.g., endorphins, enkephalins, dynorphins)
- Tachykinins (substance P)
- Pituitary (e.g., vasopressin, oxytocin)
- Gastrins (e.g., gastrin, cholecystokinin)
- Somatostatins
- Glucagon-related (e.g., vasoactive intestinal peptide)
- Pancreatic peptide-related (neuropeptide Y)
- Others (e.g., bombesin, neurotensin, bradykinin, angiotensin, calcitonin-gene-related peptide [CGRP], endothelins)

Purines
- ATP, ADP, AMP

NO

36 General Anesthetics

T. Philip Malan, Jr., Ph.D., M.D.

A GABA receptor

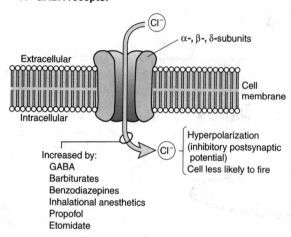

Cl⁻

α-, β-, δ-subunits

Extracellular

Cell membrane

Intracellular

Increased by:
GABA
Barbiturates
Benzodiazepines
Inhalational anesthetics
Propofol
Etomidate

Cl⁻

Hyperpolarization (inhibitory postsynaptic potential)
Cell less likely to fire

B Inhaled anesthetics

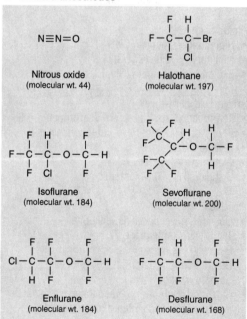

Nitrous oxide
(molecular wt. 44)

Halothane
(molecular wt. 197)

Isoflurane
(molecular wt. 184)

Sevoflurane
(molecular wt. 200)

Enflurane
(molecular wt. 184)

Desflurane
(molecular wt. 168)

C Physical characteristics of inhaled anesthetics

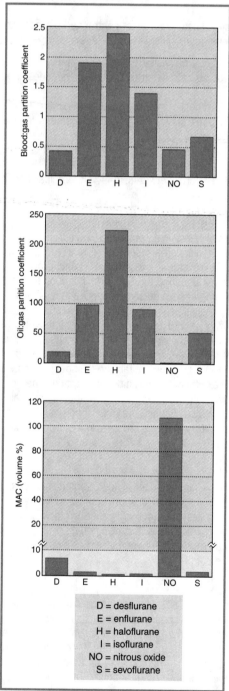

D = desflurane
E = enflurane
H = haloflurane
I = isoflurane
NO = nitrous oxide
S = sevoflurane

OVERVIEW

- Goals of a general anesthetic: (1) hypnosis (unconsciousness), (2) analgesia (freedom from pain), (3) skeletal muscle relaxation, and (4) reduction of certain autonomic reflexes.
- Anesthetic techniques: (1) inhalation anesthesia (where anesthetics are presented in the gaseous state and taken up by the lungs), (2) total intravenous anesthesia, and (3) utilizing both routes of administration.

Pharmacology

Inhaled anesthetics probably interact with hydrophobic regions of membranes. One potentially important action is facilitation of the action of the inhibitory neurotransmitter GABA at the GABA$_A$ receptor. Several intravenous anesthetics (barbiturates, benzodiazepines, etomidate, propofol) also may exert their actions by facilitating the action of GABA at the GABA$_A$ receptor. The anesthetic action of ketamine may be mediated through inhibition of the NMDA receptor.

Medicinal Chemistry

Inhaled anesthetics can be divided into two groups: anesthetic gases and volatile anesthetics. Anesthetic gases (nitrous oxide) are present in the gaseous state at room temperature and pressure. Volatile anesthetics are present as liquids at room temperature and pressure but are vaporized into gases for administration. All contemporary volatile anesthetics are halogenated hydrocarbons or halogenated ethers. A high oil:gas partition coefficient predicts high anesthetic potency. This may be because anesthetics exert their actions at hydrophobic sites. The measure of potency of inhaled anesthetics is the minimal alveolar concentration (MAC). MAC is the concentration of anesthetic in alveolar gas that prevents response to a standard painful stimulus (skin incision) in 50% of patients. Anesthetic concentration is usually expressed as volumes percent.

Pharmacokinetics

Inhaled Anesthetics. Volatile anesthetics are administered to the lungs, with consequent uptake into the systemic circulation. They are also eliminated by the lungs and do not depend on intrinsic hepatic biotransformation or renal excretion.

Intravenous Anesthetics. IV anesthetics provide a rapid onset of action. The central effect is terminated by redistribution to "peripheral" pharmacokinetic compartments. When administered for longer periods by infusion, metabolism and elimination become more important in terminating anesthetic effect.

Organ Effects

The desired effect of *inhaled anesthetics* is depression of the CNS. Another important CNS effect is increased intracranial pressure in patients with intracranial masses.

Ventilatory depression is observed with all inhaled anesthetics. All volatile anesthetics depress the cardiovascular system by producing negative inotropic effects, peripheral vasodilation, and decreases in blood pressure. Halothane can cause bradycardia, while most other volatile anesthetics produce mild tachycardia. Inhaled anesthetics, particularly halothane, can sensitize the myocardium to catecholamines, potentially causing ventricular arrhythmias.

Halogenated anesthetics inhibit the contractile response of the gravid uterus. Inhaled anesthetics cross the placenta into the fetus. Nausea and vomiting may follow general anesthesia. Patient temperature may decrease during anesthesia.

Most *sedative-hypnotic drugs* decrease cerebral metabolism and intracranial pressure. Therefore, some are used in the treatment of patients at risk for cerebral ischemia or intracranial hypertension. Most have anticonvulsant properties.

Most *intravenous anesthetics* cause dose-dependent respiratory depression. Barbiturates, benzodiazepines, and propofol cause cardiovascular depression by directly decreasing myocardial contractility and by lowering systemic vascular resistance. Others cause indirect cardiovascular depression by depressing sympathetic nervous system activity.

Toxicity and Adverse Effects

Enflurane has been associated with rare cases of renal toxicity. Halothane has been implicated in rare, unpredictable hepatic toxicity. Volatile anesthetics or succinylcholine may trigger *malignant hyperthermia*, a disorder of increased muscle metabolism, in genetically susceptible individuals. Malignant hyperthermia can be fatal, but when recognized promptly it can be effectively treated with dantrolene.

SPECIFIC INTRAVENOUS AGENTS

Barbiturates
- Thiopental (sodium pentothal), highly alkaline (pH > 10); causes tissue damage if injected extravenously
- May precipitate episodes of acute intermittent porphyria in susceptible individuals

Etomidate
- Provided in 35% propylene glycol; causes pain on injection and occasional venous inflammation
- May cause involuntary myoclonic movements during induction of anesthesia
- Causes adrenal suppression; not administered long-term

Propofol
- Supplied as egg-lecithin emulsion; causes pain on injection
- Antiemetic action, rapid emergence from anesthesia, and feeling of well-being

Ketamine
- Can be injected intramuscularly
- Increases cerebral metabolism and intracranial pressure
- Produces excellent analgesia
- May cause undesirable effects on mentation under some circumstances

Opioids and benzodiazepines
- Commonly used IV as part of the anesthetic regimen
- Opioids provide smooth emergence from anesthesia and decrease early postoperative pain
- Benzodiazepines are usually used for sedation and anxiolysis but can be used for induction of anesthesia

37 Sedative-Hypnotics

Robert B. Raffa, Ph.D.

A GABA$_A$ receptor

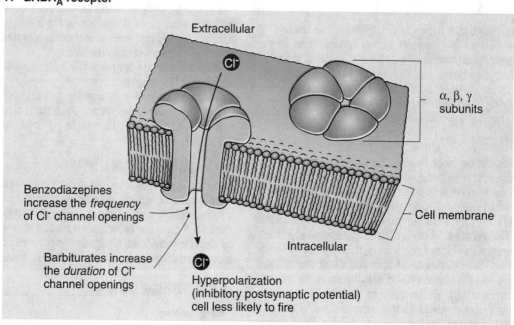

Extracellular

Cl⁻

α, β, γ subunits

Cell membrane

Intracellular

Benzodiazepines increase the *frequency* of Cl⁻ channel openings

Barbiturates increase the *duration* of Cl⁻ channel openings

Hyperpolarization (inhibitory postsynaptic potential) cell less likely to fire

B Biotransformation and elimination of benzodiazepines

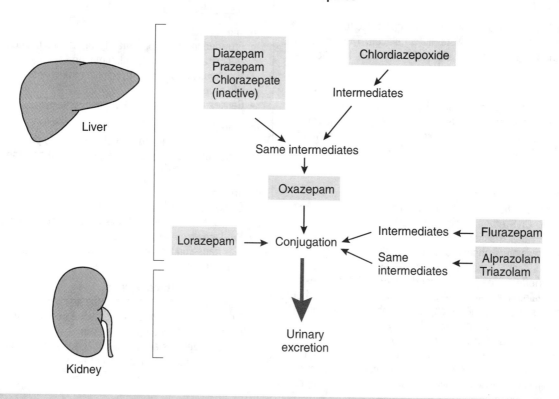

Liver

Diazepam
Prazepam
Chlorazepate
(inactive)

Chlordiazepoxide

Intermediates

Same intermediates

Oxazepam

Lorazepam → Conjugation ← Intermediates ← Flurazepam

Same intermediates ← Alprazolam Triazolam

Kidney

Urinary excretion

OVERVIEW

- When associated with acute stress, anxiety can resolve without medication, but sensitization to repeated stress can occur.
- Clinical anxieties include panic attacks, phobias, obsessive-compulsive disorder (OCD), and possibly post-traumatic stress disorder.
- Approximately 10% of the general population have clinically significant anxiety.
- Anxiety may be endogenous (genetic component not definitively established).
- Treatment includes psychotherapeutic, cognitive, behavioral, and pharmacologic interventions.
- Terminology: Sedation is a reduction of anxiety; an anxiolytic is a drug that is sedating (reduces anxiety); and a hypnotic is a drug that produces drowsiness and sleep (generally an extension of higher doses of sedatives).

Pharmacotherapy

Sedative-hypnotics have the advantages of mimicking natural relaxation and sleep, minimally affecting motor or mental functions, possessing a wide safety margin, and having a minimal effect on other organ systems. They may be used intermittently for acute anxiety attacks and chronically (4–8 weeks) for recurring symptoms. The most common means of therapy are benzodiazepines (BDZs), which were introduced in the 1960s and have replaced the barbiturates and carbamates; examples include diazepam (Valium), chlordiazepoxide (Librium), and many others. Newer drugs (e.g., buspirone [BuSpar]) offer some advantages over the BDZs, having fewer side effects and less dependence liability.

Pharmacology

GABA is a major inhibitory neurotransmitter in CNS (at about 30% of all brain synapses) that is primarily synthesized from glutamate (Glu). It occurs in CNS and some peripheral tissue (mostly in short interneurons). The $GABA_A$ receptor is mostly postsynaptic. Five subunits form Cl^- channels; increased Cl^- flux leads to hyperpolarization. Multiple combinations of the subunits occur in different brain regions and account for differences in properties of individual barbiturates and BDZs. GABA's action on the $GABA_A$ receptor complex is modulated (usually allosterically) by barbiturates, BDZs, ethanol, and other pro- and anticonvulsant substances.

Mechanisms of Action

BDZs and barbiturates bind to separate sites on the $GABA_A$ receptor complex and enhance GABA-mediated Cl^- influx by different mechanisms. BDZs might have additional anxiolytic effects on 5-HT systems. Zolpidem (Ambien) is of a different chemical class from BDZs but binds to BDZ receptors and has a similar mechanism.

Pharmacokinetics

Absorption. Most of these drugs are lipid-soluble and readily absorbed from the GI tract. Of note: Oral absorption of triazolam (Halcion) is extremely rapid; clorazepate (Tranxene) is converted to its active form (desmethyldiazepam) in stomach.

Distribution. Lipid solubility means rapid distribution to brain and other organs. Of note: Most readily pass the placenta; high plasma protein binding can lead to drug interactions.

Metabolism. (1) Barbiturates. Generally these are extensively metabolized in liver; they induce microsomal (cytochrome P-450) enzymes. (2) Benzodiazepines. These are mainly metabolized by liver microsomal enzymes; several metabolites have a long half-life. (3) Buspirone (BuSpar) and zolpidem (Ambien) undergo extensive hepatic metabolism. Fig. B shows the metabolism of some BDZs.

Toxicity

Adverse effects include excess CNS depression; decreased psychomotor function; daytime sedation; drug interactions; respiratory depression (BDZs have high therapeutic index); effects on REM sleep; liver enzyme induction (more with barbiturates); anterograde amnesia (more with BDZs); psychological or physical dependence; muscle relaxation; ataxia; tolerance may develop; withdrawal seizures (more with barbiturates). Precaution must be taken (~25% dose) with elderly, because diminished liver function increases drug accumulation.

SPECIFIC AGENTS

Benzodiazepines

Alprazolam (Xanax)	Lorazepam (Ativan)
Chlordiazepoxide (Librium)	Midazolam (Versed)
Clorazepate (Tranxene)	Oxazepam (Serax)
Clonazepam (Klonopin)	Prazepam (Centrax)
Diazepam (Valium)	Quazepam (Doral)
Estazolam (ProSom)	Temazepam (Restoril)
Flurazepam (Dalmane)	Triazolam (Halcion)
Halazepam (Paxipam)	

Benzodiazepine receptor antagonist

Flumazenil (Romazicon)

Barbiturates

Amobarbital (Amytal)	Pentobarbital (Nembutal Sodium)
Aprobarbital (Alurate)	
Butabarbital (Butisol)	Phenobarbital (Luminal Sodium)
Mephobarbital (Mebaral)	Secobarbitol (Seconal)

Other

Buspirone (BuSpar)	Meprobamate (Miltown, Equanil)
Chloral hydrate (Noctec)	
Ethchlorvynol (Placidyl)	Paraldehyde (generic)
Ethinamate (Valmid Pulvules)	Zolpidem (Ambien)
Hydroxyzine (Atarax, Vistaril)	

38 Ethanol

Robert B. Raffa, Ph.D.

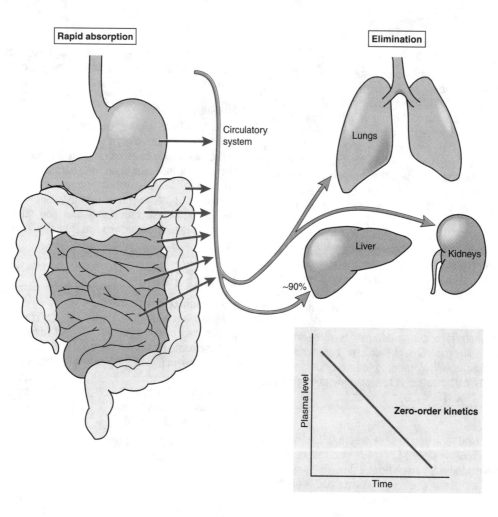

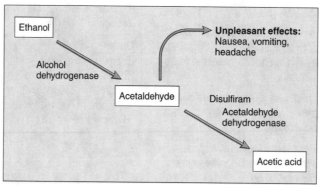

OVERVIEW

- Ethanol is a sedative-hypnotic agent, which has been used for this purpose both medically and recreationally.
- The availability of more specific agents with less associated misuse has greatly supplanted the official use of ethanol as a prescribed medication. However, the moderate consumption of ethanol has been credited with stress reduction, enhancement of aspirin's antiplatelet action, and reduced mortality.
- The abuse of ethanol can represent a significant health hazard to the imbiber and to innocent victims of the imbiber's actions.
- Concomitant use with other CNS drugs leads to additive interactions (CNS depression) or to potentiation (e.g., with vasodilators or oral hypoglycemic agents).
- Treatment of ethanol abuse is directed at aversion (disulfiram) or inhibition of craving (naltrexone).

Pharmacology

No specific receptor for ethanol has been identified. Its effect on the CNS is thought to be due to interaction with membrane proteins involved with receptor-gated ion channels or to modification of neurotransmitter function. Acute exposure enhances the action of GABA at GABA$_A$ receptors and inhibits glutamate action at the N-methyl-D-aspartate (NMDA) subtype of glutamate receptors. Enhancement of GABA (an inhibitory neurotransmitter) and inhibition of glutamate (an excitatory neurotransmitter) both lead to inhibitory effects on neuronal function. The stimulated behavior observed following ethanol ingestion is interpreted as disinhibition.

Disulfiram (generic, Antabuse) inhibits aldehyde dehydrogenase activity, giving rise to the unpleasant feelings of acetaldehyde toxicity. Naltrexone (ReVia) is an opioid antagonist that reduces craving by a mechanism not understood fully.

Pharmacokinetics

Administration and Distribution. Ethanol is a small hydrophilic molecule that is rapidly and completely absorbed following ingestion (delayed by the presence of food). Distribution is nearly complete to all tissues, with levels reaching about the same concentration as the concentration in the perfusing blood supply. Hence, the volume of distribution of ethanol approaches that of total body water. Ethanol readily crosses the blood–brain barrier.

Metabolism and Excretion. A small amount of ethanol is excreted through the lungs and in the urine, but the majority is oxidized in the liver (markedly reduced in liver disease). Its rate of disappearance normally follows zero-order kinetics. The main pathway for ethanol metabolism involves dehydrogenation (catalyzed by alcohol dehydrogenase). Alcohol dehydrogenase is located in the cytosol of liver and other (e.g., brain, stomach) cells and catalyzes the conversion of ethanol (CH_3CH_2OH) to acetaldehyde (CH_3CHO). Acetaldehyde is then oxidized to acetate (mainly by aldehyde dehydrogenase located in liver mitochondria), and acetate is further metabolized to CO_2 and H_2O. An alternative route involves the hepatic mixed-function oxidase enzymes. The latter pathway uses $NADP^+$ (instead of NAD^+) as a cofactor (hydrogen acceptor).

Toxicity and Adverse Effects

Acute

When large amounts of ethanol are consumed, NAD^+ is depleted, and the alcohol dehydrogenase system becomes saturated. Excess acetaldehyde and NADH are produced. People who have a genetic deficiency in aldehyde dehydrogenase production experience the unpleasant effects of high acetaldehyde concentrations following even moderate or low doses of ethanol.

CNS. Dose-related sedation, impaired motor function, slurred speech and ataxia, emesis, stupor, coma, respiratory depression, and death.

CV. Depression of myocardial contractility; heart abnormalities.
Smooth Muscle. Vasodilation (possible hypothermia).

Chronic

Certain persons appear to have a genetic predisposition for chronic alcohol (ab)use. Chronic alcohol consumption induces the mixed-function oxidase enzymes (resulting in increased metabolism and tolerance of ethanol), but it also decreases the rate of acetaldehyde oxidation in mitochondria. There appears to be a possible increased risk of cancer in persons who abuse alcohol.

CNS. Same as after acute administration, plus dependence and peripheral neuropathies.
Liver. Hypoglycemia, fat accumulation, hepatitis, cirrhosis.
GI. Irritation, inflammation, bleeding, and scarring can inhibit absorption of nutrients.
CV. Hypertension, anemia, myocardial infarction.
Endocrine. Gynecomastia, testicular atrophy, salt retention.
Pregnancy. Fetal alcohol syndrome (physical and mental defects).

Treatment

Aversion. Disulfiram (tetraethylthiuram disulfide) inhibits aldehyde dehydrogenase. As a consequence, the aversive effects of acetaldehyde (e.g., headache, nausea, vomiting) are experienced and serve as a deterrent to excess consumption of alcohol.

Craving. Recent studies suggest that opioid antagonists, such as naltrexone, decrease the craving that is associated with chronic alcohol consumption. Other neurotransmitter targets (e.g., serotonin, dopamine, glutamate, GABA) are under investigation. Results of clinical trials of SSRIs have been mixed. Alcoholism might be a heterogeneous disorder, requiring subtype-specific therapy.

SPECIFIC AGENTS

Aversion Therapy	Treatment of Craving
Disulfiram (generic, Antabuse)	Naltrexone (ReVia)
• Rapidly and completely absorbed from the GI tract (12 hours until peak effect)	• Oral, once a day
• Inhibition of aldehyde dehydrogenase leads to buildup of acetaldehyde	• Extensive first-pass metabolism to active and inactive metabolites
• Slow elimination rate (effect can persist for several days)	• Generally mild adverse effects at therapeutic doses
• Inhibits metabolism of several other therapeutic agents	• Potential hepatotoxicity
• Potential hepatotoxicity	

Antipsychotic Agents

Ellen E. Codd, M.S.

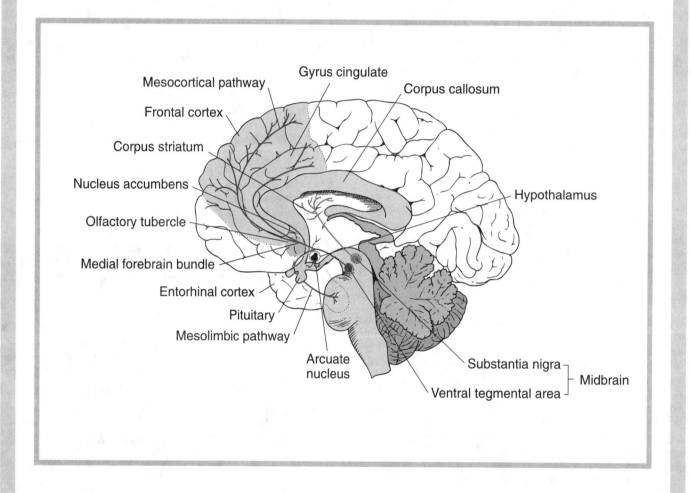

OVERVIEW

- Therapeutic uses: treatment of psychoses, especially schizophrenia.
- Mechanism of action: blockade of dopamine receptors; also often have serotonergic, adrenergic, and other CNS receptor-blocking activities, some of which contribute to therapeutic effect.
- Site of action: CNS, especially limbic areas of forebrain and basal ganglia.
- Long-term use often leads to movement disorders.
- Existing drugs are less than ideal because they lack efficacy in all disease aspects or produce unwanted side effects.
- Patient compliance is an issue.

FIRST:	extracts of *Rauwolfia*
FIRST SYNTHETIC:	**CHLORPROMAZINE** (Charpentier, 1950)
PROTOTYPICAL:	**HALOPERIDOL**
FIRST "ATYPICAL":	**CLOZAPINE**

Pharmacology

Antagonism of the dopamine D_2 receptor is common to all currently available antipsychotics (Fig.). However, blockade of several additional receptors, including other dopaminergic receptor subtypes and serotonergic, adrenergic, histaminergic, and sigma receptors, is also common and may contribute to the broadened efficacy (against negative symptoms, cognitive deficits) or reduced side-effect profiles (reduced propensity to produce extrapyramidal effects) of newer agents. The anatomy that is relevant to dopamine neurons is illustrated in the figure.

D_1-like Subtypes. D_1 has high density in forebrain; SCH23390 is used in radioactive studies. D_5 has high affinity for dopamine.

D_2-like Subtypes. D_2 has high density in striatum; typical antipsychotics have high affinity. D_3 has high density in limbic brain areas (have to do with affect). D_4 has high density in frontal cortex (cognitive area of brain); clozapine has high affinity.

Medicinal Chemistry

Most antipsychotics are multiringed structures, containing nitrogen substituent. The phenothiazines and thioxanthenes have three six-membered rings. Other antipsychotics contain a variety of components, including five- and seven-membered rings, as well as other substituents such as a fluoride (haloperidol, risperidone) or chloride (haloperidol, clozapine).

Therapeutic Usage

Antipsychotics, not particularly effective when used alone, are best used as part of a comprehensive treatment program including long-term supportive and rehabilitative therapy. Behavioral support is needed when "awakening" (awareness of loss of a portion of one's life as a result of schizophrenia) occurs on effective pharmacotherapeutic intervention, especially with the newer, "atypical" antipsychotics.

Pharmacokinetics

Administration and Distribution. Antipsychotics are usually administered orally; depot formulations (decanoate esters) are administered intramuscularly. Many of the drugs are lipophilic and become highly membrane- and protein-bound. They accumulate in the brain and are only eliminated from it slowly.

Metabolism and Excretion. The main route of metabolism is by liver microsomal oxidases. Some metabolites are active, complicating attempts to correlate drug plasma levels with therapeutic effect. Hydrophilic metabolites are excreted mainly in the urine. Some agents may induce their own metabolism.

Toxicity

CNS. The most serious side effect associated with long-term antipsychotic use is the development of movement disorders such as pseudo-Parkinsonism (muscle tremors, rigidity, spasms) and tardive dyskinesia (abnormal movements, especially facial, such as lip smacking and tongue wagging). Extrapyramidal symptoms may result from blockade of D_2 receptors in the basal ganglia.

CV. Cardiovascular side effects probably derive from the adrenergic activities of many antipsychotic compounds. The most common of these is orthostatic hypertension. Patient dosage is often increased gradually to allow accommodation to this side effect.

Other. Lethal doses of most antipsychotics are high. Other side effects are characteristic of the muscarinic activity of the compounds: faintness, palpitation, dry mouth, and constipation.

SPECIFIC AGENTS

Classic	**"Atypical"**
Chlorpromazine (Thorazine) • First synthetic antipsychotic • D_2 receptor antagonist Fluphenazine (Permitil, Prolixin) • Available also as a decanoate ester (depot formulation) Haloperidol (Haldol) • Effective against positive symptoms of schizophrenia	Clozapine (Clozaril) • Low propensity to induce extrapyramidal effects • Can cause potentially fatal agranulocytosis Risperidone (Risperdal) • 5-HT$_2$ and D_2 antagonist • "Atypical" at lower doses Olanzapine (Zyprexa) • Structural analog of clozapine • Broad receptor, binding: 5-HT$_{2A/2C}$, etc.; D_1, D_2, D_4, M_1, H_1, α_1 Quetiapine (Seroquel) • 5-HT$_2$ and D_2 antagonist

40 Anxiolytics

Richard H. Rech, Ph.D.

A Anxiolytics and CNS pharmacology

Benzodiazepine-GABA$_A$-Cl$^-$ channel ionophore

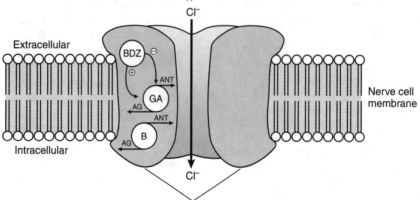

Extracellular

Nerve cell membrane

Intracellular

	Channel openers— agonists (AG)	Channel closers— antagonists (ANT)
Benzodiazepine site (BDZ)	Diazepam, alprazolam	β-Carbolines*
GABA$_A$ site (GA)	Muscimol, valproate (?)	Bicuculline
Barbiturate site (B)	Barbiturates	Picrotoxin

*β-Carbolines are more accurately termed "inverse agonists," while flumazenil is a true antagonist at BDZ receptor.

B Chemical structures

Alprazolam

Diazepam

Midazolam

C

Benzodiazepine duration of action	
Chlordiazepoxide Chlorazepate Diazepam Quazepam	Long half-life active metabolites and long duration of action
Lorazepam Alprazolam Oxazepam Midazolam	Inactive metabolites or short half-life active metabolites and short duration of action

OVERVIEW

- Benzodiazepines are currently the most effective and widely used anxiolytics.
- Mechanism of action: enhanced GABA$_A$ activity at neuronal Cl$^-$ channels with benzodiazepine receptor sites (increased inhibition).
- Site of action: widely throughout brain at benzodiazepine-GABA$_A$-Cl$^-$ channel sites.
- Therapeutic uses: multiple, depending on brain region affected—limbic system = anxiolysis; motor systems = anticonvulsant and muscle relaxant; wake-sleep controls = sedative-hypnotic; temporal lobe = amnestic.
- Problems: significant dependence liabilities; some benzodiazepines accumulate on long-term use and manifest overdose effects.

FIRST:	**CHLORDIAZEPOXIDE** (Sternbach, late 1950s)
BROAD-SPECTRUM USE:	**DIAZEPAM**
CURRENTLY FAVORED:	**ALPRAZOLAM**
INDUCTION ANESTHETIC:	**MIDAZOLAM**

Pharmacology

The primary action of benzodiazepines relates to the opening of chloride channels, coupled with γ-aminobutyric acid (GABA$_A$) receptors, on neurons of the CNS (Fig. A). The increased chloride ion concentration intracellularly inhibits neuronal discharge, thus interfering with function. The effects include release of conditioned suppression related to aversive stimuli; reduced emotional irritability; sedation, hypnosis, light anesthesia; anticonvulsant activity; muscle relaxation; and amnesia, reflecting broad influence of GABA$_A$-mediated inhibition throughout the mammalian nervous system. More recent research indicates that certain agents (alprazolam) have antipanic efficacy.

Medicinal Chemistry

The chemical structure of individual benzodiazepines varies around a 5-aryl-1,4-diazepine complex of rings with inclusion of triazolo or imidazolo rings in some examples (Fig. B). These alterations influence the selectivity of a specific agent for the various types of therapeutic actions. For example, alprazolam (a triazolo-benzodiazepine) is more selective as an anxiolytic, whereas clonazepam (more classic structure) is more selective as an anticonvulsant drug. Still, a major portion of these effects involve allosteric benzodiazepine receptors coupled to GABA$_A$–chloride channel inhibitory mechanisms. Other sites on these channels respond to barbiturates or ethanol, but the benzodiazepine influences are, for the most part, more clearly dependent on the integrity of the GABA$_A$ receptor mechanisms.

Pharmacokinetics

Administration, Distribution, and Metabolism. All benzodiazepines are highly lipophilic, though still showing considerable variances among individual agents. Most are well absorbed by all routes, although clorazepate represents a "prodrug," acting only through an active metabolite. Those converted to long–half-life active metabolites have

a long duration of action and tend to cumulate on chronic use, especially in the elderly (chlordiazepoxide, diazepam) [Fig. C]. Those metabolized to inactive metabolites directly by glucuronidation (oxazepam, temazepam, lorazepam) have intermediate durations and are not prone to accumulate. Some (alprazolam, triazolam, midazolam) form short–half-life active metabolites and thus have short to intermediate durations with less tendency to accumulate (see Fig. C). There is little tendency for this class to induce hepatic microsomal enzymes, so chronic use is not associated with accelerated metabolism to any extent. Oral contraceptives and cimetidine, among other drugs, inhibit metabolism of benzodiazepines biotransformed by oxidative processes but not those directly glucuronidated.

Toxicity

Essentially all side effects and toxic reactions of benzodiazepines refer to effects on the CNS. As expected from a drug class with broad inhibitory activity on brain neurons, dizziness, apathy, fatigue, ataxia, increased reaction time, and clouding of mental faculties may occur. Thus, operating a motor vehicle, piloting an aircraft, or using various types of machinery while under medication may be hazardous. The elderly are often more susceptible. In some patients, complaints of headache, blurred vision, diarrhea, nausea and vomiting, and incontinence have been reported.

Although physical and psychological dependency liabilities of benzodiazepines are less than those of barbiturates and other CNS depressants, they may be troublesome in a certain category of patients. Withdrawal signs similar to those associated with alcohol and barbiturates are seen (irritability, sweating, tremors) but generally are less intense.

Occasionally benzodiazepines induce a prominent disinhibition, releasing hostility and rage, particularly short-acting agents (triazolam, alprazolam) administered in larger doses. This type of effect may include restlessness, hallucinations, and hypomania. Overall, however, the benzodiazepines incur much less risk of fatal overdose, since vital functions are little affected in most subjects. Nevertheless, combination with other depressants (barbiturates, alcohol) can lead to severe respiratory and cardiovascular depression. Combining a benzodiazepine with valproate has induced psychotic behavior.

41 Antidepressant Agents

Michael Williams, Ph.D., D.Sc.

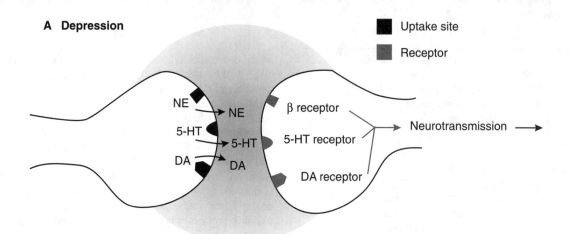

A Depression

Uptake site

Receptor

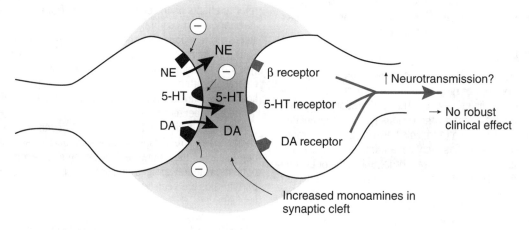

B Acute antidepressant action

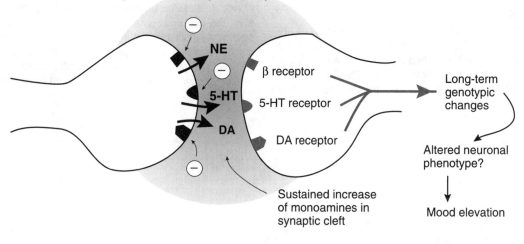

C Chronic antidepressant effect (2-3 weeks)

OVERVIEW

- Antidepressants improve the quality of life of individuals who suffer from depression and generally show a reduced interest in nearly all regular activities, have insomnia or hypersomnia, and evidence recurrent suicidal ideation. Depressed individuals have difficulty functioning effectively in society.
- While there may be an underlying genetic basis, environmental factors (e.g., stress, personal trauma) are thought to play an overwhelming role in precipitating depressive episodes.
- Mechanism of action: All known classes of antidepressant act by increasing monoamine concentrations in the synaptic cleft, effectively facilitating neurotransmission processes dependent on serotonin (5-HT), norepinephrine (NE), and to a lesser extent, dopamine (DA). As there is a delay in days to weeks in onset of the beneficial, mood-elevating effects of antidepressants, it is postulated that longer-term, adaptive changes occur at the level of the genome that leads to phenotypic changes in neuronal pathways downstream.
- Sites of action: Tricyclic antidepressants (TCAs) block the uptake of the monoamines, NE, and 5-HT; selective serotonin reuptake inhibitors (SSRIs) block presynaptic 5-HT uptake increasing synaptic 5-HT levels; serotonin norepinephrine reuptake inhibitors (SNRIs) have a similar mechanism of action to the TCAs with a reduced incidence of other receptor-related actions, such as antimuscarinic and antiadrenergic actions; monoamine oxidase inhibitors (MAOIs) block the effects of the monoamine oxidizing enzymes, MAO-A and MAO-B.
- Therapeutic uses: Antidepressants produce a sense of well-being and mood elevation in depressed patients, allowing a renewed interest in day-to-day activities and a diminution in suicidal tendencies.
- Unmet medical need: Time to onset for most antidepressants is 1–2 weeks. In severely depressed patients this permits a continuing window of suicide ideation that can prove fatal. A more rapid-onset antidepressant would be a major breakthrough. Similarly, there is a group of patients refractory to the present classes of antidepressant who would benefit from a new agent.

FIRST:	**LITHIUM** (1948)
FIRST SYNTHETIC:	**IPRONIAZID** (1957)
MOST WIDELY USED:	**FLUOXETINE** (1987)

Pharmacology

Antidepressants block the reuptake of the monoamines, 5-HT, NE, and to a lesser extent DA, or inhibit the monoamine-catabolizing monoamine oxides, MAO-A and MAO-B. The first antidepressants, the TCAs imipramine and chlorimimpramine (clomipramine), blocked the uptake of both NE and 5-HT and also had antimuscarinic and antiadrenergic side effects that limited their use. The second-generation compounds, the SSRIs, are selective blockers of 5-HT uptake. The third-generation compounds like venlafaxine and nefazodone also block NE and 5-HT uptake and have been dubbed SNRIs, partly to follow the nomenclature of the SSRIs and partly to differentiate them from the TCAs in terms of side-effect liability. MAO-A shows preference for 5-HT and NE, and MAO-B, phenylethylamine. By preventing metabolism, these agents increase monoamine concentrations in the synaptic cleft. Mirtazepine is described as an SSRI but acts by blocking α_2-adrenergic and 5-HT autoreceptors that are probably responsible for mediating feedback inhibition. Buproprion is an aminoketone CNS stimulant that has an unknown mechanism of action but appears to potentiate the actions of NE. See Appendix, E, for a list of specific agents.

Medicinal Chemistry

TCAs include dibenzoxazepines, dibenazepines, dibenzocycloheptadienes, and dibenzoxepins; SSRIs include phenylpiperazines, araalkylketones, tetrahydronapthalenamines, and piperazinoazepines; SNRIs include phenylpiperazines, cyclohexanols; MAOIs include phenylcyclopropylamines, and phenethylhydrazines.

Pharmacokinetics

The majority of antidepressants have half-lives of 12–22 hours. Exceptions are venlafaxine with a half-life of 4–9 hours, and fluoxetine with a half-life of 53 hours. Antidepressants are metabolized via the CYP2D6 isoform of cytochrome P-450. CYP3A4 (fluvoxamine, sertraline), 1 A2 (mirtazepine) are other key metabolic enzymes for antidepressants.

Toxicity and Side Effects

TCAs. These agents have antimuscarinic and antiadrenergic properties that result in dry mouth, blurred vision, tachycardia, sweating, orthostatic hypotension, retrograde ejaculation, sedation, confusion, and impaired cognition.

SSRIs. Side effects of these agents include mild GI discomfort, diarrhea, headache, anxiety, asthenia, and anorexia.

SNRIs. Somnolence, dry mouth, nausea, dizziness, constipation, asthenia, confusion, abnormal vision, postural hypotension, abnormal ejaculation, priapism are possible side effects.

MAOIs. Irreversible MAOIs produce a "cheese" effect when consumed together with tyramine-rich foods like cheese, yeast products (e.g., beer), chocolate, or with sympathomimetic drugs (OTC medications containing phenylpropanolamine or dextromethorphan) that can result in a hypertensive crisis. Newer MAOIs in development, such as befloxatone (Synthelabo, phase II), are reversible and show no signs of the cheese effects seen with classic MAOIs.

Treatment

The *Diagnostic and Statistical Manual of Mental Disorders*, 4th ed. (American Psychological Association, 1994) has established criteria that divide depression into major depressive episodes, dysthymia, and bipolar (manic-depressive) disorder. Depressive personality disorder and minor depression are two additional categories. Bipolar disorder is treated with lithium (Eskalith) and divalproex sodium (Depakote). Clomipramine has been approved for use in obsessive-compulsive disorder and buproprion for use in smoking cessation.

42 Agents for the Treatment of Epilepsy

Richard P. Shank, Ph.D., and Ross A. Reife, M.D.

A Voltage-gated ion channels in neurons

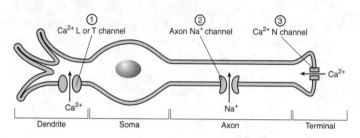

B GABA-mediated inhibitory synaptic transmission

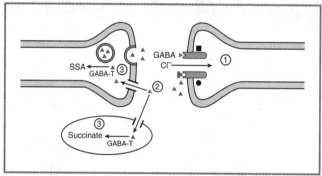

C Glutamate-mediated excitatory synaptic transmission

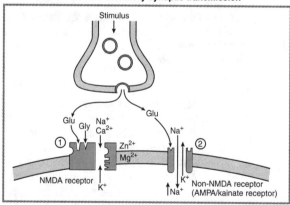

SOME ANTICONVULSANT MECHANISMS

Mechanism	Anticonvulsant Agents
Ca^{2+}-channel blockade (Fig. A—1 and 3)	Ethosuximide, gabapentin, phenobarbital (?), phenytoin (?)
Na^+-channel blockade (Fig. A—2)	Phenytoin, carbamazepine, valproic acid, lamotrigine, topiramate, gabapentin (?)
$GABA_A$ receptor positive modulation (Fig. B—1)	Diazepam, clonazepam, clobazam, phenobarbital, topiramate, primidone
$GABA_A$ transport (uptake) inhibition (Fig. B—2)	Tiagabine
Promote GABA synthesis or inhibit metabolic degradation (Fig. B—3)	Vigabatrin, valproic acid (?), gabapentin
Negative modulation of glutamate NMDA receptor (Fig. C—1)	Several experimental drugs
Negative modulation of glutamate AMPA/kainate receptor (Fig. C—2)	Topiramate

OVERVIEW

- Drugs for treating epilepsy are referred to as either anticonvulsants or antiepileptic drugs (AEDs). They prevent seizures but do not correct the underlying pathologic condition.
- AEDs can prevent clinical seizures by raising seizure threshold or blocking seizure spread from its focus.
- AEDs are classified clinically by the types of seizures they block.
- Some mechanisms for anticonvulsant activity include negative modulatory effects on voltage-gated Na^+ or Ca^{2+} channels in neurons, positive modulatory effects on the activity of the inhibitory neurotransmitter GABA, and negative modulatory effects on glutamate-activated cation channels (NMDA or α-amino-3-hydroxy-5-methylisoxazole-4-propionic acid [AMPA]/kainate receptors).
- All AEDs have the potential to cause transient CNS-related side effects, such as impaired motor coordination.

Epilepsy

Epilepsy is a disorder of the brain characterized by recurrent seizures—paroxysmal events arising from the synchronized, abnormal activity of cerebral neurons. Such an event can be associated with motor signs, sensory symptoms, autonomic symptoms, psychic symptoms, or a combination of these. In addition, there may be an impairment (or loss) of consciousness. Clinical seizures are broadly categorized as partial onset (having their origin in a limited part of the brain), generalized onset (originating diffusely in both hemispheres simultaneously), and unclassifiable.

Epileptic syndromes are defined and classified by clusters of signs and symptoms that generally occur together in a patient with recurrent seizures, such as the types of seizures, their anatomy and pathology, the age of onset, precipitating factors, severity, chronicity, and pattern of recurrence. The cerebral localization of seizures is part of the classification of epileptic syndromes: localization-related (i.e., focal, local, or partial) epilepsies, generalized epilepsies, undetermined (whether focal or generalized) epilepsies, or a special syndrome (e.g., Lennox-Gastaux). The epileptic syndromes are also classified by etiology: idiopathic, cryptogenic, or symptomatic.

Pharmacology

AEDs are classified by the types of seizures they block. No single AED has been demonstrated to be effective against all seizure types. With available AEDs the seizures of approximately 70% of patients are effectively controlled, but nearly half of these patients require two or more AEDs to be completely free of seizures.

Medicinal Chemistry

All currently used AEDs are small organic molecules, usually with a molecular weight between 200 and 400. AEDs are diverse structurally and are not classified by this criterion.

Mechanisms of Action

The mechanism underlying the activity of most AEDs is not fully established. Several AEDs appear to interact with voltage-gated Na^+ or Ca^{2+} channels in neurons to cause a use-dependent blockade, that is, they negatively modulate the channel-gating process (open-close cycle) to prevent the channels from generating action potentials at a high frequency for extended periods of time (Fig.). Several other AEDs enhance the activity of the inhibitory neurotransmitter GABA by either allosterically modulating $GABA_A$ receptors or by increasing the concentration of GABA in synaptic terminals and the synaptic cleft. A few AEDs appear to negatively modulate glutamate-gated cation (primarily Na^+) channels. Some AEDs may positively modulate voltage-gated K^+ channels, but this has not been clearly demonstrated.

Pharmacokinetics

For the major AEDs, the parent compound accounts for most or all anticonvulsant efficacy. Several are extensively metabolized in the liver and may induce the synthesis of metabolic enzymes. Because AEDs are often prescribed in combination, the effects of an AED on the pharmacokinetics of other AEDs can be an important consideration in designing the dosing regimen.

Toxicity

All AEDs have the potential to cause CNS-related side effects. In many cases these effects can be reduced by initiating therapy at a low dose and gradually escalating the dose. Most of the currently approved AEDs can cause potentially serious adverse effects, including teratogenicity.

SPECIFIC AED AGENTS EFFECTIVE IN MAJOR EPILEPSY SYNDROMES

Drug (brand name)	Partial Onset Seizures (56%)[a]	Generalized Tonic-clonic (35%)[a]	Generalized Absence (5%)[a]
Phenytoin (Dilantin)	Yes	Yes	No
Carbamazepine (Tegretol)	Yes	Yes	No
Valproate (Depakene)	Yes	Yes	Yes
Phenobarbital	Yes	Yes	No
Ethosuximide (Zarontin)	No	No	Yes
Clonazepam (Klonopin)[b]	Yes	Yes	Yes
Gabapentin (Neurontin)	Yes	Yes[c]	Yes[c]
Lamotrigine (Lamictal)	Yes	Yes	Yes
Topiramate (Topamax)	Yes	Yes	Yes
Vigabatrin (Sabril)	Yes	Yes	

[a] Prevalence in total patient population.
[b] Generally limited to short-term therapy because of a propensity for anticonvulsant tolerance to develop.
[c] This is based on published preliminary reports.

43

Agents for the Treatment of Parkinson's Disease
Sabri Markabi, M.D., Herbert Faleck, M.D., and Lynn D. Kramer, M.D.

A Main neurotransmitters involved in Parkinson's disease (PD)

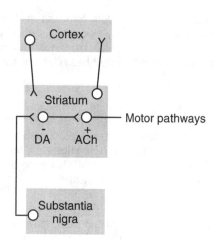

B Human brain: main structures involved in PD

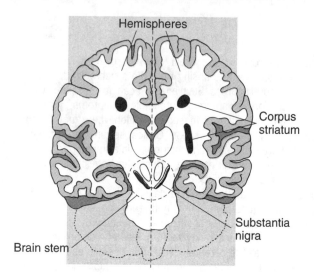

C Important catabolic pathways of L-dopa

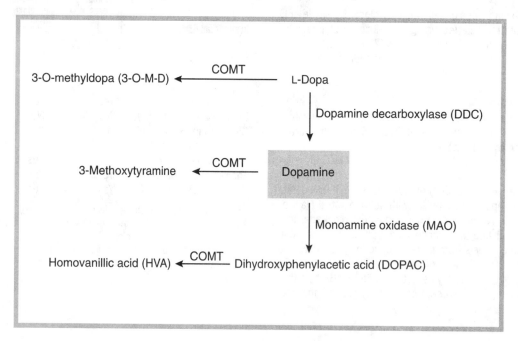

OVERVIEW

- First described by Sir James Parkinson in 1817, idiopathic Parkinson's disease is a chronic neurodegenerative condition affecting approximately 1% of adults over the age of 60 years. The disease is observed in all ethnic groups and in all socioeconomic classes.
- Clinical features: Hypokinesia (slowness and poverty of movement), muscular rigidity, resting tremor, and loss of postural reflexes; unilateral onset with gradual bilateral progression of symptoms; end stage is a rigid akinetic state with shortened life expectancy.
- Neurochemistry: The degeneration of brain dopaminergic neurons, especially the nigrostriatal dopaminergic system, results in an imbalance between the inhibitory (dopaminergic) and the excitatory (cholinergic) system.
- The different therapeutic interventions aim at restoring the balance by enhancing the dopaminergic transmission, reducing the cholinergic activity, or both.
- Pharmacotherapy: Replacement therapy with levodopa, the chemical precursor of dopamine (DA), has become the mainstay of therapy and continues to be the most effective symptomatic therapy to date. Other prodopaminergic drugs act either as direct DA agonists (e.g., bromocriptine, pergolide) or as inhibitors of enzymes responsible for DA catabolism (e.g., MAO inhibitors [MAOIs], catechol-O-methyltransferase [COMT] inhibitors). Anticholinergic agents are used to increase the relative hypoactivity of brain DA by alleviating the relative overactivity of ACh.

Pharmacology

Levodopa (L-Dopa). Pharmacologically inactive, levodopa exerts its effect after being transformed to DA via the enzyme dopa decarboxylase (DDC). This enzyme is present both centrally and peripherally.

DA Agonists. DA agonists mimic the actions of DA. These agents are used primarily as adjuncts to levodopa or as monotherapy They are generally less effective than levodopa.

COMT Inhibitors. The inhibition of COMT activity is a promising new strategy to decrease the peripheral metabolism of levodopa and to enhance its striatal availability.

MAOIs. DA is oxidized by MAO-B to dihydroxyphenylacetic acid. The inhibition of MAO-B results in increased cerebral DA bioavailability.

Anticholinergic Drugs. These competitive muscarinic receptor blockers reduce Parkinson's disease symptoms by alleviating the relative overactivity of ACh secondary to DA depletion in the striatum. Their action on the peripheral vegetative system is responsible for adverse effects. They are considered adjunctive therapy, used most often to treat tremor.

SPECIFIC AGENTS

Levodopa	MAOIs
L-Dopa and carbidopa (Sinemet)	Selegiline (Eldepryl)
DA Agonists	**Anticholinergics**
Bromocriptine (Parlodel)	Trihexyphenidyl (Artane)
Pergolide (Permax)	Biperiden (Akineton)
Amantadine (Symmetrel)	Diphenhydramine (Benadryl)
Pramipexole (Mirapex)	Benztropine mesylate
(Cogentine)	

Pharmacokinetics

Levodopa. There is considerable inter- and intrasubject variability in absorption of levodopa. The metabolism is extensive and rapid. To maximize the amount available to the brain, it is now formulated and administered almost exclusively with a selective peripheral DDC inhibitor, such as carbidopa or benserazide. Even so, only 5%–10% of orally administered levodopa reaches the brain.

Levodopa is rapidly redistributed from the plasma compartment to other tissues. The distribution half-life is about 10 minutes. The elimination half-life is about 40–80 minutes.

COMT Inhibitors. The major therapeutic benefit of COMT inhibition results from the smoother plasma concentration time profile of levodopa, allowing for its more extended delivery to the brain.

Toxicity and Adverse Effects

Levodopa

Peripheral. Digestive disorder, anorexia, and nausea and vomiting occur early and usually diminish a few weeks after treatment onset. Slow titration and administration with food are preventive measures.

Cardiovascular. Orthostatic hypotension may occur with or without clinical symptoms. In elderly patients it may induce falls. Other effects include rare, brief high blood pressure episodes and arrhythmias. Dose reduction is usually effective in managing these adverse effects.

CNS. Abnormal movements (dyskinesias) and motor fluctuations (on-off periods are frequent. Maintaining the lowest effective doses of levodopa may prevent or delay the appearance of motor dysfunction. Prolactin and growth hormone modifications may occur as a result of action on the hypothalamus.

Psychiatric. These adverse effects occur particularly in elderly patients and include depression, visual hallucinations, and confusion.

DA Agonists

CNS. Similar to levodopa.

Peripheral. Similar to levodopa.

Anticholinergic Drugs

Peripheral. Mucosal dryness, accommodation disorders, constipation, and dysuria.

CNS. Frequent in elderly patients, these include confusion, agitation, and memory disorder.

Other Therapeutic Approaches

Symptomatic. Treatment of symptoms or comorbid conditions associated with Parkinson's disease (e.g., depression) is important. Physical therapy is used to improve activities of daily life.

Surgery. Thalamotomy has been proposed for the most disabled patients with tremor. A newer approach is the striatal implants of DA-containing tissues to relieve Parkinson's disease symptoms.

A Structure of amyloid precursor protein APP-695

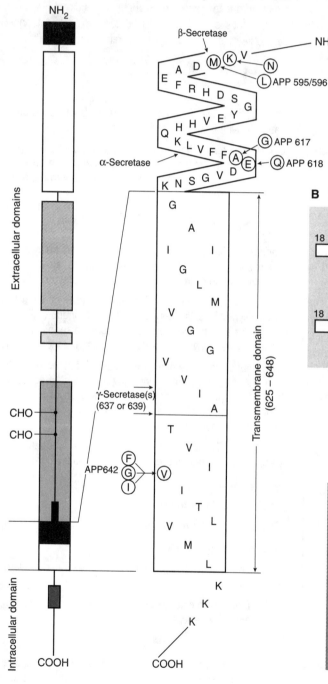

B Metabolic processing of APP-695

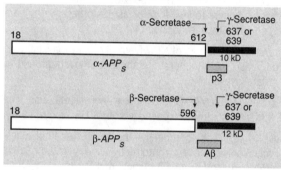

C Structural and functional domains of APP-695

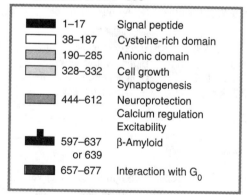

	Residues	Domain
	1–17	Signal peptide
	38–187	Cysteine-rich domain
	190–285	Anionic domain
	328–332	Cell growth Synaptogenesis
	444–612	Neuroprotection Calcium regulation Excitability
	597–637 or 639	β-Amyloid
	657–677	Interaction with G_0

Targeting Amyloid Precursor Protein Metabolites for Therapy

In the mid-1980s, the publication of the amino acid sequence of the β-amyloid (Aβ) peptide, the principal protein component of the neuritic plaques that occur universally in Alzheimer's disease brain, led to the cloning of the complementary DNA (cDNA) encoding the β-amyloid precursor protein (APP), from which Aβ is derived. This protein and its metabolites play a vital role in the etiology of Alzheimer's disease, making it a rational target for new pharmacologic therapies aimed at treating the disease.

APP Structure and Function

The 40–42 amino acid peptide Aβ that is deposited pathologically in Alzheimer's disease brain is part of the much larger APP, which is a 695–770 amino acid transmembrane protein whose site of action in the brain may be the synapse. APP has a large extracellular N-terminus and shorter cytoplasmic C-terminus (Fig. A). The first 28 amino acids of Aβ lie outside the membrane, while the remainder of Aβ is within the membrane bilayer. A protease called α-secretase cleaves between amino acids 16 and 17 of Aβ (Figs. A, B), which results in the release of secreted forms of APP (APPs) from the cell surface. This cleavage precludes the formation of Aβ. A second enzyme, termed β-secretase, cleaves APP at amino acid 596, which is the N-terminus of Aβ. β-Secretase cleavage releases the amyloidogenic C-terminal 100 amino acids of APP (C100). Further cleavage of C100 by a γ-secretase releases the 40–42 amino acid peptide Aβ. Amino acids 1–16 of Aβ, which constitute the C-terminus of APPs, may contribute to the known neurotrophic activities of these molecules. The C-terminus of APPs has neuroprotective activities that are mediated by stabilization of intracellular calcium levels and regulation of membrane excitability. In addition, APP may promote cell proliferation and stimulate neurite outgrowth and synaptogenesis. APP is thought to be a signaling protein that carries information from the exterior to the interior of neurons, consistent with the finding that C-terminal amino acids interact with the small G protein G_o.

Pathology of Metabolic Derivatives of APP

Cleavage of APP by β-secretase releases the C-terminal fragment C100, which has been proposed to be the primary agent of neurodegeneration in Alzheimer's disease. An alternative view (the amyloid hypothesis) is that Aβ is the smoking gun. $A\beta_{1-40}$ is the major species secreted from cultured cells and found in the CSF of both normal and afflicted individuals, while the 42-amino-acid-long $A\beta_{1-42}$ is the major component of amyloid depositions. It has been proposed that the latter plays the more important role in amyloid deposition and neurodegeneration in Alzheimer's disease.

Genetics of Alzheimer's Disease

Except for having a later age of onset, so-called sporadic Alzheimer's disease (90%–95% of cases) is identical in phenotype to familial Alzheimer's disease. Three genes cause approximately 90% of cases of familial Alzheimer's disease. The first, encoding APP, accounts for only a few percent of cases, while approximately 70% result from dominant mutations in genes encoding the homologous integral membrane proteins presenilin-1 (PS-1) and presenilin-2 (PS-2) on chromosomes 14 and 1, respectively. There is some evidence that familial Alzheimer's disease mutants of the presenilins alter metabolic processing of APP, increasing the production of Aβ. Both late-onset familial Alzheimer's disease and sporadic Alzheimer's disease have a strong association with apolipoprotein E (ApoE) allele ε4, located on chromosome 19. The risk for Alzheimer's disease in individuals homozygous for ε4 is greatly increased over that of an individual homozygous for ε2, with the age of onset advanced by 10–20 years, whereas ε3/ε3 individuals have an intermediate risk for Alzheimer's disease.

Pharmacologic Therapy for Alzheimer's Disease

Present. The current drugs enhance cholinergic function to ameliorate symptoms by inhibiting acetylcholinesterase. Presently available are tacrine (Cognex) and donepezil (Aricept).

Future. One target is enhancement of α-secretase to produce more of the protective fragment. Such an intervention would, in addition, inhibit the β-secretase cleavage of APP that generates C100. Proponents of the amyloid hypothesis have developed pharmacologic agents that inhibit γ-secretase cleavage at amino acid 42 of Aβ or that combat the extracellular aggregation of the increased $A\beta_{1-42}$. Alzheimer's disease may be caused, alternatively, by a disruption of the normal signaling function of APP. Peptides that modify the interaction of familial Alzheimer's disease APP with G_o may be useful for treating the disease. Finally, another potential therapy for Alzheimer's disease may be the introduction of the ApoEε2 gene product into the brains of ε4/ε4 individuals.

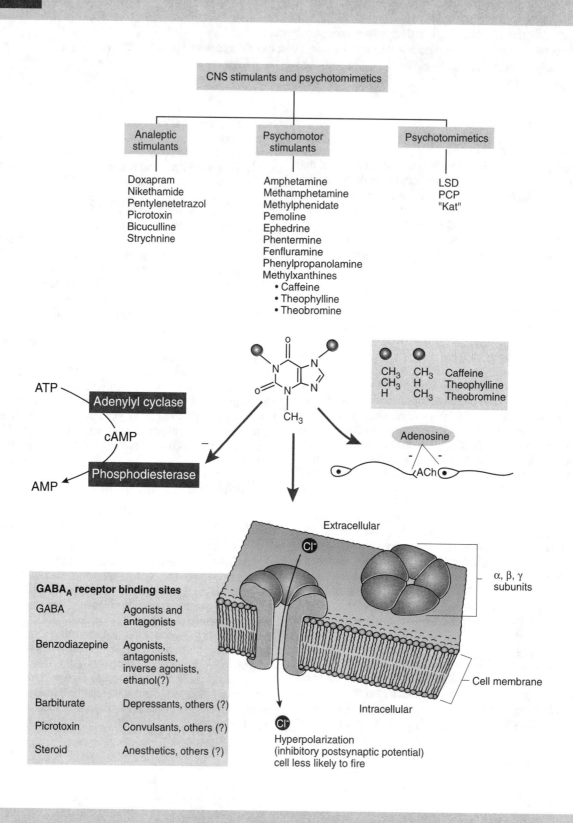

CNS stimulants and psychotomimetics

Analeptic stimulants

Doxapram
Nikethamide
Pentylenetetrazol
Picrotoxin
Bicuculline
Strychnine

Psychomotor stimulants

Amphetamine
Methamphetamine
Methylphenidate
Pemoline
Ephedrine
Phentermine
Fenfluramine
Phenylpropanolamine
Methylxanthines
• Caffeine
• Theophylline
• Theobromine

Psychotomimetics

LSD
PCP
"Kat"

CH_3	CH_3	Caffeine
CH_3	H	Theophylline
H	CH_3	Theobromine

ATP

Adenylyl cyclase

cAMP

Phosphodiesterase

AMP

Adenosine

ACh

Extracellular

Cl⁻

α, β, γ subunits

Cell membrane

Intracellular

Cl⁻
Hyperpolarization
(inhibitory postsynaptic potential)
cell less likely to fire

GABA_A receptor binding sites

GABA	Agonists and antagonists
Benzodiazepine	Agonists, antagonists, inverse agonists, ethanol(?)
Barbiturate	Depressants, others (?)
Picrotoxin	Convulsants, others (?)
Steroid	Anesthetics, others (?)

OVERVIEW

- CNS stimulation can occur as the result of the normal physiologic function of some endogenous neurotransmitters (e.g., excitatory amino acids such as glutamic acid). It also can occur as the result of drug administration, either as the intended effect or primary action of the drug (e.g., caffeine) or as an adverse effect (numerous examples).
- CNS stimulation falls along a continuum from alertness to nervousness or anxiety to convulsions.
- The possible mechanisms of a CNS stimulant action on neurotransmitters include: potentiation or enhancement of excitatory neurotransmitters, depression or antagonism of inhibitory neurotransmitters, and presynaptic control of neurotransmitter release.
- Psychotomimetics profoundly alter thought, mood, or perception without marked psychomotor stimulation or depression.

CNS Stimulants

Analeptics (Convulsants and Respiratory Stimulants)

Analeptics have been used to treat cases of overdose of CNS depressants, coma, respiratory failure and to promote arousal from anesthesia. Their use is an extreme measure of limited effectiveness and carries the risk of producing convulsions. They may be either plant alkaloids (e.g., picrotoxin, strychnine) or synthetics (e.g., doxapram, pentylenetetrazol). Most are orally absorbed, and most are metabolized by hepatic P-450 enzymes.

Adverse Effects. Most can produce uncoordinated tonic-clonic convulsions. Strychnine can produce opisthotonos. Treatment involves mechanical support, barbiturates, or benzodiazepines.

Psychomotor Stimulants

These may be classified as *amphetamine-like compounds* and methylxanthines. The therapeutic uses of amphetamine and related compounds include: the treatment or prevention of mental fatigue; promoting weight loss (limited by tolerance and abuse liability); treatment of narcolepsy (a disorder characterized by precipitous onset of daytime sleep, cataplexy (a sudden loss of muscle tone), and nightmares that persist after wakening; and treatment of hyperkinetic syndrome and attention deficit disorder, conditions characterized by hyperactivity, inability to concentrate, and a high degree of impulsive behavior. *Methylxanthines* are chemically related, biologically active substances commonly found in coffee (caffeine), tea (theophylline), and cocoa (theobromine). The degree of CNS stimulation is caffeine > theophylline > theobromine. Therapeutic uses include the treatment of overdoses of CNS depressants, treatment of alcohol intoxication (effectiveness ?), and enhancing alertness (but unaffected physical fatigue can lead to accidents). Other, non-CNS applications include use as diuretic and treatment of asthma and headaches caused by cerebrovascular constriction.

Mechanisms of Action. Amphetamine-like compounds have a direct action as monoamine receptor agonists and indirect ones of stimulation of monoamine neurotransmitter release, inhibition of reuptake, and inhibition of MAO. Proposed mechanisms of the *methylxanthines* include inhibition of phosphodiesterase (results in an increase in cAMP levels), pharmacologic antagonism of adenosine receptors, and competitive interaction with benzodiazepine site on $GABA_A$ receptor.

Pharmacokinetics. Amphetamine-like compounds generally have good oral absorption, with a considerable portion excreted unchanged; since they are weak bases, acidification of urine enhances excretion. *Methylxanthines* have good oral absorption and extensive metabolism to uric acid derivatives (but do not aggravate gout).

Adverse Effects. Amphetamine-like compounds with acute low dose may produce euphoria, dizziness, tremor, irritability, insomnia; with acute high dose, headache, angina pain, arrhythmias; a chronic high dose may induce a schizoprenia-like psychotic reaction. Psychological

and physical dependence can develop; withdrawal usually is mild, typically including prolonged sleep, fatigue, hunger (hyperphagia), depression. Adverse effects of *methylxanthines* include nervousness; insomnia; delirium; excess cardiovascular or respiratory stimulation; diuresis; and possibly dependence, though this remains to be proven.

STIMULANTS

Doxapram (Dopram)
Nikethamide (Coramine)
Pentylenetetrazol (Metrazol)
Amphetamine (Benzedrine)
D-amphetamine (Dexedrine)
Methamphetamine (Methedrine, etc.)
Methylphenidate (Ritalin)
Pemoline (Cylert)
Fenfluramine (Pondimin)

Psychotomimetics

Psychotomimetics can be classified on the basis of whether they have structural or functional relationship to known neurotransmitters. The following are examples of compounds that have potential use to gain insight into psychotic behavior and its treatment.

Related to Known Neurotransmitters

Lysergic Acid Diethylamide (LSD). An ergot alkaloid, it was synthesized in 1938 and produces hallucinations and other alterations of perception (e.g., distortion of sights and sounds, sounds confused as sights), disconnected and illogical thoughts, and possible paranoid delusions ("bad trips"). It was once marketed with the suggestion that psychiatrists try it to understand what their psychotic patients were experiencing.

Psilocybin and Psilocin. Psilocybin and psilocin are obtained from a fungus (*psilo* = bald, *cybe* = head). Synthesized in 1958, they have effects similar to LSD but are less potent.

Mescaline. Mescaline is obtained from a cactus (peyote) and has effects similar to LSD but is less potent. It produces artificial psychosis similar to acute schizophrenia.

Unrelated to Known Neurotransmitters

Phencyclidine (PCP). PCP was synthesized in 1956 and sold as an intravenous anesthetic. It produces analgesia; it is an analog of ketamine. PCP produces disorientation, hallucinations, and stereotypical behaviors; deaths have been reported.

Methcanthinone ("Kat," "Jeff"). "Kat" was synthesized in 1950s as possible appetite suppressant but has not been marketed. It has the characteristics of amphetamine; deaths have been reported.

Directions: For each of the following questions, choose the **one best** answer.

1. Which of the following is an MAO inhibitor?

(A) Imipramine

(B) Doxepin

(C) Nefazodone

(D) Fluvoxamine

(E) Phenelzine

2. A characteristic of neurotransmission in the CNS *and* the periphery includes which one of the following?

(A) Fewer neurotransmitters

(B) Less variety of neurotransmitters

(C) Cotransmitters within the presynaptic neuron

(D) More complicated neural networks

3. Sporadic (i.e., nonfamilial) Alzheimer's disease is estimated to account for about what percent of all cases?

(A) < 10%

(B) 10%–50%

(C) 50%–90%

(D) > 90%

4. What adverse effect is more likely in a patient taking a BDZ anxiolytic than in one taking a barbiturate?

(A) Decreased psychomotor performance

(B) Anterograde amnesia

(C) Respiratory depression

(D) Induction of microsomal enzymes

(E) Withdrawal seizures

5. Which enzyme is inhibited by the drug disulfiram (Antabuse)?

(A) Alcohol dehydrogenase

(B) Ethanol dehydrogenase

(C) Aldehyde dehydrogenase

(D) Acetaldehyde dehydrogenase

6. What is the most common type of epilepsy?

(A) Partial onset seizures

(B) Primary generalized tonic-clonic seizures (formerly grand mal)

(C) Generalized absence seizures (formerly petit mal)

(D) Lennox-Gastaux syndrome

(E) Epilepsy caused by a genetic disorder

7. The term for the phenomenon in which a drug produces the opposite effect as does the endogenous ligand is

(A) up-regulation

(B) down-regulation

(C) partial agonism

(D) inverse agonism

8. Which of the following best describes the mechanism of action of BDZs?

(A) $GABA_A$ receptor agonist

(B) $GABA_B$ receptor agonist

(C) $GABA_A$ receptor antagonist

(D) $GABA_B$ receptor antagonist

(E) Enhancement of GABA-mediated Cl^- influx

9. Tolerance is most likely to develop to which of the following anticonvulsants?

(A) Phenytoin

(B) Valproate

(C) Clonazepam

(D) Carbamazepine

(E) Topiramate

10. The typical BDZ has which of the following characteristics?

(A) It is a $GABA_A$ receptor agonist.

(B) It is a $GABA_A$ receptor antagonist.

(C) It allosterically enhances GABA action.

(D) It decreases Cl^- conductance.

11. Which of the following intravenous anesthetics is believed to be mediated through the *N*-methyl-D-aspartate (NMDA) receptor?

(A) Barbiturates

(B) BDZs

(C) Etomidate

(D) Ketamine

(E) Propofol

12. Replacement therapy for Parkinson's disease involves the use of

(A) levodopa

(B) bromocriptine

(C) amantadine

(D) selegiline

13. Which of the following psychotomimetics is structurally related to the dissociative anesthetic drug ketamine?

(A) LSD

(B) Mescaline

(C) PCP

(D) Psilocybin

(E) "Kat"

14. Antagonism of which of the following receptors is thought to be responsible for the production of extrapyramidal symptoms, a side effect of lengthy treatment with certain antipsychotics?

(A) D_1

(B) D_2

(C) D_3

(D) D_4

(E) 5-HT_2

15. Which of the following effects applies to halothane but not to most other volatile anesthetics?

(A) Ventilatory depression

(B) Negative inotropic effect

(C) Peripheral vasodilation

(D) Bradycardia

(E) Decrease in blood pressure

16. Which of the following statements regarding carbidopa is true?

(A) When combined with L-dopa, it increases the level of levodopa in the brain.

(B) It increases the peripheral adverse effects of levodopa.

(C) It decreases central adverse effects of levodopa.

(D) It decreases the amount of levodopa in the brain to about 75%.

17. Which of the following is a mechanism by which anticonvulsants prevent seizures?

(A) Use-dependent positive modulation of voltage-gated Na^+ channels

(B) Inhibition of the enzyme that synthesizes GABA (glutamate decarboxylase, GAD)

(C) Blockade of voltage-gated Na^+ and Ca^{2+} channels by plugging up the channels

(D) Positive modulation of the excitatory neurotransmitter glutamate by inhibition of its uptake (transport) into synaptic terminals and astrocytes

(E) Positive allosteric modulation of $GABA_A$–receptor-mediated Cl^- flux

18. Which represents the target for presently available pharmacotherapy for Alzheimer's disease?

(A) Acetylcholinesterase

(B) Aβ

(C) APP

(D) ApoE

19. Which of the following is a mechanism of action of CNS stimulants?

(A) Antagonism of $GABA_A$ receptor in the brain

(B) Antagonism of inhibitory neurotransmitters in the spinal cord

(C) Increase of norepinephrine release

(D) Blockade of Cl^- channels in the brain

20. Which of the following statements about ethanol is true?

(A) It is poorly absorbed from the GI tract.

(B) It has first-order kinetics of elimination.

(C) It is metabolized in the liver and other tissues.

(D) An ethanol receptor has been cloned.

21. Which antidepressant has been approved for treating obsessive-compulsive disorder?

(A) Desipramine

(B) Clomipramine

(C) Mirtazepine

(D) Phenelzine

(E) Tranylcypromine

22. Benzodiazepine toxicity could logically be treated with which of the following agents?

(A) Alprazolam

(B) Flumazenil

(C) Flurazepam

(D) Phenobarbital

PART IV: ANSWERS AND EXPLANATIONS

1. The answer is E.

Phenelzine is an inhibitor of the enzyme monoamine oxidase (MOA). Imipramine and doxepin are tricyclic antidepressants (TCAs), nefazadone is a selective norepinephrine reuptake inhibitor (SNRI), and fluvoxamine is a selective serotonin reuptake inhibitor (SSRI).

2. The answer is D.

Cotransmitters are a feature of neurotransmission in both the periphery and the CNS. Choices A and B are incorrect because the CNS has a greater number of neurotransmitters (more than 40); a greater variety of neurotransmitters, such as peptides, nonpeptides, and NO; and more complicated neural networks.

3. The answer is D.

About 5%–10% of cases of Alzheimer's disease are familial, occuring as an autosomal dominant trait. The rest are apparently sporadic in etiology. (Familial Alzheimer's disease is phenotypically identical to Alzheimer's disease except for a later age of onset.)

4. The answer is B.

All the adverse effects listed apply to both types of drugs in certain situations or in individual patients, but decreased psychomotor performance, respiratory depression, induction of microsomal enzymes, and withdrawal seizures are more commonly associated with barbiturates than with BDZs.

5. The answer is C.

Disulfiram inhibits the enzyme aldehyde dehydrogenase, which catalyzes the conversion of acetaldehyde to acetate following conversion of ethanol to acetaldehyde by alcohol dehydrogenase. Alcohol dehydrogenase is a cytosolic enzyme that contains zinc and catalyzes the first step of ethanol metabolism to acetaldehyde (NAD^+ is a cofactor).

6. The answer is A.

More than 50% of patients with epilepsy are classified as having partial onset seizures. Some of these patients can have secondarily generalized seizures. Primary generalized tonic-clonic seizures is not a universally accepted term. When used, it usually represents tonic-clonic seizures that cannot be found to have a focal onset, that is, they are not secondarily generalized. Approximately one-third of all patients with epilepsy have this type of seizure. Generalized absence seizures (formerly petit mal) occur primarily in children and account for about 5% of the epilepsy patient population. Lennox-Gastaux syndrome is a severe form of epilepsy that develops in young children and accounts for less than 2% of the patient population. The prevalence of epilepsy caused by a genetic disorder has not been established, but it is generally estimated to be between 10% and 30%. Epilepsy appears to arise most frequently from an insult or injury to the brain during the first 20 years life.

7. The answer is D.

When a drug produces an effect opposite to that produced by the endogenous ligand (neurotransmitter), it is said to be an inverse agonist. Chronic administration of CNS-active drugs usually leads to some compensatory response, which results in a change in receptor number or transduction. An increase in the receptor number is termed up-regulation; a decrease in the receptor number is termed down-regulation. Partial agonism refers to a drug that has less efficacy (less intrinsic activity) than a full agonist.

8. The answer is E.

BDZs modulate the tonic GABA-mediated Cl^- influx into neurons. The resultant hyperpolarization has an inhibitory influence on neuronal activity. The BDZs do not bind directly to the same site on the $GABA_A$ receptor as does GABA; they bind to specific BDZ receptors within the large $GABA_A$ receptor ion–channel macromolecular complex.

9. The answer is C.

Tolerance to an anticonvulsant can develop for at least two reasons: a marked increase in the rate at which the drug is metabolized after repeated dosing (pharmacokinetics-induced tolerance) or a homeostatic adjustment related to the mechanism of action of the anticonvulsant drug (pharmacodynamic-induced tolerance). A marked tolerance does not develop to most marketed anticonvulsant drugs. This includes phenytoin, valproate, carbamazepine, and topiramate. A propensity for the development of tolerance to the anticonvulsant activity of clonazepam often limits its usefulness for treating epilepsy. The nature of the tolerance that develops to clonazepam is not understood, but it may be related to drug-induced changes in the functional types of $GABA_A$ receptors expressed in some regions of the brain.

10. The answer is C.

BDZs are a broad class of compounds with anxiolytic activity produced primarily by allosteric modulation (enhancement) of GABA activity at $GABA_A$ receptors. BDZs do not bind to the identical site on the $GABA_A$ receptor complex as does GABA; hence, they do not act as either $GABA_A$ receptor agonists or antagonists. They enhance the action of GABA at the $GABA_A$ receptor, which results in an increase, not a decrease, in Cl^- conductance.

11. The answer is D.

The barbiturates, BDZs, etomidate, and propofol are believed to exert their anesthetic effect by facilitating the action of GABA at the $GABA_A$ receptor complex (Cl^- influx). The anesthetic action of ketamine is believed to be mediated through inhibition of the NMDA receptor.

12. The answer is A.

Levodopa is a chemical precursor to dopamine, which is the neurotransmitter deficient in critical brain regions (substantia nigra and corpus striatum) of Parkinson's disease patients. An important feature of levodopa is its ability to pass the blood–brain barrier. Bromocriptine and amantadine are both dopamine agonists and ameliorate Parkinson's disease symptoms by direct dopamine receptor activation. Selegiline inhibits MAO-B, an enzyme that metabolizes dopamine.

13. The answer is C.

PCP (phencyclidine, or "Angel Dust") was synthesized in 1956 and sold as an intravenous anesthetic. It is a ketamine analog and has analgesic activity. It also produces disorientation, hallucinations, and stereotypical behaviors. Deaths have been reported. It has high-affinity binding on neurons in frontal cortex and the hippocampus, effects on the NMDA Glu receptor channel (at low doses), and effects on dopamine reuptake and other neurotransmitter sites. LSD (lysergic acid diethylamide) is an ergot alkaloid synthesized in the 1930s. It produces hallucinations and other alterations of perception. It was once marketed with the suggestion that psychiatrists try it in order to understand better what their psychotic patients were experiencing. Mescaline (related to amphetamine) is obtained from Mexican cactus (peyote) and has effects similar to LSD but is less potent. Psilocybin is obtained from a fungus, was synthesized in 1958, and has effects similar to LSD but is less potent. "Kat" (methcathinone) was synthesized in the 1950s as a possible appetite suppressant but was not marketed.

14. The answer is B.

Extrapyramidal symptoms are neurologic events that result from long-term and high-dose treatment with typical antipsychotics. They are thought to be due to blockade of dopamine D_2 receptors in the basal ganglia. Blockade of the other receptors listed is characteristic of the newer, "atypical" antipsychotics and may either reduce the occurrence of neurologic side effects or enhance therapy of the negative symptoms of schizophrenia.

15. The answer is D.

Ventilatory depression is observed with most volatile anesthetics, and nearly all depress the cardiovascular system by producing negative inotropic effects, peripheral vasodilation, and decrease in blood pressure. Halothane can cause bradycardia, but most other volatile anesthetics produce mild *tachy*cardia.

16. The answer is A.

The advantage of a combination of carbidopa with levodopa, as in Sinemet, is enhanced levels of levodopa reaching the brain. Even when used in combination with carbidopa, only about 5%–10% of orally administered levodopa reaches the brain. Carbidopa is an inhibitor of dopa decarboxylase but does not penetrate the blood–brain barrier readily. Peripheral adverse effects are thus reduced, but central adverse effects can be increased.

17. The answer is E.

Positive allosteric modulation of GABA$_A$ receptors increases the functional activity of GABA, thereby reducing neuronal excitability. Positive modulation of Na$^+$ channels would tend to increase the frequency of the firing of action potentials. This would increase the overall excitability on neurons, resulting in a proconvulsant effect. Anticonvulsants that act on voltage-activated Na$^+$ channels exert a negative modulatory effect that limits the frequency at which the channels can be activated. These anticonvulsants are termed *use-*, or *state-dependent* Na$^+$-channel blockers. Inhibiting glutamate decarboxylase reduces the rate of the formation of the inhibitory neurotransmitter GABA, thereby reducing its functional activity. This indirectly increases neuronal excitability and therefore tends to exacerbate seizures. Compounds that plug up voltage-activated Na$^+$ channels or Ca^{2+} channels are too toxic to be useful anticonvulsants, although some are useful as local anesthetics. Inhibiting the uptake of glutamate would increase the neuroexcitatory activity of glutamate, which would tend to exacerbate seizures.

18. The answer is A.

Presently available pharmacotherapy focuses primarily on amelioration of symptoms by using acetylcholinesterase inhibitors (e.g., tacrine [Cognex] and donepezil [Aricept]). Future pharmacotherapy will probably target the peptides that are associated with Alzheimer's disease, such as Aβ and APP or ApoE.

19. The answer is C.

Amphetamine and related compounds stimulate the release of monoamine neurotransmitters (e.g., norepinephrine), inhibit reuptake, and inhibit enzymatic degradation by MAO. CNS stimulation can result from the opposite of the other mechanisms listed. For example, CNS stimulation by some compounds results from the antagonism of the inhibitory amino acid neurotransmitter GABA in the brain by antagonism of the GABA$_A$ binding site (e.g., bicuculline), by allosteric modulation (e.g., pentylenetetrazole, possibly the methylxanthines), or by blocking the Cl$^-$ channel (e.g., picrotoxin). In the spinal cord, the inhibitory amino acid neurotransmitter Gly is antagonized by strychnine, a specific, competitive, postsynaptic antagonist, and by tetanus toxin, which blocks Gly release.

20. The answer is C.

A major pathway of ethanol metabolism is catalyzed by the enzyme alcohol dehydrogenase, which is located in liver and other tissue (e.g., brain, stomach). Ethanol is rapidly and extensively absorbed from the GI tract, and its rate of disappearance normally follows zero-order kinetics. A specific receptor for ethanol has not been identified. Ethanol is thought to produce its effects on the CNS by an interaction with membrane proteins involved with receptor-gated ion channels or by modification of neurotransmitter function.

21. The answer is B.

Clomipramine has been approved for the treatment of obsessive-compulsive disorder.

22. The answer is B.

Flumazenil is a benzodiazepine (BDZ) derivative that blocks the BDZ-binding site on GABA$_A$ receptors. Hence, it acts as an antagonist and can be used to treat cases of BDZ overdose. Alprazolam and flurazepam are BDZ agonists and could worsen the toxicity. CNS depressants such as phenobarbital would not be used because they potentiate the effects of BDZs.

PART V
Treatment of Pain

46 NSAIDs and Acetaminophen

Robert B. Raffa, Ph.D.

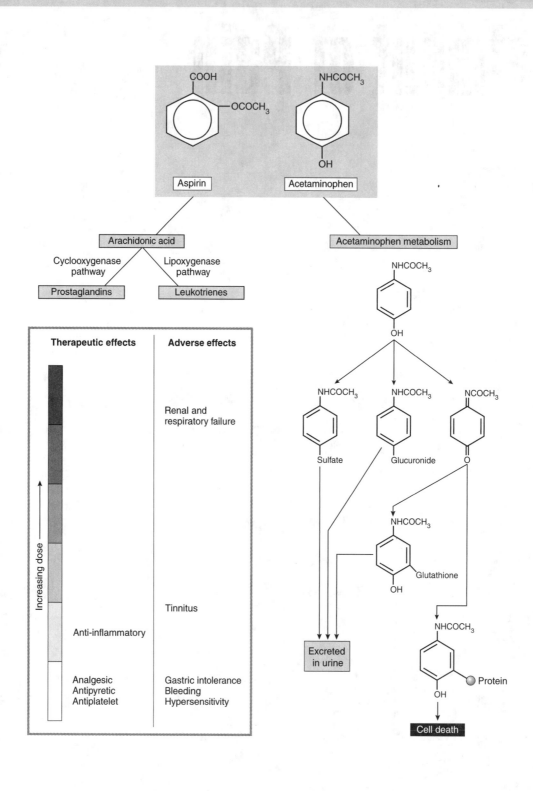

OVERVIEW

- Mild to moderate levels of pain are typically treated with nonopioid (i.e., nonmorphine-like) analgesics (analgesics are compounds that relieve pain).
- The two most-used categories are the NSAIDs and acetaminophen (the major metabolite of phenacetin).
- There are several chemical classes of NSAIDs, and all are believed to produce analgesia by inhibition of the cyclooxygenase enzyme that gives rise to biosynthesis of certain prostaglandins that cause pain (e.g., PGE_2, $PGF_{2\alpha}$, PGI_2).
- The mechanism of action of acetaminophen is not known but is thought to have a significant CNS component (as might the NSAIDs).
- The most common serious adverse effects of the NSAIDs include GI bleeding (potentially fatal) and possible drug-drug interactions resulting from high plasma protein binding. The most serious adverse effects of acetaminophen involve hepatotoxicity, resulting from intentional overdose or excess ethanol ingestion.

NSAIDs

Mechanisms of Action

NSAIDs have four major actions: (1) anti-inflammatory (against almost all causes), (2) analgesic, (3) antipyretic (reduce fever, but not normal temperature), and (4) antiplatelet. All are believed to be related to NSAID-induced decrease of prostanoid synthesis via inhibition of the cyclooxygenase pathway of arachidonic acid metabolism:

- Anti-inflammatory: Decrease in vasodilator PGs (e.g., PGE_2, PGI_2) results, indirectly, in decreased edema. The accumulation of inflammatory cells is not reduced significantly.
- Analgesic: Decreased PGs mean less sensitization of nociceptive nerve endings to mediators such as bradykinin and 5-HT. (Relief of common headache probably is secondary to decreased PG-mediated vasodilation.)
- Antipyretic: Centrally mediated; partly the result of decrease in PG response to cytokines (e.g., interleukin-1).
- Antiplatelet: Most NSAIDs induce reversible inhibition of thromboxane synthesis. Aspirin's action, however, is irreversible.

The different effects can occur at different doses. For example, an analgesic effect can be obtained at doses that are below those that are anti-inflammatory.

Cyclooxygenases. COX-1 is expressed in most tissues, is constitutively active, and is necessary for cytoprotection in the GI tract. COX-2 is induced in inflammatory cells; it is believed to be the enzyme for production of prostanoid mediators of inflammation. Most all of the commonly used NSAIDs are either more selective for COX-1 (e.g., aspirin) or are nonselective. It has been hypothesized that a COX-2 inhibitor would be analgesic and anti-inflammatory but would not produce GI ulceration. The first of this class to receive FDA approval is celecoxib (Celebra).

Pharmacokinetics

Aspirin (acetylsalicylic acid), like other weak acids ($HA \leftrightarrow H^+ + A^-$), is readily absorbed in stomach (low pH), but most of an oral dose is absorbed in the upper portion of the small intestine. Gastric irritation is decreased by raising the pH. Plasma protein binding is high (possible drug-drug interactions). Excretion is primarily through kidney (alkalinization of urine significantly increases excretion). The other NSAIDs are generally well absorbed orally (ketorolac is available as an intramuscular injection), are highly plasma-protein bound, undergo hepatic metabolism, and are excreted in the urine. Some NSAIDs (e.g., naproxen and piroxicam) have long half-lives (12–24 hours), permitting less frequent dosing.

Adverse Effects

The most common adverse effects of the NSAIDs are GI bleeding and renal damage. GI bleeding may be due to inhibition of COX-1.

Overdose of aspirin produces salicylism—tinnitus, vertigo, headache, fever, and change in mental status. Aspirin has been associated with increased risk of Reye's syndrome in children with viral infections.

SOME COMMON NSAIDs

Aspirin
Diclofenac (Voltaren)
Diflunisal (Dolobid)
Etodolac (Lodine)
Fenoprofen (Nalfon, generic)
Flurbiprofen (Ansaid, Ocufen)
Ibuprofen (Motrin, Advil, Nuprin, others, generic)
Indomethacin (Indocin, others, generic)
Ketoprofen (Orudis, others)
Ketorolac (Toradol)
Meclofenamate sodium (Meclomen, generic)
Mefenamic acid (Ponstel)
Nabumetone (Relafen)
Naproxen (Naprosyn, Anaprox, Aleve)
Oxaprozin (Daypro)
Piroxicam (Feldene, others)
Sulindac (Clinoril, others)
Tolmetin (Tolectin)

Acetaminophen

Acetaminophen has two major therapeutic actions: (1) analgesic and (2) antipyretic. Acetaminophen is not clinically anti-inflammatory (therefore, is *not* an NSAID) and does not have antiplatelet activity.

Mechanism of Action

The mechanism is largely unknown, but it might be due to (1) inhibition of a CNS-specific type of cyclooxygenase, (2) inhibition of COX-2, but only under conditions present in the CNS (and not the periphery), or (3) some other CNS action.

Pharmacokinetics

Acetaminophen is rapidly absorbed from the GI tract, 20%–50% plasma protein bound, and is excreted mainly in urine. Metabolism is primarily through hepatic glucuronidation (children have less capacity).

Toxicity

Generally acetaminophen is very well tolerated at therapeutic doses. Potentially lethal hepatic injury occurs at high doses, resulting from increased $[Ca^{2+}]_i$, activation of Ca^{2+}-dependent endonuclease, and resultant DNA fragmentation.

47 Local Anesthetics

Robert B. Raffa, Ph.D.

A Nerve characteristics

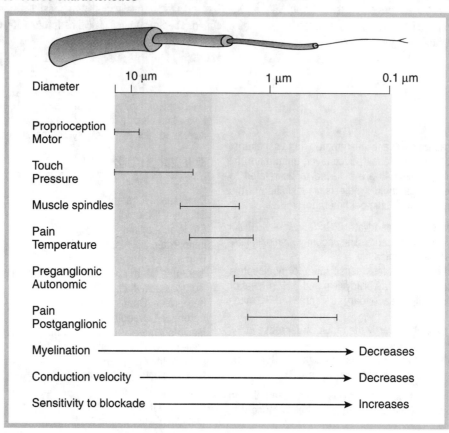

| Diameter | 10 μm | 1 μm | 0.1 μm |

Proprioception Motor

Touch Pressure

Muscle spindles

Pain Temperature

Preganglionic Autonomic

Pain Postganglionic

Myelination ⟶ Decreases

Conduction velocity ⟶ Decreases

Sensitivity to blockade ⟶ Increases

B Local anesthetic action

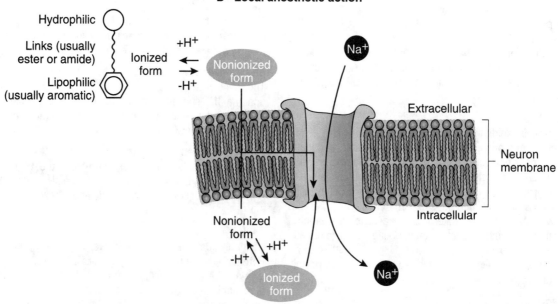

Hydrophilic

Links (usually ester or amide)

Lipophilic (usually aromatic)

Ionized form

$+H^+$
$-H^+$

Nonionized Form

Na$^+$

Extracellular

Neuron membrane

Nonionized form

$-H^+$ $+H^+$

Ionized form

Intracellular

Na$^+$

OVERVIEW

- Local anesthetics provide temporary, but complete, analgesia. The choice of agent usually is based on the desired duration of action.
- Mechanism of action: reversible block of impulse conduction along nerve axons (by blocking Na^+ influx).
- Site of action: neuronal (or other) membranes that utilize Na^+ channels for the generation of action potentials.
- Therapeutic uses: block of pain sensation; block of vasoconstrictor impulses.
- Repeated injection can lead to tachyphylaxis. Systemic absorption can lead to toxicity.

FIRST:	**COCAINE** (Köller, 1884)
FIRST SYNTHETIC:	**PROCAINE** (Einhorn, 1905)
MOST WIDELY USED:	**LIDOCAINE** (Löfgren, 1943)

Pharmacology

Local anesthetic molecules penetrate the cell membrane and diffuse across it. They exert their effect (inhibition of Na^+ influx) by an action on the inner (cytoplasmic) side or within Na^+ channels. The reversible inhibition of Na^+ influx results in temporary block of impulse conduction (action potential) along the neuron.

Medicinal Chemistry

Most local anesthetics are weak bases (partly lipid soluble and partly water soluble), allowing (1) penetration through lipid membranes and (2) access to the receptors located within channel via the cytoplasmic side. The effectiveness of local anesthetics (because of the requisite membrane penetration) is a function of pH and hence is decreased at sites of infection.

Neuronal Sites of Action

The mechanism of action of local anesthetics does not limit their effects to neurons that transmit pain sensation. Rather, the relative pain selectivity follows the order of neuron sensitivities:

- Smaller axons before larger axons
- Myelinated axons before nonmyelinated axons of same diameter
- Rapidly firing axons before resting axons

In large mixed nerves, motor nerves surround sensory nerves and pain selectivity might not be achieved (i.e., side effects observed).

Pharmacokinetics

Administration and Distribution. Local anesthetics are usually administered by injection at or near the intended target site. The spread or systemic absorption of local anesthetics (representing potential toxicity) can be reduced by coadministration of vasoconstrictor agents (this precaution might not be needed if the drug is highly lipid soluble or if the anesthetic is itself a sympathomimetic, such as cocaine).

Metabolism and Excretion. Ester local anesthetics are metabolized primarily by plasma cholinesterases, whereas amide local anesthetics are metabolized primarily by liver enzymes. (Note: metabolism by liver enzymes is a potential source of drug-drug interactions, so that a drug's half-life will increase in liver disease or in conditions of decreased hepatic blood flow.) The excretion of most local anesthetics occurs predominantly in the urine.

Toxicity

CNS. Usually the most important adverse effects, these may be lightheadedness or sedation, restlessness, nystagmus, convulsions, coma, respiratory depression (especially with procaine).

CV. Vasodilation (all except cocaine), disturbances of electrical function at high doses; intravenous bupivacaine may produce arrhythmias and hypotension; cocaine (abuse levels) may produce severe hypertension, cerebral hemorrhage, arrhythmias, myocardial infarction.

Other. A metabolite of prilocaine can cause methemoglobinemia. Metabolites of ester local anesthetics can cause allergic reactions (not observed with metabolites of amide local anesthetics).

SPECIFIC AGENTS

Esters	Amides
Procaine (teneric, Novocain)	Lidocaine (generic, Xylocaine, others)
• Short acting	• Most widely used local anesthetic
• First synthetic (1905)	
• Low potency; slow onset; short action limits use	• Almost any application where intermediate duration is needed
Cocaine (generic)	Bupivacaine (generic, Marcaine, Sensorcaine)
• Medium duration	
• Primarily for upper respiratory tract: combined anesthetic and vasoconstrictor action (shrinking of mucosa)	• Long duration
	• Popular for labor or postoperatively
• Schedule II drug	• More CV toxicity than lidocaine
Tetracaine (Pontocain)	Etidocaine (Duranest)
• Long duration (use in spinal anesthesia)	• Preferential motor block
	Prilocaine (Citanest)
• Potent, but more toxic (slow metabolism)	• Little vasodilation, less toxic than lidocaine
Benzocaine (generic)	
• Topical only	• Metabolite can produce methemo-globinemia
• Sustained action with less systemic absorption	
• Methemoglobinemia	

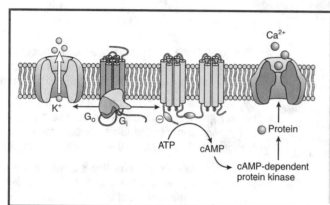

Cellular mechanisms of opioid action

- Coupled to G_i and G_o proteins
- Direct actions on ion channels
  α/β subunit $\rightarrow$ K^+ channels
- Indirect actions on ion channels
  inhibit adenylyl cyclase
  activation of phospholipase A_2 pathway

Net effects:
- Increase K^+ conductance $\rightarrow$
  hyperpolarize neurons
- Decrease Ca^{2+} conductance $\rightarrow$
  decrease neurotransmitter release
- Decrease Na^+ conductance $\rightarrow$
  decrease spontaneous firing rate

Physiologic mechanisms of opioid analgesia

Peripheral:
- Inhibits release of substance P (SP) from primary afferents $\rightarrow$
  prevents secondary activation

Spinal:
- Inhibits release of substance P and glutamate from
  primary afferents $\rightarrow$
  prevents activation of second order neurons

Supraspinal:
- Activates descending norepinephrine and 5-HT systems $\rightarrow$
  inhibits pain transmission from the spinal cord
- Activates the limbic system $\rightarrow$
  mental clouding, euphoria

Peripheral mechanisms

Primary activation

Secondary activation

Spinal mechanisms

Supraspinal mechanisms

Periaqueductal gray

Ascending system to thalamus and limbic system

Descending system

Midbrain

Ventral medulla

Spinal cord

TERMINOLOGY

- Analgesia: absence of pain without loss of consciousness (termed *antinociception* in animals).
- Opiates: natural products of poppy plant; primarily codeine, morphine, and thebaine (a precursor of semisynthetics, e.g., etorphine and naloxone).
- Opioids: opiate-like compounds.
- Narcotic: means "producing sleep"; archaic in reference to opioids; usually refers to a controlled substance (in which "narcotic analgesic" is acceptable).
- Endorphins: endogenous "morphine-like" peptides from hypothalamus and anterior pituitary (e.g., β-endorphin).
- Enkephalins: endogenous opioid pentapeptides (met- and leu-enkephalin).
- Sensation: physical component (awareness) of a noxious (nociceptive) sensory stimulus.
- Perception: affective component of pain (i.e., reactivity) [contextual].
- Tolerance: the pharmacologic effect diminishes with multiple administrations of a constant dose or the dose must be increased to maintain a given level of pharmacologic effect. (See Appendix, F, for characteristic effects of opioids.)

Pharmacology

Endogenous Opioid Peptides. Endogenous opioid polypeptides (e.g., β-endorphin, met- and leu-enkephalin, dynorphin) and their receptors mediate multiple functions of the nervous system, GI tract, temperature, immune and stress homeostasis, and feelings of pleasure and reinforcement (necessary for learning and social interaction). Opioid analgesics mimic the physiologic effects produced by the endogenous opioids.

Opioid Receptors. The three classes of receptors (each with at least two subtypes) are: μ (β-endorphin), δ (met- and leu-enkephalin), and κ (dynorphins). They are differentially expressed in various CNS and peripheral sites. All opioid receptors are transmembrane G-protein–coupled (7 TM GPC), and all are linked with cAMP, Ca^{2+}, or K^+ flux. Their anatomic localization suggests that opioids produce analgesia by inhibiting the release of substance P and other neurotransmitters from the presynaptic nerve terminals of primary afferent neurons. A second action involves the activation of descending inhibitory norepinephrine and 5-HT pathways, which modulate the incoming signal. Opioid receptors also mediate opioid-induced adverse effects.

Pharmacokinetics

Absorption. Most opioids are absorbed via all routes of administration. First-pass hepatic metabolism limits the oral potency of opioids subject to glucuronidation at C3 (e.g., morphine, hydromorphone, oxymorphone); enzyme levels vary considerably in individuals. Opioids can cross the placental barrier and may cause respiratory depression in the fetus; chronic maternal use can result in physical dependence in the newborn. The blood–brain barrier is crossed more readily by C3-substituted opioids such as codeine and heroin.

Metabolism. Compounds with free OH (e.g., morphine) undergo hepatic glucuronidation. Esters (e.g., heroin, meperidine) are hydrolyzed by tissue esterases. Metabolites can be active (e.g., morphine-6-glucuronide) and can accumulate with chronic dosing or in hepatic or renal disorders. Codeine and heroin are biotransformed into morphine in the CNS.

Excretion. Opioid excretion occurs mainly in the urine (renal failure can prolong action).

Routes of Administration. All are possible and used. Slow-release forms are available (e.g., MS Contin). Spinal target is increasing in use to increase therapeutic index. Patient-controlled analgesia (PCA) pumps are increasing in use. Patches exist for opioids with proper physiochemical properties, and there are "lollipops" for pediatric use.

Clinical Pharmacology

Analgesia. Opioids are most effective against severe, constant pain, less effective against sharp, intermittent pain, and have questionable effectiveness against neuropathic pain. They should be part of the WHO analgesic "ladder." Pain needs to be treated adequately; that is, pain may increase with disease progression. (See Appendix, F, for specific agents.)

Toxicity

Toxic effects are mostly an extension of pharmacology, the most serious being respiratory depression; all are rapidly reversed by naloxone (intravenous).

Drug Interactions. Opioids interact with CNS depressants, antipsychotics, tricyclic antidepressants, antihistamines, and MAOIs.

Cautions and Contraindications. Those for whom opioids may be contraindicated include patients with head injuries (respiratory depression increases CO_2, leading to cerebral vasodilation, increasing intracranial pressure); those pregnant (fetal dependence); patients with impaired pulmonary, renal, or hepatic function (impaired metabolism and excretion). Patients with adrenal insufficiency (Addison's disease) and hypothyroidism (myxedema) have prolonged and exaggerated responses.

Opioid Tolerance, Dependence, Withdrawal, Abuse

Tolerance is easily demonstrable in preclinical tests, but clinical relevance is controversial (e.g., perhaps pain is worsening; how important is tolerance in a dying patient?). *Dependence* is the psychological or physical craving or discomfort (withdrawal) that accompanies abstinence or antagonist administration. It develops with nearly all classes of drugs, probably as a compensatory response of the body. *Withdrawal*, abstinence-induced or antagonist-precipitated, consists of multiple symptoms, often the opposite of opioid-induced effects, that are highly uncomfortable but not life-threatening. It can be avoided by incremental decrease in dose. Opioid *abuse* (misuse) is rare among patients in pain.

Agents for the Treatment of Migraine and Chronic (Neuropathic) Pain

Robert B. Raffa, Ph.D.

A Migraine

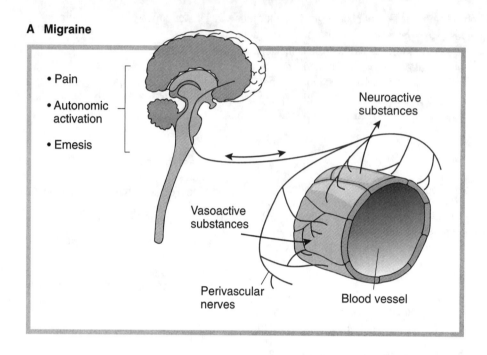

- Pain
- Autonomic activation
- Emesis

Neuroactive substances

Vasoactive substances

Perivascular nerves

Blood vessel

B Chronic pain

Possible changes

Neuronal loss
Receptor expression
Receptor distribution
Neuronal reorganization
Sprouting
"Wind-up"
Mix with sympathetic fibers
Change in ion channel number
Change in ion channel function
Receptor induction
Ion channel induction
Demyelination
Receptor transduction processes
Threshold to stimuli adaptation
Loss of inhibitory control, etc.

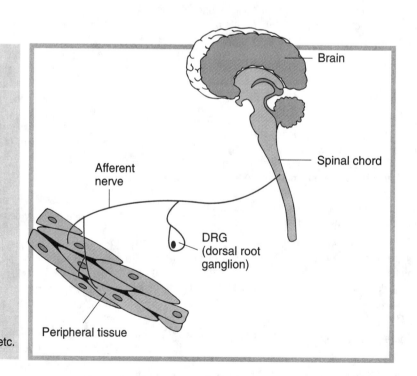

Brain

Spinal chord

Afferent nerve

DRG (dorsal root ganglion)

Peripheral tissue

OVERVIEW: MIGRAINE

Migraine consists of periodic, usually unilateral, pulsatile headaches, sometimes associated with aura. It is a familial disorder that usually begins in childhood or early adulthood and tends to decrease in frequency in later life. There are two general possible causes: (1) some humoral disturbance that alters vascular responsiveness, which in turn elicits pain, or (2) a neurologic disturbance originating in the brain or meninges, resulting in pain and vasomotor changes. More specifically, migraine could be due to vascular changes triggered by 5-HT (serotonin) release, to a neuronal abnormality similar to cortical spreading (2 mm/min) depression, or to excess activity of peptidergic nerve terminals in meningeal vessels. The release of 5-HT also leads to a local inflammatory response around extracellular vessels and the release of other mediators (e.g., bradykinin and prostaglandins) that act on nociceptive nerve terminals, causing pain and releasing neuropeptides, which further reinforce and prolong the pain (Fig. A). Afferent nerve terminals in blood vessel walls may become hypersensitive to vascular distention (Fig. B), thus accounting for the fact that many antimigraine drugs are vasoconstrictors. There is no consensus on the cause of the cerebral vasoconstriction associated with the aura.

Antimigraine Drugs

For Acute Attack. Besides analgesics (NSAIDs, acetaminophen, etc.), sumatriptan (Imitrex), approved for oral use in 1995 by the FDA, is a short-acting, 5-HT$_{1D}$ agonist. Its mechanism of action is related to presynaptic autoreceptor inhibition of 5-HT release. Adverse effects include coronary-artery vasospasm. Other triptans are now also available.

OVERVIEW: CHRONIC [NEUROPATHIC] PAIN

Chronic is the term used by many pain specialists to describe a type of persistent pain that is not associated with obvious or residual tissue damage or inflammation and hence outlasts its physiologic usefulness. Neuropathic pain is a form of chronic pain associated with diseases that affect nerves (e.g., diabetic, optic, peripheral neuropathies). Distinguishing features of this type of pain include hyperalgesia (excessive sensitivity to pain), allodynia (experience of pain to an ordinarily painless stimulus), and relative unresponsiveness to conventional analgesic drugs (Fig. B).

Possible physiologic changes in chronic pain include:
* Increased excitability of the nociceptive primary afferent neuron
* Altered phenotype of pain-transmission neurons (i.e., expression of new or more neurotransmitter receptors, ion channels, etc.)
* Structural changes in neuronal connectivity, such as loss of spinal interneurons, rearrangements of nerve processes in the spinal cord (dorsal horn), or proliferation of sympathetic fibers into sensory ganglia
* Some alteration of central processing of nociceptive input

Drug Treatment Strategies

The following classes of drugs are used:
* Opioids: usefulness debated; side effects often limit use
* Tricyclic antidepressants: amitriptyline (generic, Elavil, others) [NMDA receptor antagonist]; side effects include sedation and antimuscarinic effects
* Anticonvulsants: carbamazepine (generic, Tegretol) [NMDA receptor antagonist; Na$^+$-channel block] and phenytoin (generic, Dilantin, others) [Na$^+$-channel block]
* Antiarrhythmics: mexiletine (Mexitil) [Na$^+$-channel block]
* Local anesthetics: lidocaine (Xylocaine), tocainide (Tonocard)
* NSAIDs and combinations

50 Agents for the Treatment of Gout

Paul A. Insel, M.D.

A Uric acid formation and allopurinol action

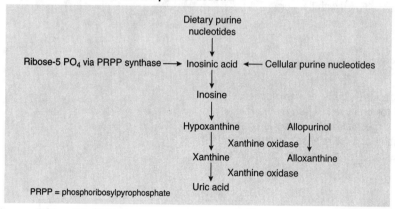

Dietary purine nucleotides

Ribose-5 PO$_4$ via PRPP synthase ⟶ Inosinic acid ⟵ Cellular purine nucleotides

Inosine

Hypoxanthine   Allopurinol

Xanthine oxidase ↓

Xanthine   Alloxanthine

Xanthine oxidase

Uric acid

PRPP = phosphoribosylpyrophosphate

B Hyperuricemia: determinants, consequences, and drug targets

Drug	Target		Target	Drug
Allopurinol	Increased uric acid production		Acute gout	NSAIDS
				Colchicine (esp. prophylaxis)
		Hyperuricemia		Corticosteroids
Uricosurics (probenecid, sulfinpyrazone)	Decreased uric acid excretion		Chronic uric acid deposition (chronic gouty arthritis, tophi, uric acid nephropathy)	Allopurinol

C Pathogenesis of gouty arthritis

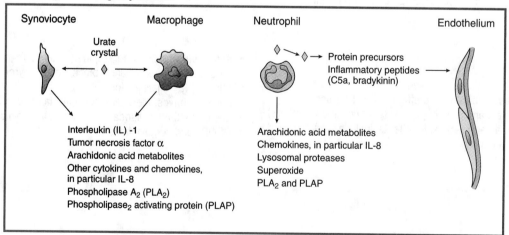

Synoviocyte   Macrophage   Neutrophil   Endothelium

Urate crystal

Protein precursors
Inflammatory peptides (C5a, bradykinin) ⟶

Interleukin (IL) -1
Tumor necrosis factor α
Arachidonic acid metabolites
Other cytokines and chemokines, in particular IL-8
Phospholipase A$_2$ (PLA$_2$)
Phospholipase$_2$ activating protein (PLAP)

Arachidonic acid metabolites
Chemokines, in particular IL-8
Lysosomal proteases
Superoxide
PLA$_2$ and PLAP

OVERVIEW

- Gout is a crystal-induced disease in which monosodium urate crystals are deposited in tissues—most important clinically, in joints—from hyperuricemic extracellular body fluids. Urate crystals in joints are phagocytosed by macrophages and synoviocytes, leading to the release of cytokines, inflammatory mediators, and molecules that enhance adhesion of leukocytes to endothelial cells, activation of polymorphonuclear leukocytes, and release of inflammatory mediators from the leukocytes.
- Gout is manifested as acute arthritis and urate deposition in joints, subcutaneous tissue (tophi), and kidney (renal stones or deposits in renal parenchyma).
- Gout can be primary, from inborn metabolic disorders with enhanced uric acid formation or decreased uric acid excretion, or secondary to acquired hyperuricemic states (e.g., myeloproliferative disorders with increased nucleic acid turnover).
- Uric acid is the product of xanthine oxidase acting on xanthine and, in turn, hypoxanthine derived from ingested or endogenously produced purines.
- Factors that contribute to hyperuricemia include high-purine diet, alcohol consumption, renal disease, and certain drugs (e.g., thiazide, loop diuretics).
- Drugs used for gout include those that decrease formation of uric acid via blockade of xanthine oxidase (allopurinol), increase excretion of uric acid by the kidney (e.g., probenecid, sulfinpyrazone), treat acute gouty arthritis (e.g., NSAIDs, colchicine, corticosteroids), or are prophylactic against acute gout (e.g., colchicine, NSAIDs).

Pharmacology

Allopurinol. An analog of hypoxanthine, allopurinol and its primary metabolite alloxanthine (oxypurinol) both inhibit xanthine oxidase and thereby block formation of uric acid. It is thus rational therapy for patients who overproduce uric acid either as a primary metabolic abnormality or with secondary hyperuricemia. Attacks of acute gout can occur during initiation of treatment with allopurinol and prophylactic treatment with colchicine may be required.

Colchicine. An alkaloid originally isolated from *Colchicum autumnale*, colchicine has an anti-inflammatory action, particularly for the treatment and prevention of acute gouty arthritis. This action is attributed to colchicine's ability to promote depolymerization of fibrillar microtubules in polymorphonuclear leukocytes and thereby phagocytosis of urate crystals and the release of proteins and inflammatory mediators. Colchicine is most useful as a prophylactic agent to prevent acute gouty attacks in patients with chronic gout or on initiation of treatment with allopurinol or uricosuric agents. It is also effective in treatment of acute gouty arthritis, but its use in this setting has largely been supplanted by NSAIDs.

NSAIDs. A variety of NSAIDs, other than salicylates, are useful in treatment of acute gouty arthritis because of their ability to block activation of inflammatory cells and formation of inflammatory mediators, in particular, cyclooxygenase products. Salicylates are contraindicated because they can decrease urate excretion, especially at lower doses, and they block the action of uricosuric agents.

Corticosteroids. Intraarticular injections of corticosteroids can be used in acute gouty arthritis. Systemic corticosteroid therapy is used when NSAIDs and colchicine are contraindicated or ineffective.

Uricosuric Agents. These agents are most appropriate for patients whose hyperuricemia results from decreased renal excretion of uric acid.

Probenecid. A lipid-soluble benzoic acid derivative, probenecid inhibits organic acid transport and, in the case of uric acid, absorption by the urate-anion exchange system in the proximal tubule. Probenecid blocks the tubular secretion of organic acids, including that of penicillin, related antimicrobials, and glucuronide metabolites of several NSAIDs. Probenecid is used in the treatment of chronic gout along with liberal fluid intake to prevent formation of uric acid stones. Since an acute gouty attack can occur in patients begun on treatment with probenecid, colchicine or a NSAID should be coadministered.

Sulfinpyrazone. Structurally related to the NSAID phenylbutazone, this agent inhibits renal tubular reabsorption of uric acid. Sulfinpyrazone lacks the anti-inflammatory effects of phenylbutazone but has an antiplatelet effect.

Pharmacokinetics

Allopurinol. Well absorbed orally, allopurinol has a plasma half-life of approximately 3 hours. It is largely metabolized to alloxanthine, which has a plasma half-life of about 24 hours in patients with normal renal function and a longer half-life in patients with decreased glomerular filtration.

Colchicine. Colchicine can be administered orally or intravenously; GI side effects may be dose-limiting, especially after oral administration. The drug is extensively metabolized and primarily excreted in the feces.

Probenecid. Completely absorbed after oral administration, probenecid is generally well tolerated.

Sulfinpyrazone. Well-absorbed orally and highly bound to plasma albumin, this anionic drug (pK_a 2.8) can displace other anionic drugs at binding sites on albumin.

Toxicity and Adverse Effects

Allopurinol. Allopurinol has important drug interactions with mercaptopurine and azathioprine by decreasing their metabolism and thus requiring a decrease in dosage of those drugs when combined with allopurinol. Allopurinol is well tolerated by most patients; hypersensitivity reactions, especially skin rash, are the most common adverse effects.

Colchicine. Colchicine can cause GI side effects, including hemorrhagic gastroenteritis, especially after oral administration. Other side effects are bone marrow depression and neuromyopathy.

Probenecid. Its principal toxicities are GI irritation, especially in patients with a history of peptic ulcer disease, and hypersensitivity reactions.

Sulfinpyrazone. GI irritation, a particular problem in patients with peptic ulcer disease, is the principal side effect. Uric acid stones and urate deposition within the kidney can also occur, especially during initiation of therapy; thus, the drug should be used along with a liberal fluid intake.

Directions: For each of the following questions, choose the **one best** answer.

1. Which of the following is a correct statement about sumatriptan?

(A) It is a 5-HT$_{1D}$ antagonist.

(B) It is not approved for oral use.

(C) It enhances 5-HT release.

(D) Adverse effects include coronary-artery vasospasm.

(E) It is long acting.

2. Which of the following drugs is most useful in treating acute gout?

(A) Allopurinol

(B) Aspirin

(C) Colchicine

(D) Probenecid

3. Which of the following actions of NSAIDs is believed to be related to the inhibition of thromboxane synthesis?

(A) Anti-inflammatory

(B) Analgesic

(C) Antipyretic

(D) Antiplatelet

4. All of the following drugs are matched correctly with an adverse effect EXCEPT

(A) acetaminophen: GI bleeding

(B) acetaminophen: hepatotoxicity

(C) aspirin: tinnitus and vertigo

(D) NSAIDs: GI bleeding

(E) NSAIDs: renal damage

5. The molecular target of opioids is

(A) membrane pores

(B) ligand-gated ion channels

(C) 7 transmembrane G-protein–coupled receptors (7 TM GCPRs)

(D) cytoplasmic receptors and transcription

6. Which of the following drugs is more effective in treating migraine than neuropathic pain?

(A) Amitriptyline

(B) Carbamazepine

(C) Mexiletine

(D) Propranolol

7. The major mechanism of action of local anesthetics is believed to involve

(A) Na$^+$ channels

(B) Ca^{2+} channels

(C) external membrane receptors

(D) the resting state of Na$^+$ channels

8. The duration of the local anesthetic effect of procaine would most likely be prolonged by

(A) warming of the injection site

(B) coinjection of norepinephrine

(C) liver disease

(D) diuresis

9. Which of the following agents is an opioid receptor antagonist?

(A) D-Propoxyphene

(B) Fentanyl

(C) Methadone

(D) Codeine

(E) Naloxone

1. The answer is D.

Sumatriptan is an agonist, not antagonist, at the 5-HT_{1D} subtype of serotonin receptor, thereby inhibiting 5-HT release. It is short acting and was approved for oral use in 1995.

2. The answer is C.

Allopurinol blocks the formation of uric acid and does not aid in the treatment of acute gout. Colchicine promotes phagocytosis of urate crystals and thus inhibits acute gout. Probenecid inhibits the reabsorption of uric acid in the proximal tubule of the kidney but does not aid in the management of acute gouty arthritis. Aspirin, like other salicylates, decreases urate secretion (especially at lower doses) and increases serum urate.

3. The answer is D.

The antiplatelet action of NSAIDs is thought to result from the inhibition of thromboxane synthesis. The other three actions are believed to be related to NSAID-induced decrease of prostanoid synthesis via inhibition of the cyclooxygenase pathway of arachidonic acid metabolism. The anti-inflammatory action is probably due to a decrease in vasodilator prostaglandins and, hence, decreased edema. The analgesic action is probably due to decreased sensitization of nociceptive nerve endings to mediators such as bradykinin and 5-HT. The antipyretic action is probably centrally mediated and partly caused by a decrease in prostaglandin response to cytokines.

4. The answer is A.

Acetaminophen generally is not associated with significant GI bleeding even at high doses. The major toxic effect of acetaminophen involves hepatotoxicity. The most common adverse effects of the NSAIDs are GI bleeding and renal damage. Aspirin overdose produces salicylism, which includes tinnitus and vertigo.

5. The answer is C.

All known opioid receptors are members of the 7 TM GPCR superfamily, and all are linked with cAMP production or with Ca^{2+} or K^+ flux. The receptors mediate the therapeutic effects (e.g., analgesia) and opioid-induced adverse effects (e.g., constipation). They are located throughout the CNS and the periphery (e.g., the GI tract). Three types have been cloned (μ, δ, κ) and subtypes of each have been postulated.

6. The answer is D.

Propranolol, although better known for other therapeutic uses, is more effective in the treatment of migraine. In the case of neuropathic pain, the use of opioid analgesics such as morphine is often limited because the high doses required are often accompanied by limiting side effects. Alternatives include: tricyclic antidepressants, such as amitriptyline (NMDA receptor antagonist); anticonvulsants, such as carbamazepine (NMDA receptor antagonist and Na^+-channel blocker), and antiarrhythmics, such as mexiletine (Na^+-channel blocker).

7. The answer is A.

Local anesthetics inhibit Na^+ influx by an inhibitory action on Na^+-channel function. The effect is selective for Na^+, not Ca^{2+}, channels. Most local anesthetics produce their effect on the intracellular (cytoplasmic) side of the nerve membrane or within the Na^+ channel. Local anesthetics have a lower affinity for the resting state than for the active state of Na^+ channels.

8. The answer is B.

Norepinephrine produces vasoconstriction, thus reducing the passage of procaine into the bloodstream (away from the site of action). Warming the injection site produces vasodilation and thus increased passage into the bloodstream (systemic absorption). Procaine, an ester local anesthetic, is metabolized primarily by plasma cholinesterases, not liver enzymes. The excretion of most local anesthetics is predominantly via the urine, hence diuresis (if it had any effect) would decrease the duration of action.

9. The answer is E.

Naloxone (Narcan) is an opioid receptor antagonist. All of the other drugs are opioid receptor *agonists*. D-Propoxyphene (Darvon) is related chemically to methadone. It is relatively weak given alone, so it is used in combination with other opioid or nonopioid analgesics. Fentanyl (Sublimaze) is a highly potent opioid agonist available as a patch (Duragesic) and as oral lozenges. Methadone is *not* an opioid receptor antagonist, despite its use in treating opiate addicts, which is based on other aspects of its pharmacology. Codeine is a well-known analgesic and antitussive agent.

PART VI
Chemotherapy

A β-Lactamases and β-lactamase inhibitors

β-Lactam ring

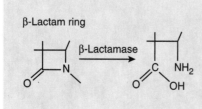

β-Lactamase

β-Lactamases cleave β-lactam ring, inactivating the antibiotic

Secreted into periplasm of gram-negative bacteria

Secreted into extracellular milieu by gram-positive bacteria

Clavulanic acid, a competitive inhibitor of many β-lactamases

COOH

B β-Lactam antibiotics: general structures

Penicillin

Cephalosporin

Carbapenem

Monobactam

C β-Lactams inhibit transpeptidation reactions

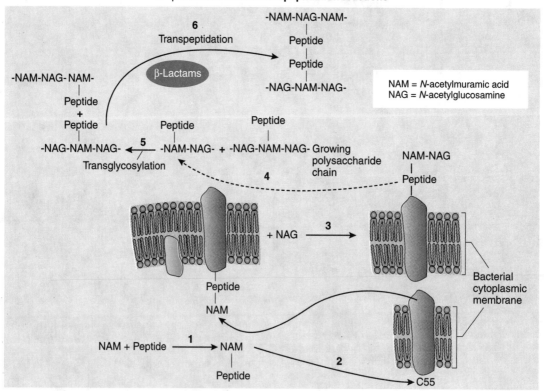

NAM = N-acetylmuramic acid
NAG = N-acetylglucosamine

OVERVIEW

- Penicillins, cephalosporins, carbapenems, and monobactams are members of a family of antibiotics that contain a β-lactam ring in their chemical structure and are one of the most useful and successful classes of antibiotics.
- Therapeutic uses: The treatment or prevention of infectious diseases caused by bacteria. The β-lactams currently available vary in their spectrum of activity; some may kill both gram-positive and gram-negative bacteria, whereas others may have a more limited spectrum of activity.

Pharmacology

β-Lactams have proven to be remarkably safe antibiotics. The early penicillins had minimal direct toxicity. Their major complications were allergic or immune-mediated reactions. The development of the newer penicillins and cephalosporins has introduced new problems in direct, nonallergic toxicity; however, these antibiotics still retain a favorable chemotherapeutic index.

Mechanism of Action

The β-lactams inhibit a set of transpeptidation reactions (Fig. C) that catalyze the final cross-linking reactions in the biosynthesis of peptidoglycan, a component of the bacterial cell wall that is essential for its survival: (1) NAM is linked to pentapeptide in the cytoplasm of the cell; (2) NAM-peptide attaches to a lipid carrier (C55); (3) NAG is linked to the NAM-peptide in the cytoplasm; (4) NAG-NAM peptide is released from C55 outside the cytoplasmic membrane; (5) NAG-NAM is linked to the growing polysaccharide chain (transglycosylation); and (6) peptide cross-links are formed (transpeptidation). β-Lactams also bind to and inhibit the action of other bacterial cytoplasmic membrane proteins that have a role in peptidoglycan synthesis and turnover. These transpeptidases and transglycosylases are referred to as penicillin-binding proteins (PBPs). The net result of β-lactam action is the stimulation of endogenous bacterial enzymes called autolysins that degrade peptidoglycan, causing cell lysis and death.

Medicinal Chemistry

More than 50 years after the discovery of penicillin, the β-lactams continue to provide useful products for the treatment of diverse infections. At least 40 products are marketed worldwide. Major thrusts of the medicinal chemistry are to synthesize compounds with improved spectrum and potency of antibacterial activity, resistance to β-lactamases, long half-life, and safety. The table below shows representative antibiotics commonly used for treatment. Many derivatives are increasingly stable to β-lactamases (e.g., imipenem). β-Lactamase inhibitor combinations (e.g., amoxicillin–clavulanic acid) successfully treat infections caused by β-lactamase-producing bacteria.

Pharmacokinetics

Metabolism, tissue distribution, and elimination rates of the β-lactams may vary widely among members of this large group of compounds. Urinary excretion is the prime route of elimination for β-lactams, although biliary excretion and metabolism contribute to the elimination of several. For most, urinary excretion involves both glomerular filtration and renal tubular secretion. Kidney dysfunction or the coadministration of probenecid cause dramatic changes in drug elimination. Clinical efficacy is related to the time the drug serum concentration remains above the minimum inhibitory concentration.

Toxicity and Adverse Effects

Allergic and Immune-mediated. These are usually the most important adverse effects and include anaphylactic reactions, hemolytic anemia, and neutropenia; cross-hypersensitivity among β-lactams may occur up to 10% of the time.

CNS. Myoclonic activity, confusional states, and seizures (especially with carbapenems) are more common in patients with CNS disorders and compromised renal function.

GI. Diarrhea and pseudomembranous colitis (overgrowth of *Clostridium difficile* with toxin production) may occur.

Other. Bleeding associated with coagulation test abnormalities, disulfuram-like reactions with alcohol ingestion, and elevation of liver transaminase levels may occur.

Resistance

Bacterial resistance to antibiotics such as β-lactams has become a major worldwide health problem. One of the major causes of resistance to β-lactam antibiotics is hydrolysis of the β-lactam ring by bacterial enzymes (β-lactamases). Other resistance mechanisms include bacteria with reduced permeability to the drug and cells with altered PBPs that have a much lower affinity for β-lactams (e.g., methicillin-resistant *Staphylococcus aureus*).

SPECIFIC AGENTS

Penicillins	Cephalosporins	Other β-Lactams
Oral administration		
Penicillin G	Cephalexin	
Ampicillin	Cefaclor	
Amoxicillin	Cefuroxime axetil	
Oxacillin	Cefixime	
Parenteral administration		
Methicillin	Cefazolin	Aztreonam[a]
Piperacillin	Defamandole	Imipenem[b]
Ticarcillin	Cefuroxime	Meropenem[b]
Azlocillin	Cefotaxime	
	Cefoxitin	
	Cefotetan	
	Ceftazidime	
	Ceftriaxone	

[a] monobactam
[b] carbapenem

Folate Antagonists: Sulfonamides and Trimethoprim

Charles R. Craig, Ph.D.

A

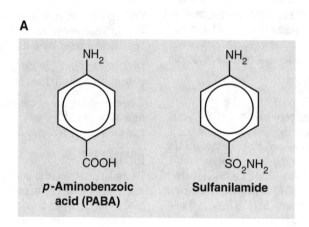

p-Aminobenzoic acid (PABA)

Sulfanilamide

B Synthesis of tetrahydrofolate from PABA in bacteria showing site of action of sulfonamides and trimethoprim

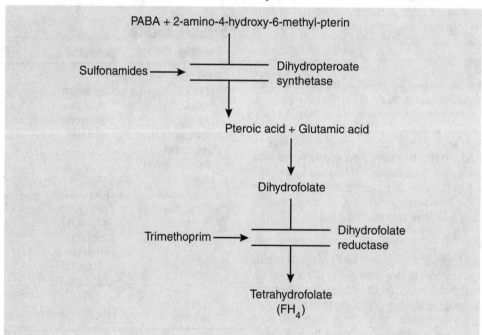

PABA + 2-amino-4-hydroxy-6-methyl-pterin

Sulfonamides ⟶ | Dihydropteroate synthetase

Pteroic acid + Glutamic acid

Dihydrofolate

Trimethoprim ⟶ | Dihydrofolate reductase

Tetrahydrofolate (FH$_4$)

OVERVIEW

- The sulfonamides are structurally related to *p*-aminobenzoic acid (PABA); this is particularly apparent when comparing the structure of one compound, sulfanilamide, with the structure of PABA (Fig. A).
- Mechanism of action: Both the sulfonamides and trimethoprim inhibit synthesis of folic acid. However, they act at two different sites, thus making the combination more effective than either agent alone in many instances.
- Site of action: The drugs act on enzymatic pathways involved in the synthesis of folic acid (Fig. B). Since humans are unable to synthesize folic acid and must obtain it from dietary sources and since bacteria must synthesize folic acid to survive, the use of sulfonamides, trimethoprim, and particularly of the combination is an excellent example of selective toxicity.
- Therapeutic uses: The sulfonamides were the first useful chemotherapeutic agents; they have been used effectively against a variety of microorganisms for many years. The development of resistant organisms and agents with fewer side effects has caused them to be used less often at the present time. However, the combination of sulfonamides and trimethoprim continues to be widely used for a variety of bacterial infections as well as for the treatment of *Pneumocystis carinii* infection. Although organisms do not develop resistance as quickly to the combination, bacterial resistance does occur and limits the combination's usefulness.

Pharmacology

The sulfonamides competitively inhibit the incorporation of PABA into folic acid. Trimethoprim acts at a second step in the synthesis of folic acid (see Fig. B) and competitively inhibits dihydrofolate reductase; this inhibits the conversion of dihydrofolic acid to tetrahydrofolic acid.

Medicinal Chemistry

There are a large number of sulfonamides on the market; within the group there are major differences in the chemistry. The prototype sulfonamide is sulfanilamide. Trimethoprim is a weak base and therefore accumulates intracellularly.

Pharmacokinetics

Administration and Distribution. Most sulfonamides are rapidly absorbed from the GI tract and are therefore administered orally. Peak blood levels are usually seen 2–3 hours after oral administration. There are some sulfonamides that are poorly absorbed from the GI tract, and these may be used against organisms within the GI tract. Some sulfonamides are used only topically. Trimethoprim is well absorbed from the GI tract; its half-life is approximately 11 hours.

Metabolism and Excretion. The sulfonamides and trimethoprim are degraded by metabolic processes, primarily in the liver. The unchanged parent compound as well as metabolic products are ultimately excreted in the urine.

Clinical Uses

The sulfonamides are rarely the drug of first choice. They are, however, useful in a variety of bacterial infections if the causative organism is susceptible to the drug, as in infections of the urinary tract and lower respiratory tract. They are also of some use in the treatment of infections caused by *Nocardia* and *Chlamydia trachomatis*. Topically active sulfonamides (Sulfamylon Cream) are helpful in preventing infections in burn patients.

Trimethoprim is rarely used alone; it is most frequently combined with sulfamethoxazole. This combination is used in a variety of infectious diseases, including otitis media; prostatitis; and urinary, intestinal, and lower respiratory tract infections caused by susceptible bacteria. The combination has been used with some success in the treatment and prevention of the pneumonitis caused by the protozoan, *P. carinii*. This pneumonitis is a frequent late consequence of AIDS, as well as occurring in other situations in which the immune system has been compromised.

Resistance. Bacteria rapidly become resistant to sulfonamides and to trimethoprim. Resistance to the combination is slower to develop; nevertheless, resistance has markedly decreased the effectiveness of these agents.

Toxicity

The most common adverse effects are hypersensitivity reactions. These take the form of rashes, drug fever, and eosinophilia. Skin rashes are particularly common in patients with compromised immune systems. Because these drugs are eliminated by hepatic drug metabolism and excreted via the kidneys, their use is contraindicated in patients with severe hepatic or renal disease.

SPECIFIC AGENTS

Sulfonamides	Sulfonamides and Trimethoprim
Sulfadiazine and sulfisoxazole • examples of short-acting sulfonamides Sulfamethoxazole • intermediate-acting sulfonamide • most often used in combination with trimethoprim Mafenide (Sulfamylon Cream) • topically active sulfonamide • often used in burn patients	Trimethoprim • most often used in combination with sulfamethoxazole as Septra or Bactrim

Protein Synthesis Inhibitors: Erythromycins
Robert B. Raffa, Ph.D.

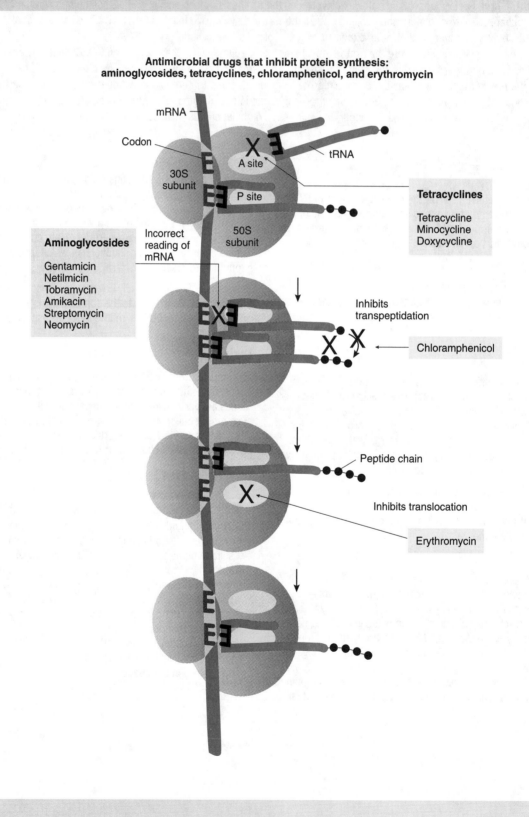

Antimicrobial drugs that inhibit protein synthesis: aminoglycosides, tetracyclines, chloramphenicol, and erythromycin

mRNA

Codon

30S subunit

A site

P site

50S subunit

tRNA

Tetracyclines

Tetracycline
Minocycline
Doxycycline

Aminoglycosides

Gentamicin
Netilmicin
Tobramycin
Amikacin
Streptomycin
Neomycin

Incorrect reading of mRNA

Inhibits transpeptidation

Chloramphenicol

Peptide chain

Inhibits translocation

Erythromycin

OVERVIEW

- These drugs interfere selectively with the mechanism(s) involved in protein synthesis in various microorganisms. Their selectivity derives from the different ribosomal subunits in bacterial and mammalian cells.
- Various modes of action are possible, depending on whether the drugs interfere with binding of tRNA, reading of mRNA, transpeptidation, or translocation.
- Major drug (chemical) classes include aminoglycosides, macrolides, and tetracyclines.
- Aminoglycosides are mostly bactericidal; the others are mostly bacteriostatic.
- Strains of bacteria resistant to all of these drug classes develop.

Pharmacology

Aminoglycosides. Diffuse across the outer membrane through porin channels (a process enhanced synergistically by penicillin or vancomycin) and bind to the 30S subunit of bacterial ribosomes (but not the 40S subunit present in mammals). Irreversible and lethal inhibition of protein synthesis occurs by interference with the proper attachment of mRNA, misreading of the mRNA (incorporation of incorrect amino acid sequences), and other actions.

Macrolides. Bind to the 50S subunit of bacterial ribosomes and block formation of the initiation complex and the translocation step.

Tetracyclines. Enter cells by passive and active transport, bind reversibly to the 30S subunit of bacterial ribosomes, and block the binding of aminoacyl-tRNA to the acceptor site on the mRNA-ribosome complex, thereby preventing addition of amino acids to the growing peptide.

Medicinal Chemistry

Aminoglycosides. Consist of three characteristic portions: a hexose ring, a glycosidic link, and amino sugars. Various analogs have different degrees of resistance to degradation by bacterial enzymes.

Macrolides. Characterized by a large macrocyclic lactone ring (hence, macrolide), typically containing 14 or 16 carbon atoms. Deoxy sugars are attached to the lactone ring.

Tetracyclines. So named because of their characteristic four 6-membered C-rings connected linearly. They can chelate divalent metal ions (which can interfere with their absorption or activity).

Pharmacokinetics

Aminoglycosides. Poor oral absorption and highly polar, so they do not readily penetrate CNS or eyes in the absence of inflammation. They are usually administered intravenously and are cleared by the kidney (in the absence of renal impairment).

Macrolides. Susceptible to stomach acid. Food interferes with oral absorption, and large amounts are excreted in the bile and feces. They have limited access to the CNS.

Tetracyclines. Oral absorption depends on the drug (can be 30%–100%); can be affected by food, divalent cations, dairy products, or alkaline pH. Typically 40%–80% is plasma protein–bound. They are excreted mainly in bile (enterohepatic circulation) and urine (an exception is doxycycline, which is less affected by renal insufficiency).

Susceptible Bacteria

Aminoglycosides. Mostly used against gram-negative enteric bacteria (anaerobic bacteria generally are resistant). They are used with β-lactams to include gram-positive strains and for synergistic therapeutic interaction.

Macrolides. Act on gram-positive or gram-negative bacteria, depending on the drug. Pneumonia caused by *Mycoplasma*, legionnaire's disease, chlamydia infections, diphtheria (*Corynebacterium diphtheriae*), and whooping cough (*Bordetella pertussis*) are treated with macrolides.

Tetracyclines. Effective against many gram-positive and gram-negative bacteria, including *Borrelia*, *Chlamydia*, *Mycoplasma*, *Rickettsia* spp., and some spirochetes.

Resistance

Bacterial resistance to each drug category can develop. It can be induced within an individual organism or can develop as a result of preferential growth of inherently resistant organisms when competing organisms are killed. The latter occurs when antimicrobial therapy is stopped prematurely in an individual patient or when antimicrobials are overutilized in the general population.

Toxicity

Aminoglycosides. Nephrotoxicity and ototoxicity (permanent in small percent of patients), neuromuscular block (high doses or combination with nicotinic ACh receptor antagonists), and hypersensitivity reactions (infrequent).

Macrolides. GI intolerance is usually the major reason for discontinuance. Reversible acute cholestatic hepatitis, thrombophlebitis, and drug-drug interactions by interference with hepatic metabolism are other possible side effects.

Tetracyclines. Uncommon hypersensitivity reactions (e.g., skin rash, fever), local irritation (oral, intravenous, or intramuscular administration), hepatic dysfunction (particularly in pregnancy), and in children, discoloration of teeth and depressed bone growth.

SPECIFIC AGENTS

Aminoglycosides
Amikacin (generic, Amikin); gentamicin (generic, Garamycin); neomycin (generic, Mycifradin) netilmicin (Netromycin); paromomycin (Humatin); streptomycin (generic); tobramycin (generic, Nebcin)

Macrolides
Azithromycin (Zithromax); clarithromycin (Biaxin); erythromycin (generic, Ilotycin, Ilosone, E-Mycin, Erythrocin, others)

Tetracyclines
Demeclocycline (Declomycin); doxycycline (generic, Vibramycin, others); methacycline (Rondomycin); minocycline (Minocin); oxytetracycline (generic, Terramycin); tetracycline (generic, Achromycin V, others)

54 Agents for the Treatment of Urinary Tract Infections

William A. Petri, Jr., M.D., Ph.D., and Christopher D. Huston, M.D.

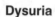

Dysuria

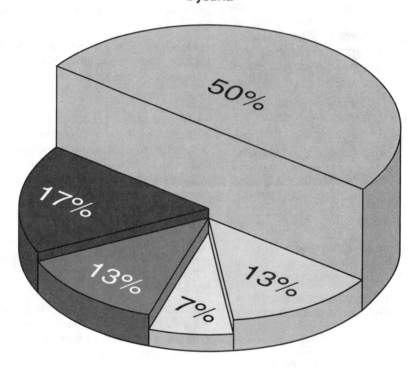

13%	Unknown
7%	*Chlamydia* urethritis
13%	Vaginitis
17%	UTI $\leq 10^5$ bacteria/mL
50%	UTI $\geq 10^5$ bacteria/mL

OVERVIEW

- Antibiotic and antifungal drugs are used to cure urinary tract infections (UTIs) by selectively targeting microbial processes or structures.
- Antiseptic drugs are used to cure or chronically suppress UTIs by virtue of their activation in the urine to broadly toxic compounds such as formaldehyde.
- Analgesic agents act to treat the symptoms of UTIs.
- Antimuscarinic agents are used to treat detrusor overactivity, which can mimic the symptoms of UTIs.

Pharmacology

Antibiotics. Quinolones inhibit bacterial DNA gyrase. Examples include nalidixic acid, norfloxacin, ciprofloxacin, and ofloxacin. Trimethoprim-sulfamethoxazole blocks sequential steps in folate metabolism in bacteria. β-lactams, such as the cephalosporins and penicillins, inhibit bacterial cell wall (peptidoglycan) synthesis.

Antifungals. Fluconazole inhibits biosynthesis of ergosterol for the cytoplasmic membrane of susceptible fungi. The antifungal activity of amphotericin B is believed to result from the drug-binding ergosterol in the membrane of fungi, causing the formation of pores or channels.

Antiseptics. Methenamine decomposes in acid urine to formaldehyde, acting as a urinary tract antiseptic. Urea-splitting bacteria that alkalinize the urine, such as *Proteus*, are usually resistant. Nitrofurantoin is a synthetic nitrofuran that is reduced by bacteria to a highly reactive intermediate thought to be responsible for the ability of the drug to damage DNA.

Analgesics. Phenazopyridine is an azo dye that is a urinary tract analgesic.

Antimuscarinics. These agents, such as tolterodine, are used for the treatment of urinary frequency, urgency, and incontinence caused by bladder (detrusor) overactivity.

Pharmacokinetics

Administration and Distribution

Antibiotics. The quinolones, β-lactam antibiotics such as amoxicillin and cephalexin, and trimethoprim-sulfamethoxazole are absorbed from the GI tract.

Antifungals. Fluconazole is absorbed from the GI tract. Amphotericin B must be administered IV or locally to the bladder via irrigation.

Antiseptics. Methenamine is orally absorbed and renally excreted. Acidification of the urine with mandelic acid or hippuric acid promotes the generation of formaldehyde from methenamine. Nitrofurantoin is well absorbed from the GI tract, with 40% of the drug rapidly eliminated in the urine. The presence of the drug turns the urine brown.

Analgesics. Phenazopyridine is absorbed from the GI tract.

Antimuscarinics. These drugs are also absorbed from the GI tract.

Metabolism and Excretion

Antibiotics. Some quinolones are renally cleared (ofloxacin, norfloxacin, ciprofloxacin), others are not (nalidixic acid). Amoxicillin, cephalexin, and trimethoprim-sulfamethoxazole are renally excreted.

Antifungals. Fluconazole is renally excreted. Amphotericin B is extensively bound to protein. Metabolism of the drug appears to be unchanged in patients with renal failure and with hepatic disease.

Antiseptics. Methenamine decomposes in water at acidic pH to formaldehyde and ammonia. It is nearly completely eliminated in the urine. Nitrofurantoin is reduced by bacteria to an active intermediate in the urine.

Analgesics. Phenazopyridine is excreted in the urine and colors the urine red or orange.

Antimuscarinics. Tolterodine, one of the new muscarinic receptor antagonists, is rapidly absorbed from the GI tract, metabolized in the liver, and excreted in the urine.

Side Effects and Toxicity

Antibiotics. Side effects of the quinolones include nausea, abdominal discomfort, headache, and dizziness. Rarely, hallucinations and seizures have occurred in patients also receiving theophylline or an NSAID, and photosensitivity reactions can occur. All quinolones can cause arthropathy and are not recommended for prepubertal children and pregnant women. Trimethoprim-sulfamethoxazole toxicities include dermatologic reactions, nausea, vomiting, stomatitis, and, less commonly, cholestatic hepatitis, headache, depression, hallucinations, anemia, granulocytopenia, renal insufficiency, and Henoch-Schönlein purpura. β-lactam toxicities include hypersensitivity reactions, bone marrow depression, hepatitis, antibiotic-associated colitis, and CNS toxicity including seizures, hallucinations, and headaches.

Antifungals. Fluconazole increases the plasma levels of many drugs, including phenytoin, zidovudine, rifabutin, cyclosporin, warfarin, sulfonylureas, and to a lesser extent terfenadine. Nausea and vomiting, diarrhea, abdominal pain, rash, and headache are side effects. Rarely, hepatic failure and Stevens-Johnson syndrome have been associated with fluconazole use. Amphotericin B causes fever and chills upon infusion and a dose-dependent azotemia in most patients. Hypotension accompanied by hypokalemia may occur, requiring potassium supplementation.

Antiseptics. Methenamine degradation to formaldehyde produces ammonia as a by-product; therefore it should not be given to patients with hepatic insufficiency. High doses of methenamine may result in painful micturition, albuminuria, hematuria, and rashes. Methenamine mandelate should not be given to patients with renal insufficiency because of crystalluria from the mandelate moiety. Nitrofurantoin toxicity is increased in patients with renal insufficiency. Toxicity includes nausea, vomiting, diarrhea, and hypersensitivity reactions (chills, fever, leukopenia, granulocytopenia, hemolytic anemia in patients with glucose-6-phosphate dehydrogenase deficiency, acute pneumonitis, pulmonary fibrosis), various neurologic disorders (headache, vertigo, drowsiness, nystagmus, polyneuropathies with demyelination), hepatocellular damage, and cholestatic jaundice.

Analgesics. Phenazopyridine causes gastrointestinal upset in up to 10% of patients. Overdose can result in methemoglobinemia.

Antimuscarinics. Limited usefulness due to antimuscarinic adverse effects, including dry mouth, cognitive impairments, and cardiac effects; should not be used in patients with narrow angle glaucoma.

55 Antimycobacterial Agents

Steven P. Gelone, Pharm.D.

Drug	Dose (mg/kg)	Maximum Daily Dose	Adverse Effects	Comments	Preg-nancy	CNS TB Disease	Renal Insufficiency
First-line agents							
Isoniazid	5	300 mg	Liver functions; hepatitis; peripheral neuropathy; drowsiness	Hepatitis risk increases with age and alcohol consumption; pyridoxine (vitamin B$_6$) can prevent peripheral neuropathy	Safe	Good penetration	No change in dose
Rifampin	10	600 mg	GI upset; rash; flu-like syndrome; bleeding problems	Drug interactions; colors bodily fluids orange; may permanently discolor soft contact lenses	Safe	Good penetration	No change in dose
Pyrazinamide	15 – 30	2 g	Hepatitis; rash; GI upset; joint aches; hyperuricemia	Treat hyperuricemia only if patient has symptoms	Avoid	Good penetration	
Ethambutol	15	2.5 g	Optic neuritis	Not recommended for children too young to be monitored for vision changes unless TB is drug resistant	Safe	Penetrates i.m. only	Prolong dosing interval
Streptomycin	15	1 g	Ototoxicity; renal toxicity	Avoid or reduce dose in patients > 60 years old	Avoid	Penetrates i.m. only	Follow serum levels
Second-line agents							
Capreomycin	15 – 30	1 g	Ototoxicity; renal toxicity	After bacteriologic conversion, may reduce dosage to 2–3 times per week	Avoid	Penetrates i.m. only	Prolong dosing interval
Kanamycin	15 – 30	1 g	Ototoxicity; renal toxicity	After bacteriologic conversion, may reduce dosage to 2–3 times per week	Avoid	Penetrates i.m. only	Prolong dosing interval
Ethionamide	15 – 20	1 g	GI upset; hepatotoxicity; hypersensitivity; metallic taste; bloating	Start with low dosage and increase as tolerated; may cause hypothyroid condition, especially with PAS	Do not use	Good penetration	No change until Clcr <10, then 50% of dose daily
P-Aminosali-cyclic acid (PAS)	150	12 g	GI upset; hypersensitivity; hepatotoxicity; sodium load	Start with low dosage and increase as tolerated; monitor cardiac patients for sodium load	Safe	Penetrates	Incomplete data
Cycloserine	15 – 20	1 g	Psychosis; convulsions; headaches; rash	Start with low dosage and increase as tolerated. Pyridoxine may decrease CNS effects; avoid in patients with seizure history	Avoid	Good penetration	Prolong dosing interval
Amikacin	15 – 20		Renal toxicity; ototoxicity	Not approved by FDA for TB treatment	Avoid	Penetrates i.m. only	Follow serum levels

Note. Ototoxicity = vestibular dysfunction, hearing loss, dizziness; i.m. = inflamed meninges; Clcr = creatinine clearance.

OVERVIEW

- Therapy of mycobacterial disease constitutes a diverse group of antimicrobial agents.
- Therapeutic agents differ markedly in chemistry, mechanism of action, pharmacokinetics, adverse reactions, and bactericidal versus bacteriostatic effects.
- Antimycobacterial agents can be classified according to their spectrum of activity: (1) *Mycobacterium tuberculosis*, (2) atypical mycobacteria including *M. avium* complex, and (3) *M. leprae*.

First-Line Agents

Isoniazid (Nydrazid). Also known as isonicotinic acid hydrazide or INH. Bactericidal against rapidly growing *M. tuberculosis* and bacteriostatic against nonreplicating organisms. Its mechanism of action is inhibition of oxygen-dependent synthetic pathways of mycolic acid synthesis. When INH is administered alone, resistance to it tends to emerge. Well absorbed orally or intramuscularly and is distributed throughout the body. CSF levels may approach serum concentrations in the presence of inflamed meninges. Metabolism occurs initially by N-acetyltransferase. Diminished acetylation is inherited as an autosomal recessive trait. Most notable serious toxicity is hepatitis, correlated with age. INH is an inhibitor of the cytochrome P-450 enzyme system and can potentiate the effect or toxicity of drugs metabolized via this system. Indicated for all forms of TB. Always combine with at least one other agent. It is the prophylaxis regimen of choice in patients who have been exposed to TB.

Rifampin (Rifadin). Inhibits DNA-dependent RNA polymerase. Bactericidal against susceptible *M. tuberculosis* strains comparable to INH activity and is active against intracellular, slowly replicating bacilli and somewhat active against nearly dormant organisms in necrotic foci. Well absorbed orally and widely distributed. CSF concentrations range from undetectable in uninfected individuals to 50% of serum concentrations with meningeal inflammation. Excretion is primarily into the GI tract. Dosage adjustment is necessary for liver dysfunction but not for renal impairment. Major toxicity is hepatotoxicity. GI upset is frequent. Bodily fluids appear orange (soft contact lenses will be permanently discolored). A potent inducer of hepatic cytochrome P-450 enzyme activity, rifampin results in many clinically significant drug interactions, and its metabolism is autoinduced. Indicated for all forms of TB and should always be employed in combination with other agents.

Pyrazinamide (PZA). An analog of nicotinamide. Possess bactericidal activity against metabolically active tubercle bacilli that is maximally achieved at an acid pH. PZA is well absorbed orally, widely distributed, and crosses inflamed meninges. It is metabolized by the liver, and metabolites are excreted mainly by the kidneys. The most common adverse effects are nausea and vomiting. Uric acid retention is common, and photosensitivity reactions may occur. PZA is included in the initial regimen of short-course chemotherapy for TB.

Ethambutol (Myambutol). A synthetic, orally available agent. Bacteriostatic against tubercle bacilli. Its mechanism of action is unknown. It is well absorbed and widely distributed. It crosses inflamed meninings. The major toxicity is retrobulbar neuritis. It is used as part of combination therapy for the treatment of TB.

Streptomycin. An aminoglycoside antibiotic introduced in the 1940s as the first drug to reduce TB mortality. Given that it requires parenteral administration, other agents have replaced it in most situations.

Second-Line Agents

p-Aminosalicyclic Acid (PAS). Impairs folate synthesis. Its absorption is incomplete and erratic. Its major toxicity is GI intolerance that is often severe. It has been associated with a lupus-like state and a mono-nucleosis-like syndrome.

Cycloserine (Seromycin). Inhibits cell wall formation. Readily absorbed orally and distributed throughout the body. Cycloserine can cause peripheral neuropathy or CNS dysfunction.

Ethionamide (Trecator-SC). A derivative of isonicotinic acid. Bacteriostatic against *M. tuberculosis*, presumably by inhibition of oxygen-dependent mycolic acid synthesis. Well absorbed and distributed throughout the body. Interferes with the acetylation of isoniazid. GI distress with nausea and vomiting occur frequently.

Capreomycin (Capastat). A polypeptide antibiotic, obtained from *Streptomyces capreolus*. Active against most strains of *M. tuberculosis* including drug-resistant strains. There is no cross-resistance between streptomycin and capreomycin.

Treatment of Leprosy

Dapsone. Diaminodiphenylsulfone (dapsone), like other sulfone derivatives, inhibits dihydropteroate synthetase, which decreases folate synthesis. Weakly bactericidal against *M. leprae*. Well absorbed orally and distributed throughout the body. Dapsone is acetylated, with 70%–80% excreted as metabolites in urine. Adverse effects include dose-dependent hemolysis, which is worse in those with underlying glucose-6-phosphate dehydrogenase (G6PD) deficiency. Sulfone syndrome can occur, usually within 5–6 weeks after initiation of therapy, characterized by fever, jaundice, dermatitis, and lymphadenopathy. Dapsone is one of the principal agents used to treat both multibacillary and paucibacillary *M. leprae* infection.

Clofazimine (Lamprene). A phenazine dye. Its action may relate to iron chelation, with resulting production of nascent oxygen radicals intracellularly. Weakly bactericidal against *M. leprae*. A delay of approximately 50 days ensues before tissue antimicrobic activity is demonstrated. It is largely unmetabolized. Billary excretion appears to be the major route of excretion. GI side effects, including anorexia, diarrhea, and abdominal pain, are most common. Skin pigmentation is common. Clofazimine is used to treat multibacillary infection.

Thalidomide (Thalomid). This synthetic glutamic acid derivative, marketed in Europe in the 1950s as a sedative, recently has been approved by the FDA for treatment of leprosy.

56 Antifungal Agents

Steven P. Gelone, Pharm.D.

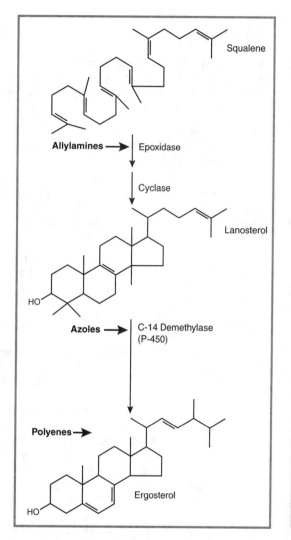

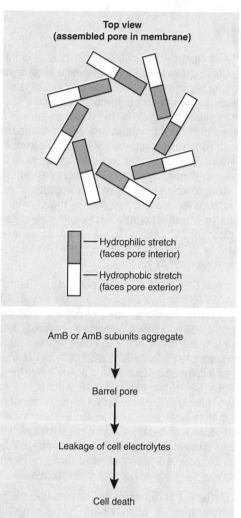

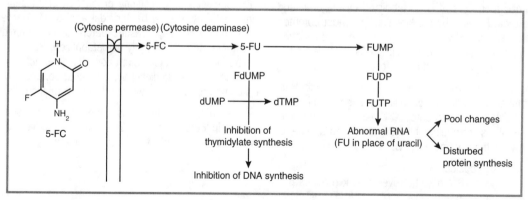

OVERVIEW

- Fungal infections in humans range from superficial and cutaneous to deeply invasive and disseminated.
- Over the past 20 years the incidence of fungal infections has dramatically increased, paradoxically as a result of advances in medical practice, including organ transplantation.
- Three major groups of antifungal compounds are in clinical use: polyene antibiotics, azole derivatives, and allylamines.

Polyene Antibiotics

Amphotericin B (AmB) and Nystatin. AmB is active against most pathogenic fungi. It remains the cornerstone of therapy for patients with invasive fungal disease. Not absorbed orally or intramuscularly. The commercial product is a micellar suspension. Primary mechanism of action is binding to ergosterol, the principal sterol present in the cell membrane of sensitive fungi. Binding disrupts the membrane, possibly secondary to the formation of pores composed of aggregates of AmB and sterol, and increases membrane permeability to protons and monovalent cations that ultimately leads to cell death. AmB binds with less affinity to other sterols, such as cholesterol, which accounts for much of its toxicity to mammalian cells. High intestinal tract concentrations make AmB suitable as prophylaxis or treatment of orointestinal yeast infections. The metabolic fate of AmB is unknown. Only 5%–10% is excreted in the urine or bile. No dose modification is necessary for underlying renal or liver dysfunction. AmB causes two major types of toxicity: infusion-related reactions (IRRs) and nephrotoxicity. Recently, AmB and nystatin have been incorporated into lipid formulations that maintain antifungal activity and minimize nephrotoxicity and IRRs.

Azole Derivatives

These compounds have one or more five-membered azole rings; each ring contains two (imidazoles: clotrimazole, miconazole, ketoconazole) or three (triazoles: fluconazole, itraconazole) N atoms. They inhibit fungal cytochrome P-450 3A–mediated conversion of lanosterol to ergosterol. This leads to accumulation of 14-α-methyl-sterols and depletion of ergosterol in the fungal cell wall, resulting in altered properties, increased permeability, and inhibition of cell growth and replication.

Clotrimazole and Miconazole. Neither is significantly absorbed from the GI tract. Because of induction of microsomal liver enzymes after systemic administration, clotrimazole is used only as a topical agent. Miconazole is used mainly as a topical agent.

Ketoconazole. The first oral azole derivative. Absorption is variable and is affected by food. Highly bound to plasma proteins and penetrates poorly into CSF, urine, and saliva. Extensive hepatic biotransformation occurs; the drug is excreted mainly in the bile. Common adverse effects include nausea, anorexia, and vomiting. Cross-inhibition of mammalian steroid biosynthesis manifests as decreased testosterone levels in men and menstrual irregularities and alopecia in women. Many drug interactions occur, notably with cyclosporine, cisapride, and astemizole. Ketoconazole metabolism is significantly increased by drugs that induce hepatic enzyme function. Considered a second-line therapy to AmB or the triazole antifungals in nonmeningeal endemic mycoses and is indicated for treatment of oropharyngeal and vaginal *Candida* infection.

Fluconazole. Available in IV and oral forms. Minimally bound to serum proteins. Excellent penetration into the CSF, brain, and eye. Dose adjustment required for renal dysfunction, including hemodialysis. Fluconazole is very well tolerated. Nevertheless, interactions with astemizole, cisapride, and rifampin should be noted. The drug of choice for coccidioidal meningitis, for maintenance therapy of cryptococcal meningitis, for oropharyngeal and vaginal *Candida* infection.

Itraconazole. Structurally related to ketoconazole. Only available orally. Gastric acidity is vital for absorption (in capsule formulation). It is highly protein bound (95%). Concentrations in body tissue, including the brain, are two to ten times serum levels. Itraconazole is extensively metabolized by the liver. It is well tolerated; most adverse reactions are transient; it is devoid of effects on mammalian steroidogenesis. Several clinically important drug interactions exist. Use of lipid-lowering agents lovastatin and simvastatin is contraindicated. Itraconazole has excellent activity against dermatophyte infections; treatment of choice for sporotrichosis and nonmeningeal paracoccidioidomycosis, blastomycosis, and histoplasmosis in nonimmunosuppressed patients.

Allylamine Derivatives

Terbinafine. This and other allylamines inhibit ergosterol biosynthesis at the level of squalene epoxidase. Available as topical and oral formulations. It is 99% protein bound and is extensively metabolized. Terbinafine has excellent activity against dermatophytes; one of the treatment regimens of choice for onychomycosis. Possesses excellent in vitro activity against *Aspergillus* spp., *Fusarium* spp., many other filamentous fungi, dimorphic fungi, and *Pneumocystis carinii*. Activity is more variable against *Candida* spp. and other yeasts. Terbinafine is not metabolized via the cytochrome P-450 enzyme system; thus potential for drug interactions is diminished. Common adverse effects are diarrhea, dyspepsia, nausea, and mild elevations in hepatic transaminase levels.

Miscellaneous Compounds

Flucytosine (5-FC). Flucytosine, chemically related to fluorouracil, is available only in oral formulation. It is transported into cells by the fungus-specific enzyme cytosine permease and converted in the cytoplasm by cytosine deaminase to 5-fluorouracil (5-FU). 5-FU is phosphorylated and incorporated into RNA, where it causes miscoding and is converted to its deoxynucleoside, which inhibits thymidylate synthetase and thereby DNA synthesis. Rapidly and almost completely absorbed, negligible protein binding, and distributed throughout the body. CSF levels typically are 60%–90% of serum concentration. Approximately 90% is excreted unchanged. Dosage adjustment required for renal, but not hepatic, dysfunction. The most serious toxicity is bone marrow suppression. Monitoring serum concentrations is essential as 5-FC is usually coadministered with AmB, which will induce changes in renal function. The anticancer drug cytosine arabinoside competitively inhibits action of 5-FC; these agents should not be used concomitantly.

57 Antihelminthic Agents

Steven P. Gelone, Pharm.D.

Some Common Human Helminthic Parasites

Name	Common name	Disease-producing form/source	How infection occurs	Major disease manifestation/diagnosis
Ascaris lumbricoides	Large-intestinal roundworm	Adult worms in colon; eggs on perianal region	Eggs are transferred from hand to mouth	Perianal itching/eggs found by cellophane test
Capillaria philippinensis	Capillariasis	Source: fish	Ingestion of infected, raw fish	Malabsorption syndrome, extreme diarrhea/adults multiply and cause blockage
Echinococcus granulosus	Dog tapeworm	Source: canine species intermediate host, sheep	Accidental ingestion of eggs by close contact with an infected dog	Cough, chest pain, eosinophilia/ cyst most commonly found in liver
Schistosoma mansoni	Manson's blood fluke; swamp fever	Adult in colon; eggs trapped in liver	Organism burrows into the capillary bed of feet, legs, or arms	Granuloma formation around eggs (liver, intestine, bladder)
Strongyloides stercoralis	Threadworm	Larval migration: pulmonary signs; adults: small intestine	Infective larva penetrate host skin (usually feet)	Dermatitis, abdominal pain, moderate eosinophilia/ larvae in feces
Toxocara species	Toxocariasis; visceral larval migrans (VLM)	Source: dog, cat	Ingestion of infective larvae from soil	Eosinophilia, hepatomegaly, cough, fever, cyst in eye that mimics retinoblastoma

Representative Life Cycle Diagrams

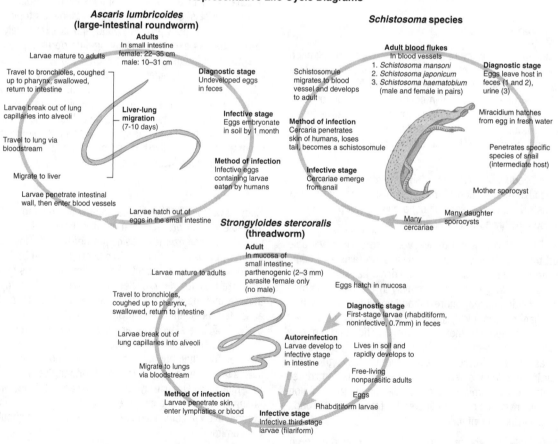

Ascaris lumbricoides (large-intestinal roundworm)

Adults
In small intestine
female: 22–35 cm
male: 10–31 cm

Larvae mature to adults

Travel to bronchioles, coughed up to pharynx, swallowed, return to intestine

Diagnostic stage
Undeveloped eggs in feces

Larvae break out of lung capillaries into alveoli

Liver-lung migration
(7-10 days)

Infective stage
Eggs embryonate in soil by 1 month

Travel to lung via bloodstream

Migrate to liver

Method of infection
Infective eggs containing larvae eaten by humans

Larvae penetrate intestinal wall, then enter blood vessels

Larvae hatch out of eggs in the small intestine

Schistosoma species

Adult blood flukes
In blood vessels
1. *Schistosoma mansoni*
2. *Schistosoma japonicum*
3. *Schistosoma haematobium*
(male and female in pairs)

Schistosomule migrates to blood vessel and develops to adult

Diagnostic stage
Eggs leave host in feces (1 and 2), urine (3)

Miracidium hatches from egg in fresh water

Method of infection
Cercaria penetrates skin of humans, loses tail, becomes a schistosomule

Penetrates specific species of snail (intermediate host)

Infective stage
Cercariae emerge from snail

Mother sporocyst

Many cercariae

Many daughter sporocysts

Strongyloides stercoralis (threadworm)

Adult
In mucosa of small intestine; parthenogenic (2–3 mm) parasite female only (no male)

Larvae mature to adults

Eggs hatch in mucosa

Travel to bronchioles, coughed up to pharynx, swallowed, return to intestine

Diagnostic stage
First-stage larvae (rhabditiform, noninfective, 0.7mm) in feces

Larvae break out of lung capillaries into alveoli

Autoreinfection
Larvae develop to infective stage in intestine

Lives in soil and rapidly develops to

Migrate to lungs via bloodstream

Free-living nonparasitic adults

Method of infection
Larvae penetrate skin, enter lymphatics or blood

Eggs

Rhabditiform larvae

Infective stage
Infective third-stage larvae (filariform)

OVERVIEW

- Helminth infection is a growing problem in the United States, likely secondary to increased travel and immigration.
- The benzimidazole derivatives constitute the largest class of antihelminthic agents.

Benzimidazole Derivatives

The mechanism of action appears to be specific, high-affinity binding to free β-tubulin in parasite cells, resulting in selective inhibition of parasite microtubule polymerization and inhibition of microtubule uptake of glucose. This appears to result in endogenous glycogen depletion. Benzimidazoles bind to β-tubulin of parasites at much lower concentrations than to mammalian β-tubulin.

Albendazole (Albenza). Albendazole is administered orally with food. Therapy has been associated with seizures or hydrocephalus (the use of concomitant corticosteroid and anticonvulsant therapy should be strongly considered). It is also indicated for the treatment of hydatid disease. Adverse effects include increases in hepatic enzymes and, rarely, effects on the bone marrow such as neutropenia.

Mebendazole (Vermox). Mebendazole is minimally absorbed from the GI tract. It is highly protein bound and eliminated via decarboxylation to an inactive metabolite. Mebendazole has a broad range of indications: for treatment of pinworm, capillariasis, and hydatid disease. Nausea, vomiting, headache, tinnitus, numbness, and dizziness have been reported. Noteworthy drug interactions include phenytoin and carbamazepine, which induce the metabolism of mebendazole and decrease levels, and cimetidine, which inhibits mebendazole's metabolism.

Thiabendazole (Mintezol). Thiabendazole is rapidly absorbed from the GI tract and can be absorbed through the skin. It is extensively metabolized via hydroxylation and subsequently conjugated with sulfuric acid or glucuronic acid. Adverse effects usually are mild and self-limited. The most frequent are anorexia, nausea, vomiting, and dizziness. Seizures, vertigo, paresthesia, and psychic disturbances may occur.

Other Agents

Ivermectin (Stromectol). A derivative of avermectin B_1, a macrocyclic lactone produced by the actinomycete *Streptomyces avermitilis.* Active in low doses against a broad range of nematodes and blood-sucking arthropod parasites. Blocks signal transmission from interneurons to excitatory motor neurons. GABA is the neurotransmitter that is blocked, but ivermectin does not appear to compete with GABA for binding and does not bind directly to the GABA binding site. It is highly protein bound and concentrates in the liver and adipose tissue. Only a small percentage is excreted in the urine. In general, ivermectin is well tolerated. When used for onchocerciasis, it may cause fever, headache, peripheral edema, tachycardia, and orthostatic hypertension. When used for strongyloidiasis, it may cause GI disturbances, pruritus, and dizziness.

Oxamniquine (Vansil). A semisynthetic tetrahydroquinine derivative used in the treatment of schistosomal infection. It causes the worms to be dislodged from their usual site of residence in the mesenteric veins to the liver, where they are retained and subsequently killed by host–tissue reactions. The dislodgment appears to occur 2–6 days after a single dose, principally as a result of contraction and paralysis of their musculature and immobilization of their suckers. There is significant interpatient variability in absorption, which may be secondary to biodegradation of the drug in the GI mucosa. Oxamniquine and praziquantel may be synergistic against *Schistosoma mansoni.* Adverse effects are usually mild. Nervous system effects are seen most commonly, with dizziness, drowsiness, and headache occurring in 30%–50% of patients. In patients with a history of seizure disorders, the drug should be used with caution.

Piperazine Citrate. Piperazine exerts its antihelminthic effect against *Ascaris lumbricoides* by blocking the stimulatory effects of ACh at the myoneural junction through hyperpolarization of the muscle membrane and suppression of spontaneous spike potentials. The paralyzed worms are expelled from the GI tract by normal peristalsis. Piperazine is well absorbed from the GI tract. Adverse effects include nausea, vomiting, diarrhea, and abdominal cramps; headache occurs occasionally. The drug may cause hemolytic anemia. The concomitant use of chlorpromazine and piperazine may cause seizures. Pyrantel pamoate and piperazine are antagonistic and should not be administered together.

Praziquantel (Biltricide). Praziquantel is a synthetic pyrazinoisoquinoline derivative structurally unrelated to other antihelminthic agents. It kills susceptible adult schistosomes and causes the dead or dying worm to be dislodged from its usual residence in the mesenteric veins to the liver, where it elicits a host–tissue reaction. The drug appears to increase the permeability of the cell membrane of the worms to calcium, which leads to paralysis. The drug has broad-spectrum activity against trematodes, such as *Schistosoma,* and cestodes (tapeworms). Praziquantel is well absorbed from the GI tract but undergoes significant first-pass metabolism. Adverse effects occur frequently but are usually mild and transient. Dizziness, headache, malaise, and abdominal pain occur in up to 90% of patients. CSF reaction (including headache, seizures, increased CSF protein, hyperthermia, meningism) may occur in the treatment of neurocysticercosis and may be minimized by the use of corticosteriods. GI reactions, especially abdominal pain, may be severe. Praziquantel distributes to breast milk. Synergy with oxamniquine against schistosomes has been described.

Pyrantel Pamoate. Pyrantel pamoate is a pyrimidine derivative. It is a depolarizing neuromuscular blocking agent that exerts its effect via release of ACh and inhibition of cholinesterase, resulting in stimulation of nicotinic receptors of susceptible helminths. Unlike piperazine, pyrantel produces depolarization of the muscle membrane and increases spike discharge frequency. The paralyzed worms are expelled from the GI tract by normal peristalsis. Pyrantel pamoate is poorly absorbed from the GI tract. It is partially metabolized by the liver. Adverse effects are usually mild, infrequent, and disappear when the drug is discontinued. Pyrantel should not be used concomitantly with piperazine, as their effects are antagonistic. It is not recommended for use in children under 2 years of age.

58 Antiviral Agents

Daniel H. Havlichek, Jr., M.D.

Sites of action of antiviral agents

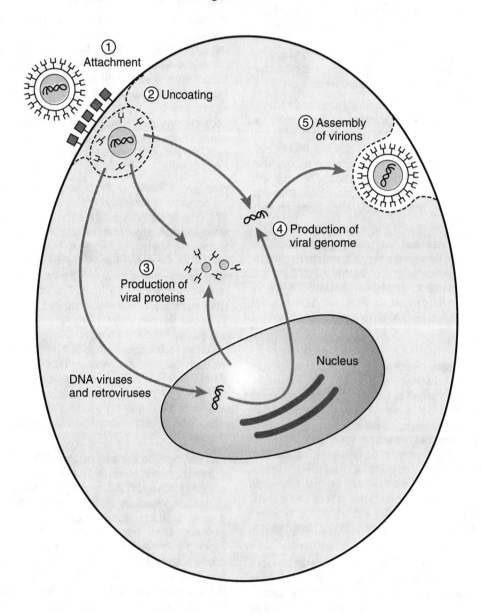

OVERVIEW

- Antiviral agents work by inhibiting any of a number of steps in viral replication.
- Antiviral agents may prevent attachment of viral particles to susceptible cells, prevent uncoating of viral particles, inhibit viral DNA or RNA synthesis, inhibit enzymes necessary for viral assembly, or modulate the immune system to slow viral growth.
- Since antiviral agents slow but do not generally stop viral growth, they work best in immunocompetent patients.
- Prolonged use of antiviral agents can result in viral resistance.

Pharmacology

An antiviral agent's usefulness is affected by its ability to penetrate infected cells specifically and to cause limited toxicity to uninfected cells. In some instances specific viral enzymes activate an antiviral agent, causing high concentrations of the active compound to accumulate inside infected cells. For example, herpes simplex virus possesses a unique thymidine kinase that monophosphorylates acyclovir and related compounds, resulting in significantly greater accumulation in infected cells.

Medicinal Chemistry

Many antiviral agents are inhibitors of DNA or RNA synthesis and are nucleic acid analogs. Examples include many inhibitors of HIV reverse transcriptase, many antiherpesvirus compounds, and ribavirin. These medications require triphosphorylation of the active compound. This is usually done by cellular kinases. Antiviral agents for influenza A prevent uncoating of the viral particles and therefore inhibit tissue damage and virus growth. Interferons act by stimulating both the immune system against the virus and the development of intracellular antiviral proteins. Since most antiviral agents are inhibitors of viral growth, an intact immune system is necessary for optimal response, and immunosuppressed patients often need chronic suppressive therapy to prevent reactivation of latent viral infections.

Pharmacokinetics

Administration and Distribution. Antiviral agents are primarily administered orally, although some agents such as foscarnet are only available intravenously. Ribavirin is administered as an aerosol for children with severe respiratory syncytial virus infection. Some compounds are extremely acid-sensitive and are formulated with antacid buffer (didanosine). Saquinavir is better absorbed with food. Compounds that resemble nucleic acids are primarily excreted by the kidney, and dosage adjustments are necessary in renal failure. Interferons are administered intralesionally or systemically. The effect of interferons is not related to their serum half-life, since their biologic effect lasts several days.

In many patients with significant immunosuppression, antiviral agents are used in combination. This is especially true in HIV-infected persons, where nucleoside reverse transcriptase inhibitors combined with protease inhibitors have significant advantages over individual agents. The role of nonnucleoside reverse transcriptase inhibitors and multiple protease inhibitors combined with nucleoside inhibitors in managing HIV infection is being investigated. HIV protease inhibitors

may affect hepatic metabolism of many other medications, and dosage adjustments are often necessary. Agents that delay the excretion of nucleic acids (probenecid) increase the serum concentration of nucleic acid antiviral agents.

Toxicity

Bone marrow suppression is a common side effect of nucleic acid analogs. This is, in general, a dose-related phenomenon. In HIV-infected persons peripheral neuropathy and pancreatitis are common side effects of nucleic acid analogs. Use of HIV protease inhibitors has been associated with bleeding in hemophiliac patients. Agents excreted by the kidney may cause renal stones, and adequate hydration should be maintained. Nucleic acid analogs are not well studied in pregnancy, and their use should be avoided unless clearly indicated. Frequent side effects of these medications also include nausea, vomiting, and headache.

Amantadine and rimantadine penetrate the blood-brain barrier and can cause nervousness and anxiety. Foscarnet binds divalent cations and can result in severe hypocalcemia or hypomagnesemia with resultant arrhythmia or seizures. Cidofovir and foscarnet can cause renal insufficiency, and ganciclovir causes bone marrow suppression. Interferons elicit an influenza-like syndrome in most persons receiving them, and this may prevent successful therapy.

SPECIFIC AGENTS

Anti-influenza agents
Rimantadine and amantadine

Antiherpesvirus agents
Acyclovir, valacyclovir, famciclovir, ganciclovir, foscarnet, cidofovir

Anti-HIV agents
Nucleoside reverse transcriptase inhibitors
  didanosine (ddl), dideoxycytidine (ddC), lamivudine (3TC), stavudine (d4T), zidovudine (ZDV, formerly AZT)
Nonnucleoside reverse transcriptase Inhibitors
  Delaviridine, nevirapine
Protease inhibitors
  Indinavir, nelfinavir, ritonavir, saquinavir

Nonspecific
Ribavirin, interferons

Antineoplastic Agents

James M. Larner, M.D.

A   Cell-cycle specific agents

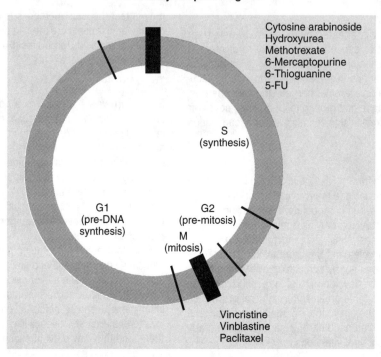

Cytosine arabinoside
Hydroxyurea
Methotrexate
6-Mercaptopurine
6-Thioguanine
5-FU

S
(synthesis)

G1
(pre-DNA
synthesis)

G2
(pre-mitosis)

M
(mitosis)

Vincristine
Vinblastine
Paclitaxel

B   Nonspecific agents and mechanism of action of all agents

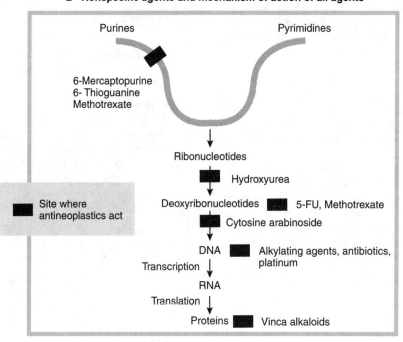

Purines

Pyrimidines

6-Mercaptopurine
6- Thioguanine
Methotrexate

Ribonucleotides

Hydroxyurea

■ Site where
antineoplastics act

Deoxyribonucleotides   5-FU, Methotrexate

Cytosine arabinoside

DNA   Alkylating agents, antibiotics,
platinum

Transcription

RNA

Translation

Proteins   Vinca alkaloids

OVERVIEW

- Cancer is a leading cause of death in the United States, second only to heart disease.
- Antineoplastic agents, along with surgery, radiation therapy, and more recently, immunotherapy and gene therapy, are the only known effective treatments for cancer.
- Chemotherapy can either be given for palliation (relief of symptoms) or with curative intent. Frequently chemotherapy is given as an adjuvant to surgery in the absence of any detectable disease with the hope of curing micrometastatic disease.
- Occasionally antineoplastic agents are given for benign hyperproliferative conditions such as severe psoriasis or rheumatoid arthritis.
- Death of rapidly dividing cells in normal tissues such as bone marrow, gonads, intestine, and hair follicles are responsible for most of the acute toxicity. Normal tissue and tumor cells undergo programmed cell death (apoptosis) or necrosis in response to chemotherapy.

Pharmacology

Antineoplastic agents have diverse mechanisms of action. In general antineoplastics are divided into the four classes: alkylating agents, antimetabolites, plant alkaloids, and antibiotics. Representative drugs from each class are discussed below. For mechanisms of action see the figure, where they are depicted in terms of cell-cycle-specific versus nonspecific mechanisms. Adaptive cellular responses to antineoplastics include not only increasing intrinsic resistance (table) but also activation of signaling pathways and cell-cycle checkpoints.

POTENTIAL MECHANISMS OF RESISTANCE

- Decrease uptake or increase efflux
- Enhance conversion to inactive metabolite
- Alter drug target
- Amplify gene or increase transcription of target protein
- Alter metabolism (GSH, etc.)
- Enhance DNA repair

Antineoplastic Agents

Alkylating Agents

Alkylating agents bind covalently to DNA (frequently the N-7 position of guanine) through a moiety that includes an ethylene ammonium ion. The resulting adducts on DNA impede both replication and transcription, leading to cell death.

Mechlorethamine. This nitrogen mustard is the prototype alklating agent and is active in lymphoma.

Melphalan. Similar to mechlorethamine. Used frequently in myeloma.

Cyclophosphamide. The most widely used alkylating agent. Can cause hemorrhagic cystitis and cardiac toxicity.

Carmustine (BCNU) and Lomustine (CCNU). Both agents are nitrosoureas and are active in CNS tumors since they cross the blood-brain barrier. Major toxicity is delayed myelosuppression.

Dacarbazine (DTIC). Useful in melanoma and Hodgkin's disease. Myelosuppression is the major toxicity.

Antimetabolites

These agents function by competing with critical precursors of DNA and RNA synthesis, thereby inhibiting cellular proliferation.

Methotrexate. Inhibits dihydrofolate reductase, depleting intracellular reduced folates necessary for DNA synthesis. Useful in leukemia, head and neck, and breast cancer.

Cytarabine. A cytidine analog highly active in acute myelogenous leukemia.

Fluorouracil (5-FU). A uracil analog that inhibits thymidylate synthase, thereby depleting dTTP and inhibiting DNA synthesis.

Mercaptopurine and thioguanine. Purine analogs useful in the treatment of leukemias.

Plant Alkaloids

Plant alkaloids are natural products that inhibit microtubular formation and topoisomerase function, thus blocking cell division and DNA replication. Topoisomerases modify the topology of DNA, allowing regions of DNA to become uncoiled to facilitate replication and transcription.

Vincristine and Vinblastine. Vincristine and vinblastine block microtubular formation, resulting in the inability of the daughter cells to segregate properly in mitosis. Both are useful in leukemias and breast and CNS tumors. The principal toxicity is peripheral neuropathy.

Paclitaxel. Originally isolated from the bark of the yew tree, paclitaxel has the opposite effect on microtubule aggregation to that of the vinca alkaloids. It stabilizes microtubular formation and impairs segregation of the daughter nuclei. It is active in lung and breast cancer. Dose-limiting toxicities are myelosuppression and peripheral neurotoxicity.

Etoposide. A topoisomerase-2 inhibitor, etoposide has activity in lung and testicular cancers, lymphomas, and leukemias. It is derived from podophyllotoxin, which was originally extracted from the mandrake plant.

Topotecan. Topotecan is a topoisomerase-1 inhibitor that is a derivative of the plant alkaloid 20(S) camptothecin. It is active in colorectal cancer but has substantial GI toxicity.

Antibiotics

The antibiotics, also natural products, were originally isolated from various species of *Streptomyces* and intercalate with DNA, inhibiting both DNA and RNA synthesis.

Daunorubicin, Doxorubicin, and Idarubicin. These anthracycline antibiotics have a tetracycline ring structure with a sugar attached by a glycosidic linkage. They are useful in a wide variety of cancers including hematologic and breast cancer and sarcomas. Cardiomyopathy is a unique toxicity of these drugs.

Bleomycin. Bleomycin causes scission of DNA. It is active in germ cell tumors and lymphomas.

Directions: For each of the following questions, choose the **one best** answer.

1. Which of the following antifungal drugs is incorporated into fungus RNA?

(A) Amphotericin B

(B) Clotrimazole

(C) Flucytosine

(D) Terbinafine

2. Which one of the following statements most accurately describes the antibacterial mode of action of β-lactam antibiotics?

(A) They bind to the 30S subunit of the bacterial ribosome and prevent the cell from synthesizing proteins.

(B) They inhibit the transpeptidation reaction that is responsible for cross-linking the peptide side chains of the polysaccharide peptidoglycan backbone.

(C) They inhibit enzymes called autolysins, which are involved in the degradation of bacterial peptidoglycan.

(D) They act as structural analogs of NAM peptides by forming an irreversible penicilloyl-enzyme complex during the final stages of transglycosylation.

(E) They inhibit bacterial growth by inhibiting bacterial β-lactamases, which belong to a group of proteins called penicillin-binding proteins (PBPs).

3. Macrolides perform which of the following actions?

(A) They bind to the 30S subunit of bacterial ribosomes.

(B) They bind to the 40S subunit of bacterial ribosomes.

(C) They bind to the 50S subunit of bacterial ribosomes.

(D) They enhance formation of the initiation complex.

(E) They enhance the translocation step.

4. Which of the following antiviral agents is only available intravenously?

(A) Foscarnet

(B) Retonavir

(C) Ribavirin

(D) Saquinavir

5. Which of the following statements regarding sulfonamides and trimethoprim is correct?

(A) The sulfonamides antagonize the actions of trimethoprim.

(B) The combination is no longer used because of serious adverse effects.

(C) There are much better choices for treating bacterial infections.

(D) They act at different sites of folate synthesis and thereby exert selective toxicity.

6. Bacterial resistance to a number of antibiotics such as β-lactams is becoming a major worldwide health problem. Which one of the following statements concerning the major causes of resistance to β-lactams is correct?

(A) Hydrolysis of the β-lactam ring structure by β-lactamases is the major cause of bacterial resistance to β-lactam antibiotics.

(B) Methicillin-resistant *Staphylococcus aureus* (MRSA) strains show reduced permeability to the drug, preventing it from passing through the cell wall and reaching its target PBPs.

(C) β-Lactamase inhibitor combinations are successful in treating MRSA infections because they have a much higher affinity for cells with altered PBPs.

(D) Carbapenems are effective against resistant bacterial strains because of their increased susceptibility to β-lactamases.

(E) β-Lactam antibiotics that stimulate bacterial autolysins become more resistant to the lytic action of the drug.

7. Methotrexate is given with several other drugs to a 7-year-old boy with acute leukemia. Although the patient originally achieves a complete remission, he develops CNS leukemia while being consolidated with methotrexate, implying that his disease is resistant to methotrexate. Which of the following observations concerning leukemia cells harvested from the CSF support the claim that this child's disease is truly resistant to methotrexate?

(A) 100x amplification of the dihydrofolate reductase (DHFR) gene by fluorescence in situ hybridization

(B) Loss of both copies of the DHFR gene by fluorescence in situ hybridization

(C) 100x amplification of the ribonucleotide reductase gene by fluorescence in situ hybridization

(D) Loss of both copies of the ribonucleotide reductase gene by fluorescence in situ hybridization

8. Which one of the following agents binds to free β-tubulin in parasite cells and inhibits microtubule polymerization and glucose uptake?

(A) Stromectol

(B) Albendazole

(C) Piperazine

(D) Biltricide

9. Hallucinations and seizures are recognized side effects of

(A) methenamine

(B) phenazopyridine

(C) quinolones

(D) fluconazole

(E) trimethoprim-sulfamethoxazole

10. Which of the following drugs has poor oral availability?

(A) Ethambutol

(B) Isoniazid

(C) Pyrazinamide

(D) Rifampin

(E) Streptomycin

11. The sulfonamide most often combined with trimethoprim is

(A) mafenide

(B) sulfadiazine

(C) sulfamethoxazole

(D) sulfisoxazole

12. The primary mechanism of action of amphotericin B and nystatin antifungals is

(A) binding to ergosterol

(B) binding to cholesterol

(C) inhibition of conversion of lanosterol to ergosterol

(D) inhibition of ergosterol biosynthesis

13. Which of the following agents penetrates inflamed meninges only?

(A) Ethambutol

(B) Isoniazid

(C) Pyrazinamide

(D) Rifampin

14. A 24-year-old woman presented with an enlarged left neck node, and a biopsy established a diagnosis of non-Hodgkin's lymphoma. She was treated with six cycles of cyclophosphamide, doxorubicin, vincristine, and prednisone (CHOP) and had a complete remission. An inexperienced physician administered three additional cycles of CHOP "just to be sure she is cured." One year later she is disease free but has shortness of breath. A chest radiograph shows an enlarged heart and evidence of congestive heart failure (CHF). A cardiac catherization shows an enlarged heart with poor ventricular function but no evidence of coronary disease. The drug most likely to produce this patient's symptoms is

(A) vincristine

(B) doxorubicin

(C) cyclophosphamide

(D) prednisone

(E) vincristine plus prednisone

15. What is the usual adverse effect responsible for discontinuance of macrolides?

(A) Nephrotoxicity

(B) Ototoxicity

(C) Gastrointestinal intolerance

(D) Discoloration of teeth

(E) Depressed bone growth

16. The best match of drug and adverse effect is

(A) amantadine: sedation, depression

(B) foscarnet: hypercalcemia

(C) interferons: flu-like symptoms

(D) nucleic acid analogs: leukocytosis

17. All of the following statements about the mechanism of action of antimicrobial agents are true EXCEPT

(A) oral amphotericin can be used for the treatment of fungal urinary tract infections (UTIs) by virtue of its forming pores or channels in fungal cell membranes

(B) oral quinolone antibiotics act via inhibition of bacterial DNA gyrase

(C) the target of orally administered β-lactam antibiotics is synthesis of the bacterial cell wall

(D) methenamine's antimicrobial activity is due to its conversion after oral administration to formaldehyde

(E) after oral administration, nitrofurantoin is activated by bacteria in the urine

PART VI: ANSWERS AND EXPLANATIONS

1. The answer is C.

Flucytosine is transported into susceptible fungal cells by the enzyme cytosine permease and is converted by cytosine deaminase to 5-fluorouracil, which is phosphorylated and incorporated into RNA, causing miscoding. Mammalian cells are less affected, since they have little or no cytosine deaminase. Amphotericin B is a polyene derivative antifungal agent, which binds to ergosterol. Clotrimazole is an azole derivative, which inhibits the conversion of lanosterol to ergosterol. Terbinafine is an allylamine derivative, which inhibits ergosterol biosynthesis.

2. The answer is B.

Peptidoglycan is an essential component of the bacterial cell wall. Most β-lactams inhibit a set of transpeptidases that catalyze the final cross-linking reactions in the synthesis of the cell wall. Binding of β-lactams to PBPs leads to the stimulation of autolysins, which attack peptidoglycan.

3. The answer is C.

Macrolides bind to the 50S subunit of bacterial ribosomes and block formation of the initiation complex and the translocation step. Aminoglycosides diffuse across the outer membrane through porin channels and bind to the 30S subunit of bacterial ribosomes (but not the 40S subunit present in mammals). Irreversible and lethal inhibition of protein synthesis occurs by interference with proper attachment of mRNA, misreading of mRNA (incorporation of incorrect amino acid sequences), and other actions. Tetracyclines bind reversibly to the 30S subunit of bacterial ribosomes and block the binding of aminoacyl-tRNA to the acceptor site on the mRNA-ribosome complex, preventing the addition of amino acids to the growing peptide.

4. The answer is A.

Foscarnet is only available as an intravenous injection. Antiviral agents are primarily administered orally; some, such as saquinavir, are better absorbed with food. Ribavirin can also be administered as an aerosol for children with severe respiratory syncytial virus infection.

5. The answer is D.

The combination of sulfonamides with trimethoprim is still widely used for treating a variety of bacterial infections as well as for treating *Pneumocystis carinii* infection.

6. The answer is A.

β-Lactamases have had a significant impact on bacterial resistance to β-lactams. This has led to chemical modification efforts producing many semisynthetic β-lactam derivatives with increased stability to β-lactamases; for example, the discovery of the β-lactamase inhibitor clavulanic acid led to amoxicillin–clavulanate combination therapy to treat infections caused by β-lactamase-producing organisms.

7. The answer is A.

Several different mechanisms exist by which cells develop resistance to antineoplastics. The target protein of methotrexate is the protein DHFR. By amplifying, the DHFR gene cells produce more DHFR protein and therefore become resistant to methotrexate. Since ribonucleotide reductase is the target of hydroxyurea, it would not be expected to amplify in response to a methotrexate challenge.

8. The answer is B.

Albendazole is an anthelminthic agent. Its mechanism of action is specific, high-affinity binding to free β-tubulin in parasite cells, resulting in inhibition of parasite microtubule polymerization and inhibition of glucose uptake.

9. The answer is C.

Patients receiving quinolone antibiotics who are also receiving theophylline or a nonsteroidal anti-inflammatory drug have been observed on rare occasions to have seizures and hallucinations.

10. The answer is E.

Streptomycin is available for intramuscular injection (although it has been administered intravenously). The requirement for parenteral administration of streptomycin has resulted in its replacement in most situations by other agents. The other antimycobacterial agents listed, ethambutol, isoniazid, pyrazinamide, and rifampin, are well absorbed orally.

11. The answer is C.

Trimethoprim is most often used in combination with sulfamethoxazole (e.g., Septra, Bactrim). Mafenide is a topically active sulfonamide useful for treatment of burn patients. Sulfadiazine and sulfisoxazole are short-acting sulfonamides.

12. The answer is A.

Ergosterol is the principal sterol in the cell membrane of sensitive fungi. Binding results in disorganization of the membrane, depolarization, increase in permeability, and cell death. The drugs also bind to cholesterol, and this accounts for much of their toxicity to mammalian cells. Inhibition of conversion of lanosterol to ergosterol is the major mechanism of action of antifungal azole derivatives. Inhibition of ergosterol biosynthesis is the major mechanism of action of antifungal allylamine derivatives.

13. The answer is A.

Ethambutol is well absorbed and distributes widely throughout the body. Little crosses normal meninges, but levels at 10%–50% of plasma levels are achieved in the presence of meningeal inflammation. The other antimycobacterial agents listed, isoniazid, pyrazinamide, and rifampin, readily cross the blood–brain barrier.

14. The answer is B.

This patient suffered from congestive cardiomyopathy, which is known to be a complication of the anthracyclines. Two forms of anthracycline cardiac toxicity exist. An acute form, which is rarely a serious clinical problem, consists of ECG changes and arrhythmias. The more serious form, from which this patient suffered, is a cumulative dose-related toxicity manifested by CHF that is unresponsive to digitalis. The mortality rate for CHF secondary to the anthracyclines is greater than 50%. Vincristine produces peripheral neuropathy, while cyclophosphamide can cause hemorrhagic cystitis. There has been recent interest in reducing anthracycline cardiac toxicity with the concomitant administration of an iron chelator.

15. The answer is C.

Macrolides such as erythromycin have a relatively low incidence of serious toxicity. Gastrointestinal intolerance is usually the major reason for discontinuance. Reversible acute cholestatic hepatitis, thrombophlebitis (intravenous), and drug–drug interactions by means of interference with hepatic metabolism of other drugs can occur. Aminoglycosides can cause nephrotoxicity and ototoxicity, neuromuscular block (high doses or combination with nicotinic ACh receptor antagonists), and infrequent hypersensitivity reactions. Tetracyclines produce uncommon hypersensitivity reactions, local irritation (oral, intravenous, intramuscular), liver dysfunction (particularly in pregnancy), and in children, discoloration of teeth and depressed bone growth.

16. The answer is C.

Interferons often elicit influenza-like symptoms that can interfere with successful therapy. Amantadine penetrates the blood–brain barrier and can cause nervousness and anxiety (not sedation and depression). Foscarnet binds divalent cations and can produce severe *hypo*calcemia or hypomagnesemia that results in arrhythmias or seizures. Bone marrow suppression is a relatively common side effect of nucleic acid analogs.

17. The answer is A.

Amphotericin is not appreciably absorbed after oral administration. Fungal UTIs can be treated with oral fluconazole or by bladder irrigation with, or intravenous administration of, amphotericin B.

PART VII
Endocrine Pharmacology

60 Hypothalamic and Pituitary Hormones

Marie C. Kerbeshian, Ph.D., and William S. Evans, M.D.

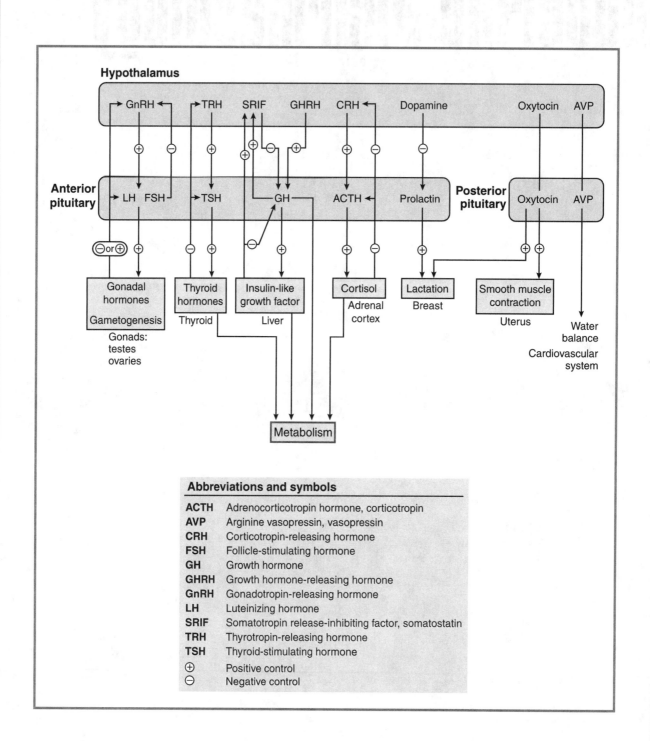

Abbreviations and symbols

ACTH	Adrenocorticotropin hormone, corticotropin
AVP	Arginine vasopressin, vasopressin
CRH	Corticotropin-releasing hormone
FSH	Follicle-stimulating hormone
GH	Growth hormone
GHRH	Growth hormone-releasing hormone
GnRH	Gonadotropin-releasing hormone
LH	Luteinizing hormone
SRIF	Somatotropin release-inhibiting factor, somatostatin
TRH	Thyrotropin-releasing hormone
TSH	Thyroid-stimulating hormone
⊕	Positive control
⊖	Negative control

- Hypothalamic peptides and biogenic amines stimulate or inhibit release of hormones from the anterior pituitary.
- Anterior pituitary hormones stimulate hormone release by peripheral target organs.
- Target organ hormones can stimulate or inhibit hypothalamic and anterior pituitary hormone release.
- Posterior pituitary (neurohypophysis) hormones are produced in hypothalamic cell bodies, transported through the cell axons to the posterior pituitary, and released into circulation.
- Clinical use of TRH, TSH, CRH, and ACTH is diagnostic and is not discussed further.

Physiology and Process

Gonadotropin-releasing hormone (GnRH) is released in a pulsatile manner from the hypothalamus; this pulsatile release is necessary for normal function. GnRH triggers the release of luteinizing hormone (LH) and follicle-stimulating hormone (FSH) from the anterior pituitary. Continuous administration of long-acting GnRH agonists down-regulates pituitary receptors and suppresses LH release.

In women, LH and FSH pulses from the anterior pituitary regulate ovarian estrogen production, follicular growth, and ovulation. In men, they stimulate testosterone production and spermatogenesis in the testes.

The hypothalamic hormones growth hormone–releasing hormone (GHRH) and somatostatin (somatotropin release–inhibiting factor, SRIF) regulate anterior pituitary secretion of growth hormone (GH). GHRH stimulates GH release; GH indirectly stimulates somatostatin release. Somatostatin then suppresses GH release. Somatostatin is also produced elsewhere (e.g., in the nervous system and the gut). It has a variety of effects depending on its site of production.

GH governs linear growth and aspects of metabolism. It stimulates the liver's production of insulin-like growth factor 1, amino acid incorporation into muscle and adipose tissue protein, and lipolysis in adipose tissue.

Hypothalamic dopamine inhibits prolactin release from the anterior pituitary.

Arginine vasopressin (AVP) is released from the posterior pituitary. It is the primary antidiuretic hormone (ADH), influencing water balance and the cardiovascular system. It stimulates the production of antihemophilic factor (factor VIII).

Oxytocin is released from the posterior pituitary. It works with prostaglandins to stimulate uterine contractions during the later stages of labor. Cervical stretch during labor acts to stimulate further release of oxytocin. Oxytocin also triggers the milk ejection reflex in lactating women.

Clinical Correlations

GnRH. Replacement is used in cases of abnormalities of the GnRH pulse generator to treat primary hypothalamic amenorrhea in women; pulsatile administration with a portable infusion pump stimulates ovulation. In men, idiopathic hypogonadotropic hypogonadism is treated with pulsatile administration, which leads to testosterone secretion and spermatogenesis.

GnRH Agonists. Continuous administration suppresses LH; it is employed for medical gonadectomy in men with advanced prostatic cancer, women with endometriosis, and children with precocious puberty. It can be coadministered with the antiandrogen flutamide to suppress the initial increase in gonadal hormones.

LH and FSH. Human menopausal gonadotropin is used to promote follicular growth and ovulation in women and spermatogenesis in men with hypothalamic or pituitary deficits. It also bypasses the normal hypothalamic-pituitary-ovarian feedback loop, which can lead to ovarian hyperstimulation and possibly multiple pregnancies.

Clomiphene citrate is a nonsteroidal stimulator of LH and FSH that avoids problems of human menopausal gonadotropin and is often the first treatment used to induce ovulation.

Urofollitropin, highly purified FSH, is given to women with polycystic ovary syndrome who do not respond to clomiphene.

GHRH and SRIF. These are not approved for therapeutic use in the United States. In trials, GHRH promotes linear growth in GH-deficient children, and SRIF decreases GH in patients with acromegaly.

Octreotide, an SRIF agonist approved for therapeutic use, treats a variety of neuroendocrine tumors.

GH. Produced by recombinant DNA technology, GH promotes linear growth in children with GH deficiency, chronic renal insufficiency, and Turner syndrome. It has no major effect on short children with normal GH levels.

Dopamine. These agonists terminate lactation from physiologic hyperprolactinemia in nonnursing postpartum women, treat pathophysiologic hyperprolactinemia from prolactin-secreting adenomas, decrease GH levels in acromegalic patients, and are used in the treatment of Parkinson's disease.

AVP and Vasopressin Tannate. AVP and vasopressin tannate are used for replacement therapy in patients with neurogenic diabetes insipidus from inadequate vasopressin production and release. They are also used to stimulate factor VIII for treatment of mild hemophilia A and mild-to-moderate von Willebrand disease.

Desmopressin, an analog with antidiuretic effects and no pressor effects, is used in patients with coronary artery disease and to maintain hemostasis before and after surgery, when bleeding is a complication of trauma.

Oxytocin. Oxytocin induces labor or augments dysfunctional labor; it is used for extended pregnancy, early rupture of membranes, and placental insufficiency. Its use requires caution because administration with prostaglandins may cause uterine rupture.

61 Thyroid and Antithyroid Agents

Alan P. Farwell, M.D.

A Feedback regulation of thyroid function

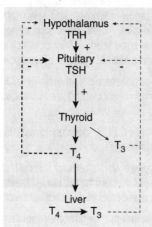

Hypothalamus
TRH
+
Pituitary
TSH
+
Thyroid
T4 → T3
Liver
T4 → T3

B Pathways of iodothyronine metabolism

Sulfation
Glucuronidation

$R = CH_2 - CH \begin{smallmatrix} COOH \\ NH_2 \end{smallmatrix}$

T4

T3

rT3

T2

T2

T2

C Site of action of antithyroid agents in the thyroid gland

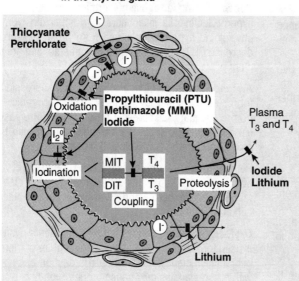

Thiocyanate
Perchlorate

Oxidation

Propylthiouracil (PTU)
Methimazole (MMI)
Iodide

I_2^0

Iodination

MIT   T4
DIT   T3
Coupling

Proteolysis

Plasma
T3 and T4

Iodide
Lithium

Lithium

D Structures of the thioureylene drugs

6-*n*-Propylthiouracil
(PTU)

$CH_3CH_2CH_2$

1-Methyl-2-mercaptoimidazole
(Methimazole)

CH_3
SH

Carbimazole

CH_3
S
$COOC_2H_5$

OVERVIEW

- Thyroid hormones are the only known iodine-containing compounds with biologic activity.
- Thyroxine (T_4) is metabolized in peripheral tissues to triiodothyronine (T_3), which binds to nuclear thyroid hormone receptors and modulates gene transcription in target tissues.
- Synthetic levothyroxine sodium is the drug of choice for thyroid hormone replacement in hypothyroidism and for thyroid hormone suppression in nodular goiter and thyroid cancer.
- Antithyroid drugs are useful to control hyperthyroidism in preparation for surgery or radioactive iodine and as definitive treatment of Graves' disease in anticipation of a remission.
- Ionizing radiation produced by sodium iodide I-131 is the treatment of choice by many endocrinologists for most forms of hyperthyroidism.

Thyroid Hormones

Background. Thyroid hormones are crucial to normal development, especially in the CNS (Porterfield and Hendrich, 1993). In the adult, thyroid hormones act to maintain metabolic stability, affecting the function of virtually all organ systems. The predominant actions are mediated via binding to nuclear receptors and modulating transcription of specific genes (Brent, 1994). In this regard, thyroid hormones share a common mechanism with steroid hormones, sex steroids, vitamin D, and retinoids, and together they make up a superfamily of nuclear receptors (Evans, 1988). Overall, 99.97% of circulating T_4 and 99.7% of circulating T_3 are bound to plasma proteins; thus, alterations in the binding capacity of these serum proteins dramatically alters the total iodothyronine content in the circulation. Only the unbound hormone has metabolic activity (Mendel, 1989).

Regulation and Metabolism. Synthesis and secretion of thyroid hormone is regulated by the anterior pituitary hormone, TSH, and TRH from the hypothalamus (Fig. A) [Bravuman and Utiger, 1996]. T_4 constitutes approximately 90% of the secreted hormone under normal conditions. T_4 deiodination in peripheral tissues, principally the liver, generates more than 80% of the transcriptionally active T_3 (Fig. B) [Leonard and Koehrle, 1996]. In addition, local production of T_3 from T_4 deiodination is important in certain tissues, such as brain and pituitary, where T_3 acts to decrease TSH secretion in a negative feedback fashion. T_4 and T_3 are further metabolized by deiodination to inactive iodothyronines (rT_3 and T_2s) or by conjugation in the liver and excretion in the bile.

Synthetic Preparations. Levothyroxine sodium (L-T_4) [Synthroid, Levoxyl, Euthyrox, Levothroid] is the drug of choice for thyroid hormone replacement. Absorption occurs in the small intestine and is variable and incomplete (Hays, 1991). Certain drugs may interfere with absorption of L-T_4, including sucralfate (Carafate), cholestyramine resin, iron supplements, and aluminum hydroxide. Because of the prolonged half-life of L-T_4 (7 days), new steady-state concentrations of T_4 are not achieved until 4–6 weeks after a change in dose.

Liothyronine sodium (L-T_3) [Cytomel, Triostat] may occasionally be used when a quicker onset of action is desired. Both L-T_4 and L-T_3 are available for IV use. Less commonly used is a mixture of these two preparations, marketed as liotrix (Thyrolar). Desiccated preparations derived from animal thyroids (Armour Thyroid, Thyrar) contain both T_4 and T_3 but have highly variable biologic activity.

Clinical Indications. The major indication for the therapeutic use of thyroid hormone is hormone replacement therapy in patients with hypothyroidism or cretinism. TSH suppression therapy with L-T_4 is indicated to decrease recurrence rates after treatment for thyroid cancer and may be helpful in decreasing the size of nontoxic goiters.

Antithyroid Agents

Compounds that interfere with the synthesis, release, or action of thyroid hormones are useful for the treatment of thyrotoxicosis resulting from hyperthyroidism, such as Graves' disease (toxic diffuse goiter) and toxic nodular goiter (Fig. C) [Farwell and Bravuman, 1996]. Adjuvant drugs are useful in controlling the peripheral manifestations, including β-adrenergic antagonists, Ca^{2+}-channel blockers, and agents that inhibit peripheral T_4 to T_3 conversion, such as dexamethasone and the iodinated radiologic agents iopanoic acid (Telepaque) and sodium ipodate (Oragrafin).

Thioureylenes. The thioureylenes belong to the family of tiomides and include propylthiouracil (PTU) and methimazole (Tapazole) [Fig. D]. The thioureylenes inhibit synthesis of the iodothyronines by inhibiting the enzyme thyroid peroxidase, which is required for the incorporation of iodine into tyrosyl residues (Taurog, 1996). The absorption of effective amounts of PTU occurs within 20–30 minutes of an oral dose. Both PTU and methimazole are concentrated in the thyroid, leading to a longer biologic half-life. Both drugs are excreted in the urine, cross the placenta, and can be found in milk. Agranulocytosis occurs with an incidence of 0.44% for PTU (idiosyncratic) and 0.12% for methimazole (possibly doserelated) and is reversible on discontinuation of the drug (Meyer-Gessner et al., 1994). The most common reaction is an urticarial papular rash that can often be managed with antihistamines or by changing drugs.

Ionic Inhibitors. These compounds are monovalent, hydrated anions of a size similar to iodine that interfere with the concentration of iodide by the thyroid gland. Thiocyanate is a dietary goitrogen that also inhibits iodide organification and that may be a contributing factor in endemic goiter. Perchlorate (ClO_4^-) is ten times more active than thiocyanate and has been used clinically to deplete iodide stores in the thyroid gland in iodine-induced hyperthyroidism and as a diagnostic test of iodide organification (Wolff, 1998). Lithium has a multitude of effects on thyroid function; its principal effect is decreased secretion of thyroid hormones.

Iodide. Iodide is the oldest remedy for thyroid disorders (Bravuman, 1994). High concentrations can inhibit essentially all aspects of iodine metabolism. In time, there is an escape from this inhibition and the hyperthyroidism often returns worse than before. The main clinical use for iodide in hyperthyroidism is in preparation for surgery and in the acute control of thyrotoxic crisis in conjunction with antithyroid drugs. Acute reaction is manifested by angioedema, skin hemorrhages, and serum sickness. Chronic intoxication (iodism) may begin as an upper respiratory illness and progress with skin lesions and lymph node and parotid gland enlargement. Most symptoms resolve after discontinuation of the iodide.

Radioactive Iodine. Sodium iodide I-131 (Iodotope Therapeutic) is rapidly trapped by the thyroid, organified, and deposited into the thyroid follicles, where it is slowly liberated, producing ionizing radiation that destroys the thyroid follicular cells. The short-lived sodium iodide I-123 is useful as an imaging agent.

62 Agents for the Treatment of Osteoporosis

Daniel D. Bikle, M.D., Ph.D.

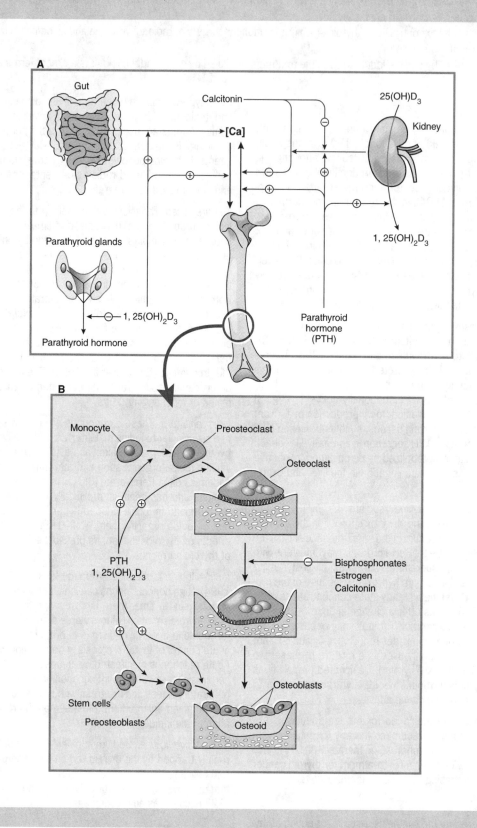

OVERVIEW

- Osteoporosis is a systemic bone disease characterized by low bone mass and microarchitectural deterioration of bone tissue leading to increased bone fragility and susceptibility to fractures.
- Osteoblasts make new bone, whereas osteoclasts resorb bone. The two processes are closely coupled during normal bone remodeling; osteoporosis develops when resorption exceeds formation.
- Bone remodeling is controlled by the calciotropic hormones: parathyroid hormone (PTH) acts to stimulate bone remodeling, calcitonin acts to suppress bone remodeling, and the active vitamin D metabolites provide adequate amounts of bone mineral (calcium and phosphate) from the diet by enhancing their absorption across the intestine.
- Agents such as estrogen and bisphosphonates reduce bone resorption and, along with calcium, are the major currently approved means of treatment.
- Fluoride stimulates bone formation, but its use in osteoporosis is not yet approved.

Pharmacology

Fig. A depicts the regulation of calcium homeostasis by the calciotropic hormones. The active metabolite of vitamin D, $1,25(OH)_2D_3$, stimulates intestinal calcium transport, blocks PTH secretion from the parathyroid glands, promotes the deposition of calcium into bone, and increases serum and urine calcium. PTH activates bone remodeling, increases calcium reabsorption from the kidney, stimulates $1,25(OH)_2D_3$ production by the kidney, and raises serum calcium. Calcitonin blocks bone resorption, increases calcium excretion and decreases serum calcium. Serum calcium increases calcitonin production and secretion while decreasing that of PTH and $1,25(OH)_2D_3$.

Fig. B illustrates the bone remodeling cycle and the sites of action of the drugs used to prevent and treat osteoporosis. Bone remodeling is initiated by activation of the osteoclast to resorb bone. In osteoporosis, the amount of bone removed exceeds the amount filled in. PTH and $1,25(OH)_2D_3$ are both able to stimulate the differentiation of preosteoclasts and preosteoblasts, and PTH in particular is able to activate the mature cells, thus increasing bone turnover. Bisphosphonates, estrogen, and calcitonin (CT), on the other hand, block the activation of osteoclasts and ultimately lead to a reduction in bone turnover.

Calciotropic Hormones

Calcitonin

Clinical Application. Calcitonin is administered subcutaneously, intramuscularly, or intranasally. Calcitonin has little toxicity but is not very potent. The half-life of human calcitonin is approximately 10 minutes; that of salmon calcitonin is approximately three times longer. The kidney is the major site of clearance.

Mechanism of Action. Calcitonin acts directly on osteoclasts to block their activity and inhibits the renal reabsorption of calcium and phosphate.

Vitamin D and Its Metabolites

Clinical Application. Vitamin D is generally used as a dietary supplement at doses of 400–800 U/day. Pharmacologic preparations of 25,000–100,000 U/day may be used when intestinal absorption is decreased. The active metabolite of vitamin D, calcitriol, or analogs such as $1\alpha\text{-}OHD_3$, have also been used in the treatment of osteoporosis, but have not been approved for this purpose in the United States. Physiologic doses of vitamin D carry little risk. However, pharmacologic doses of vitamin D or the use of active metabolites and analogs that bypass the activation steps can lead to hypercalcemia, hypercalciuria, nephrocalcinosis, and nephrolithiasis.

Mechanism of Action. Vitamin D and its metabolites stimulate the intestinal absorption of calcium and phosphate. However, receptors for calcitriol are found in many tissues including the parathyroid gland and osteoblasts; through these receptors calcitriol inhibits PTH secretion and promotes osteoblast differentiation and function.

Calcium

Clinical Application. The most commonly used oral preparations are calcium carbonate and calcium citrate used as dietary supplements to ensure 800 mg calcium a day during midlife and 1500 mg calcium a day in the elderly, when intestinal calcium transport is reduced.

Mechanism of Action. Calcium is essential for bone formation. Calcium also suppresses PTH secretion, which if increased in the face of calcium deficiency would result in net bone resorption.

Estrogen

Clinical Application. Estrogen prevents bone loss. Commonly used preparations include conjugated equine estrogens (Premarin, 0.625–1.25 mg/d), 17β-estradiol (Estrace, 1–2 mg/d), and a transdermal patch (Estraderm, 0.05–0.1 mg twice weekly). Women with a uterus should also receive concurrent or cyclic treatment with a progestin to block the hyperproliferative changes and so prevent endometrial cancer.

Mechanism of Action. Estrogen reduces bone turnover primarily by reducing bone resorption. Both osteoblasts and osteoclasts have estrogen receptors. Estrogen also promotes $1,25(OH)_2D_3$ production indirectly, perhaps by reducing serum calcium levels and raising PTH levels as a result of decreasing bone resorption.

Bisphosphonates

Clinical Application. Currently only one bisphosphonate, alendronate, is approved for use in the prevention and treatment of osteoporosis, although others are nearing approval. Alendronate is given as a 5 mg/day dose to prevent osteoporosis and as a 10 mg/day dose to treat osteoporosis. Much of the drug is bound to bone, where it persists until the bone is resorbed, giving it a long (months) biologic half-life. Nonbound drug is excreted by the kidney. Esophagitis and gastritis may result if the pill is allowed to remain in contact with the esophageal or gastric mucosa.

Mechanism of Action. Bisphosphonates are analogs of pyrophosphate in which the P-O-P bond is replaced with the nonhydrolyzable P-C-P bond. These compounds bind strongly to hydroxyapatite and block bone resorption by direct action on the osteoclast.

63 Estrogens, Progestins, and Their Antagonists

Cynthia L. Williams, Ph.D.

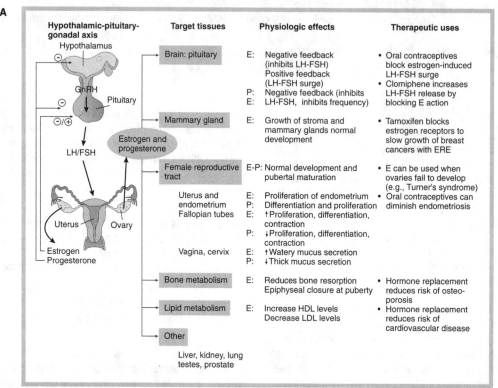

A

Hypothalamic-pituitary-gonadal axis	Target tissues	Physiologic effects	Therapeutic uses
	Brain: pituitary	E: Negative feedback (inhibits LH-FSH) Positive feedback (LH-FSH surge) P: Negative feedback (inhibits E: LH-FSH, inhibits frequency)	• Oral contraceptives block estrogen-induced LH-FSH surge • Clomiphene increases LH-FSH release by blocking E action
	Mammary gland	E: Growth of stroma and mammary glands normal development	• Tamoxifen blocks estrogen receptors to slow growth of breast cancers with ERE
	Female reproductive tract	E-P: Normal development and pubertal maturation	• E can be used when ovaries fail to develop (e.g., Turner's syndrome)
	Uterus and endometrium Fallopian tubes	E: Proliferation of endometrium P: Differentiation and proliferation E: ↑Proliferation, differentiation, contraction P: ↓Proliferation, differentiation, contraction	• Oral contraceptives can diminish endometriosis
	Vagina, cervix	E: ↑Watery mucus secretion P: ↓Thick mucus secretion	
	Bone metabolism	E: Reduces bone resorption Epiphyseal closure at puberty	• Hormone replacement reduces risk of osteoporosis
	Lipid metabolism	E: Increase HDL levels Decrease LDL levels	• Hormone replacement reduces risk of cardiovascular disease
	Other		
	Liver, kidney, lung testes, prostate		

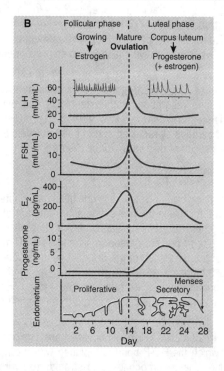

B

Follicular phase — Luteal phase

Growing → Mature **Ovulation** → Corpus luteum

Estrogen — Progesterone (+ estrogen)

LH (mIU/mL) 60 40 20 0

FSH (mIU/mL) 20 10 0

E₂ (pg/mL) 400 200 0

Progesterone (ng/mL) 10 5 0

Endometrium — Proliferative — Menses Secretory

Day: 2 6 10 14 18 22 24 28

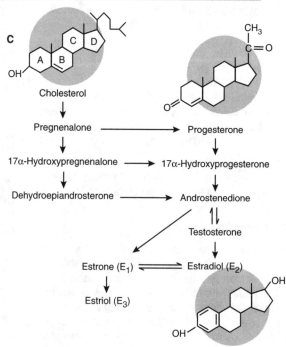

C

Cholesterol

↓

Pregnenalone → Progesterone

↓ ↓

17α-Hydroxypregnenalone → 17α-Hydroxyprogesterone

↓ ↓

Dehydroepiandrosterone → Androstenedione

⇅

Testosterone

↓

Estrone (E₁) ⇌ Estradiol (E₂)

↓

Estriol (E₃)

OVERVIEW

- Estrogen and progesterone are endogenous ovarian steroid hormones that are involved in development, growth, and puberty; control of ovulation; preparation of the reproductive tract for fertilization and implantation; and maintenance of pregnancy.
- Estrogen and progesterone also have effects on energy metabolism and calcium homeostasis.
- These steroid hormones exert their effects by binding to specific nuclear receptors, which then interact with specific DNA sequences (estrogen response elements [EREs]) to elicit changes in gene expression.

Physiology

A neuroendocrine cascade involving the hypothalamus, pituitary, and ovaries regulates estrogen and progesterone synthesis and secretion. A neurologic "clock" in the mediobasal hypothalamus fires spontaneously about once an hour, resulting in the intermittent, pulsatile release of gonadotropin-releasing hormone (GnRH). GnRH triggers the release of luteinizing hormone (LH) and follicle-stimulating hormone (FSH) from pituitary gonadotrophs. LH and FSH stimulate the graafian follicle to mature and secrete estrogen. Estrogen levels gradually rise during the follicular phase of the menstrual cycle (days 1–14). During this time, estrogen exerts a negative feedback effect on the pituitary to decrease the amount of LH released. At midcycle, estrogen levels rise dramatically and are sustained for 36 hours. Inexplicably, estrogen now exerts a positive feedback effect on the pituitary and triggers a huge release (surge) of LH and FSH that results in the rupture of the follicle and ovulation. The corpus luteum, the remnant of the ruptured graafian follicle, secretes progesterone and estrogen for a fixed period of about 14 days. If the ovum is not fertilized, the corpus luteum ceases to function, estrogen and progesterone levels decline, and the endometrium is shed (menstruation). If GnRH is delivered constantly or at a frequency slower than once an hour during the follicular phase, the LH-FSH surge is blocked, and there is no ovulation. If estrogen or progesterone are elevated early in the follicular phase, the LH-FSH surge is blocked, and ovulation is prevented. This is the primary mechanism by which oral contraceptives work.

Medicinal Chemistry

Chemical modifications of steroidal estrogens have resulted in improved oral efficacy and longer half-life. Nonsteroidal estrogens (diethylstilbestrol, [DES]) and antiestrogens (tamoxifen, clomiphene) have been developed for therapeutic use. Synthetic progestins have varying potencies at progesterone receptors. The actions of progestins at other steroid receptors contribute greatly to their side effects.

Pharmacokinetics

Estrogens and progestins are extremely lipophilic and are therefore absorbed well. The compounds are available for oral, parenteral, transdermal, or topical administration. Natural progesterone and estradiol are ineffective orally because of extensive first-pass metabolism by the liver and short half-life (minutes). Ethinyl estradiol (frequently used in oral contraceptives) is resistant to hepatic metabolism and has a long half-life (12–24 hours). Conjugated estrogens (used in hormone replacement therapies) are not absorbed until they reach the lower intestine, where they are hydrolyzed by enzymes in the colon. It is important to note that conjugated estrogens are administered in seemingly higher doses (0.625 mg/day) than oral contraceptive ethinyl-estradiol (20–35 µg/day), but because of decreased potency and bioavailability, the dose is actually much lower than that used for oral contraceptives and is associated with fewer side effects.

SPECIFIC AGENTS

Drugs	Therapeutic Uses	Mechanism of Action	Side Effects
Agonists			
Conjugated estrogens + progestins	Hormone replacement	Diminish effects of menopause: hot flashes, osteoporosis, vaginal atrophy, hypercholesterolemia	Nausea, vomiting, weight gain, migraine Increased risk of gallbladder disease *Benefit:* Reduced risk of cardiovascular disease, osteporosis
Prototypes: estrone sulfate + medroxyprogesterone acetate (MPA)			
Estrogen + progestins	Oral contraceptives	Block estrogen-induced LH surge to prevent ovulation	Mild: nausea weight gain, breakthough bleeding Severe: Increased risk of thromboembolism and cerebrovascular accident. *Benefit:* Reduced risk of endometrial cancer, ovarian cysts, or cancer
Prototypes: ethinyl estradiol or mestranol with norethindrone, norgestrel, or norgestimate			
Progestin only	Contraceptives	Blocks estrogen-induced LH surge to prevent ovulation Increase cervical mucus	Menstrual irregularities, edema, weight gain
Prototypes: norgestrel (minipill), MPA (Depo-Provera)	Postcoital contraceptive, implanted contraceptive		
Anti-estrogens			
Tamoxifen	Breast cancer treatment	Competitive partial agonist/antagonist blocks estrogen-induced growth of breast cancers that express estrogen receptors	Nauea, vomiting, hot flashes, endometrial hyperplasia (agonist action in endometrium)
Clomiphene	Infertility	Partial agonist increases LH and FSH secretion to simulate ovulation	Hot flashes, ovary hyperstimulation and enlargement
Antiprogesterone			
Mifepristone (RU-486)	Abortifacient	Competitive antagonist blocks progesterone and glucocorticoid receptors to terminate pregnancy	Pain, prolonged bleeding, diarrhea, vomiting

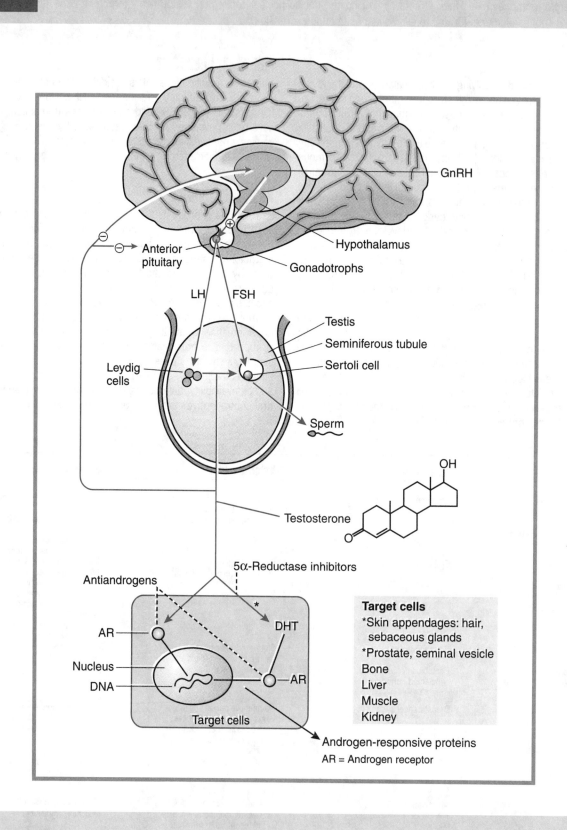

OVERVIEW

- Testosterone, the most important androgen in men, stimulates masculinization and spermatogenesis. Androgens are also produced in women, but their biologic role, other than as precursor steroids for estrogens, remains unclear.
- Mechanism of action: Androgens bind to intracellular receptors (AR), which activate androgen-regulated genes. Testosterone is converted to dihydrotestosterone (DHT) in certain target tissues by the enzyme 5α-reductase, where DHT binds to the AR. 5α-Reductase inhibitors block DHT production, and antiandrogens bind to the AR but fail to promote gene transcription.
- Therapeutic uses: Androgens are used as replacement therapy for hypogonadal men. 5α-Reductase inhibitors are used to treat benign prostate enlargement. Antiandrogens block the actions of androgens in women and men with androgen-dependent disease.
- Side effects: Dose-dependent and formulation-specific.

Pharmacology

Testosterone is produced by testicular Leydig cells and by the adrenal cortex and ovarian theca cells. Testicular testosterone production is stimulated by pituitary luteinizing hormone (LH). Testosterone also controls its own production in men by inhibiting gonadotropin-releasing hormone (GnRH) and LH secretion. Normal plasma levels are 300–1000 ng/dL for men and < 40 ng/dL for women. Most circulating testosterone is bound to plasma proteins.

Medicinal Chemistry

Esterification increases the lipid solubility of testosterone, prolonging its physical half-life. 17α-Methyl derivatives of testosterone for oral or sublingual use are metabolized more slowly than testosterone and interact directly with the AR. Transdermal systems deliver testosterone at a controlled rate into the systemic circulation, avoiding the high and low levels observed with long-acting testosterone esters.

Mechanism of Action

Androgens are steroid hormones. The AR is a member of the steroid receptor family of ligand-activated nuclear transcription factors. The receptor consists of a central DNA-binding domain, which is highly homologus with progesterone and glucocorticoid receptors, and a specific androgen-binding domain in its carboxyl terminus. Binding of the androgen to its receptor dissociates the native receptor from carrier proteins. Activated receptors dimerize and bind steroid response elements in the 5′ noncoding region of responsive genes to promote gene transcription. Negative transcriptional regulation is less well understood. Finasteride is a specific inhibitor of 5α-reductase and has no AR binding. Antiandrogens are competitive antagonists of the AR that bind but fail to activate the receptor.

Pharmacokinetics

Administration and Distribution. Testosterone esters are administered intramuscularly in an oil suspension, absorbed gradually from the intramuscular depot, and converted to free testosterone in the circulation. Doses of 150–200 mg of testosterone enanthate or cypionate maintain normal adult male levels for 10–14 days. Steroid hormones can be absorbed through the skin into the systemic circulation. Scrotal skin is at least five times more permeable to testosterone than are other skin sites.

Metabolism and Elimination. Testosterone is metabolized to 17-keto-steroids (17-KS), which are excreted into the urine. Testosterone is also conjugated to glucuronic and sulfuric acids and excreted in bile. Testosterone is metabolized to two biologically active compounds, DHT (4%) and estradiol (1%). DHT is produced by the enzyme testosterone 5α-reductase. Two functional genes encode different 5α-reductase isoenzymes. The type 2 isozyme predominates in genital tract tissues and skin appendages. The level of DHT exceeds testosterone five- to tenfold in prostate but is one-tenth as high as testosterone in plasma in men. Conversion of testosterone to estradiol (and androsterone to estrone) is catalyzed by the aromatase cytochrome P-450 enzyme. This gene is expressed not only in granulosa cells of the ovary but also in testicular Leydig cells, brain, liver, and adipose stroma.

Adverse Effects and Toxicity

Dose-dependent side effects include acne; salt and water retention with edema, weight gain, and hypertension; polycythemia; and excessive stimulation of libido. Gynecomastia may occur because of bioconversion to estradiol. Formulation-specific side effects are described below. Androgen replacement is contraindicated in men with prostate or breast cancer.

SPECIFIC AGENTS

Testosterone esters
  Unesterified natural testosterone
  Testosterone propionate
  Testosterone enanthate (Delatestryl, generic)
  Testosterone cypionate (Depo-Testosterone, generic)

Transdermal testosterone
  Scrotal patch (Testoderm)
  Nonscrotal path (Androderm, Testoderm-TTS)

Testosterone derivatives
  Methyltestosterone, fluoxymesterone

5α-Reductase inhibitors
  Finasteride (Proscar)

Androgen antagonists
  Spironolactone (Aldactone, generic)
  Flutamide (Eulexin), bicalutamide (Casodex)

65 Corticosteroids

Robert B. Raffa, Ph.D.

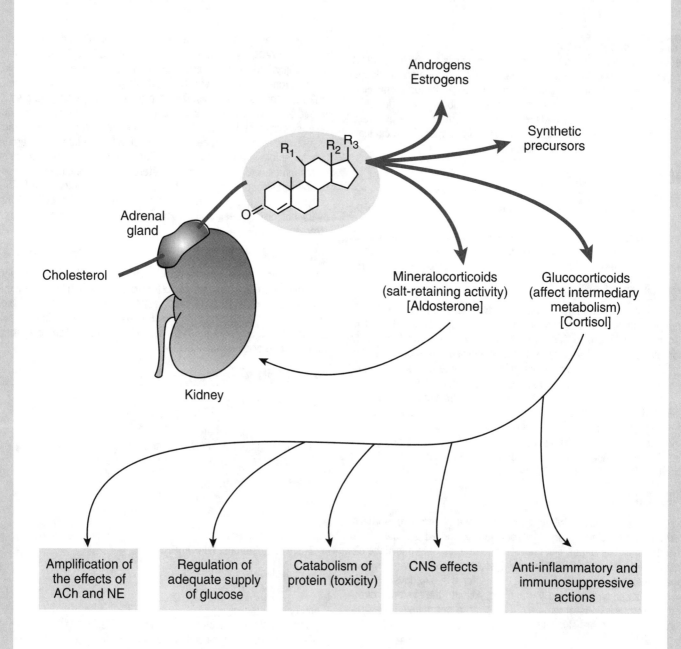

Androgens
Estrogens

Synthetic precursors

R_1 R_2 R_3

Adrenal gland

Cholesterol

Kidney

Mineralocorticoids
(salt-retaining activity)
[Aldosterone]

Glucocorticoids
(affect intermediary
metabolism)
[Cortisol]

| Amplification of the effects of ACh and NE | Regulation of adequate supply of glucose | Catabolism of protein (toxicity) | CNS effects | Anti-inflammatory and immunosuppressive actions |

OVERVIEW

- The cortex of the adrenal (suprarenal) gland synthesizes and releases a variety of bioactive substances or related structures.
- These substances are classified on the basis of their functions as androgens or estrogens, as glucocorticoids (affecting intermediary metabolism), as mineralocorticoids (affecting salt-retention activity), or as precursors to metabolic reactions.
- Cortisol (hydrocortisone) is the major natural glucocorticoid in humans. It is synthesized from cholesterol, is released under the control of ACTH, and its effects are mediated by specialized (mostly intracellular) receptors.
- Major categories of effects of endogenous or synthetic glucocorticoids include amplification of the action of some neurotransmitters such as ACh and norepinephrine, maintenance of adequate glucose supply, and anti-inflammatory and immunosuppressive actions.
- Main therapeutic uses include replacement therapy in cases of adrenal insufficiency and as anti-inflammatory or immunosuppressive agents.
- Chronic dosing induces changes that warrant monitoring. Chronic therapy should not be stopped abruptly.

Cortisol

Under the control of ACTH released from the pituitary, cortisol enters into the general circulation at a rate that is influenced by circadian rhythms, stress, disease, time of day, meals, light, levels of corticosteroid-binding globulin (CBG) in plasma, and other factors. Cortisol stimulates gluconeogenesis, so that energy demand and supply are matched, and modulates lipogenesis and lipolysis. Detrimentally, cortisol promotes catabolism of muscle protein and bone (resulting in osteoporosis or inhibition of growth). There is a high density of steroid receptors in the limbic system of the brain. A significant number of depressed patients have elevated cortisol levels or atypical circadian variations in the levels. Possible therapeutic use of glucocorticoids for a variety of CNS disorders is currently under investigation.

Medicinal Chemistry

Synthetic corticosteroids are usually derivatives of cholic acid from animals or steroid sapogenins from plants. They consist of a four-ring corticosteroid backbone. Substitutions on this backbone result in synthetic agents with a spectrum of receptor affinity and pharmacokinetics. For example, half-life can be increased by halogenation at the C9 position (B ring), unsaturation of the Δ1-2 bond (A ring), methylation at C2 or C16 (D ring), and hydroxylation at C11 (C ring).

Mechanism of Action

Cortisol and corticosteroids produce many of their effects through widely distributed glucocorticoid receptors, not members of ion-channel or G-protein–coupled receptor families, that are located intracellularly and bind ligands that are transported to the cell by CBG. The ligand-receptor complex (dimerized) enters the nucleus and regulates transcription at specific portions of DNA. The gene product (a protein), up- or down-regulated, brings about the observed response to the hormone.

Pharmacotherapy

The most obvious use of corticosteroids is cortisol-replacement therapy in cases of adrenal insufficiency. In addition, they are used to correct excess ACTH production (through a negative feedback loop) in response to depressed synthesis of cortisol. The dexamethasone suppression test is used for the diagnosis of Cushing's syndrome and to aid diagnosis of clinical depression. Fetal lung maturation requires cortisol. Hence, corticosteroids given to the mother reduce the incidence of respiratory distress syndrome in premature infants. They are also used in many conditions involving an inflammatory component. The drugs inhibit the deleterious actions of leukocytes and tissue macrophages; inhibit synthesis of prostaglandins, leukotrienes, and cytokines; inhibit activity of kinins and endotoxins; inhibit histamine release; and enhance neutrophil activity. Immunosuppressant action of the corticosteroids derives from inhibition of components of the immune response. These properties make glucocorticoids useful for the treatment of lymphocytic leukemias and for the inhibition of organ transplant rejection.

Pharmacokinetics

Glucocorticoids are available for aerosol, surface (dermatologic), and oral administration and in formulations offering a wide selection of potencies, half-lives, or specific levels of plasma protein binding, or route of metabolism or elimination.

Adverse Effects and Toxicity

Acute treatment with even moderately high doses is generally well tolerated by most patients, although behavioral changes and acute peptic ulcer are possible. Chronic treatment may result, in a drug-induced Cushing's disease. More serious consequences of protein catabolism (e.g., muscle wasting) and diversion of substrates for glucose production place significant strain on multiple systems resulting in a wide range of adverse effects (e.g., growth retardation, osteoporosis, diabetes) and potentially life-threatening adrenal suppression, and consequently enhanced susceptibility to otherwise innocuous stressors. Particularly with chronic therapy, an increase in intraocular pressure is relatively common, cataracts may develop, and slight-to-serious mental changes are possible.

REPRESENTATIVE GLUCOCORTICOIDS

Beclomethasone—aerosol formulations (Beclovent, Vanceril)

Betamethasone—oral, parenteral, topical formulations (Ceslestone)

Cortisone—oral, parenteral (Cortone Acetate, generic)

Dexamethasone—oral, injectable, topical (Decadron, others, generic)

Fludrocortisone—oral, injectable, topical (Florinef Acetate)

Hydrocortisone (= cortisol)—oral, parenteral, topical formulations (Cortef, generic)

Prednisone—(Meticorten, others, generic)

66 Insulin and Hypoglycemic Agents

Stephen N. Davis, M.D.

Sites and mechanisms of action of therapeutic agents used in the treatment of diabetes mellitus

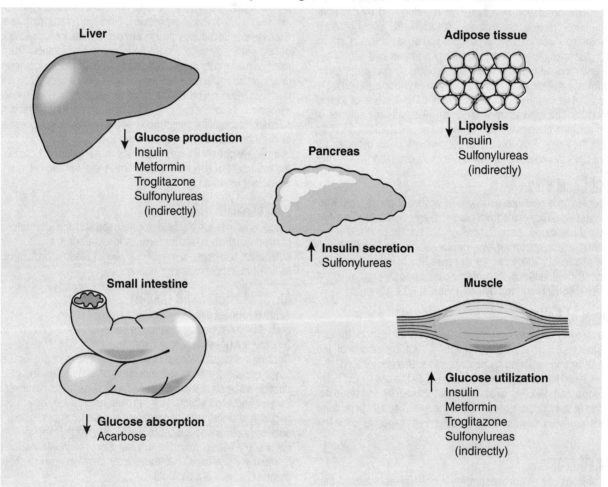

Liver

↓ **Glucose production**
Insulin
Metformin
Troglitazone
Sulfonylureas
   (indirectly)

Adipose tissue

↓ **Lipolysis**
Insulin
Sulfonylureas
   (indirectly)

Pancreas

↑ **Insulin secretion**
Sulfonylureas

Small intestine

↓ **Glucose absorption**
Acarbose

Muscle

↑ **Glucose utilization**
Insulin
Metformin
Troglitazone
Sulfonylureas
   (indirectly)

OVERVIEW

- Diabetes mellitus is classified into three main categories: type 1, type 2, and gestational diabetes.
- Insulin is the treatment of choice for type 1 and gestational diabetes.
- Oral hypoglycemic agents are now the initial treatment of choice for type 2 diabetes.

Pathophysiology of Diabetes Mellitus

Diabetes is an absolute or relative lack of insulin. Definitions based on blood glucose have changed (June 1997) and are shown in the table below. Insulin exerts its hypoglycemic effects by (1) inhibiting endogenous glucose production (primarily from liver) and (2) stimulating glucose removal from the circulation (primarily skeletal muscle). In diabetes there is unrestrained glucose production and severely blunted glucose utilization by tissues. Type 2 diabetes is also characterized by insulin resistance: key tissues (liver, pancreas, muscle, adipocytes) normally involved in carbohydrate homeostasis have blunted physiologic responses to insulin (Fig.) [Howey et al., 1996].

BLOOD GLUCOSE DEFINITIONS OF ABNORMAL CARBOHYDRATE TOLERANCE

Condition	Normal	Impaired Glucose Tolerance	Diabetes
Fasting	< 110 mg/dL	110–125 mg/dL	≥ 126 mg/dL
Non-fasting	< 140 mg/dL	140–199 mg/dL	≥ 200mg/dL

Pharmacology

Insulin release from pancreatic beta cells is stimulated by glucose, amino acids, fatty acids, glucagon-like peptide 1, gastrin, secretin, vasoactive intestinal peptide, α_2-adrenergic receptor antagonists, and vagal stimulation. β_2-Adrenergic receptor antagonists inhibit release. Insulin binds to specific cell surface receptors and promotes glucose entry into cells by a family of transporters (Glut 1–Glut 7). Once inside a cell, insulin exerts diverse effects on intermediary metabolism.

Insulin Therapy in Type 1 and Type 2 Diabetes

Currently available human insulin preparations are classified as rapid-acting (regular and lispro) or intermediate-acting (NPH, lente, and ultralente). Human lispro (Lys [28], Pro [29] insulin) has been recently introduced as the first ultra short-acting insulin analog (Howey et al., 1996). Lispro action can start within 15 minutes after injection and will last 2–3 hours. Consequently, lispro should be injected immediately prior to a meal, rather than the 20–30 minutes earlier usually recommended for regular insulin.

Oral Therapeutic Agents for Type 2 Diabetes

Recently, metformin (Glucophage) [Bailey, 1992], acarbose (Precose) [Chiasson et al., 1994], troglitazone (Rezulin) [Saltiel and Olefsky, 1996], repaglinide (Prandin), and glimepiride (Amaryl) [Matthews and Riddle, 1996] have been approved for use in type 2 diabetes. These agents can be used in conjunction with subcutaneous insulin therapy, in combination with each other, or as monotherapy. Metformin and sulfonylureas have very similar effects on lowering fasting and postprandial glucose levels. Metformin, unlike sulfonylureas, does not promote weight gain and produces substantial reductions in triglycerides and low-density lipoprotein (LDL) cholesterol. Metformin and sulfonylureas work powerfully in combination and produce dramatic reductions in glucose levels of type 2 diabetic patients. Metformin, however, should not be administered to patients with renal, hepatic, pulmonary, or cardiac failure (Defronzo and Goodman, 1995).

Acarbose, when used in doses of 75 mg three times a day or lower, appears to be a very safe drug. Although acarbose has less glucose-lowering potential than the other newer oral agents, because of its safety profile, it may be considered first-line therapy in the elderly.

Glimepiride is a new long-acting sulfonylurea that may be used once a day. It produces less hypoglycemia in type 2 patients compared to glyburide and is associated with lower insulin levels during exercise in type 2 patients compared to previous sulfonylureas. This mimics the normal physiologic response and helps prevent hypoglycemia.

Repaglinide is a new oral hypoglycemic agent of the meglitinide class. Repaglinide causes insulin secretion from pancreatic beta cells, and thus its mode of action is similar to sulfonylureas.

SPECIFIC ORAL AGENTS FOR USE IN TYPE 2 DIABETES

Agent	Mechanism of Action	Metabolism/Excretion	Adverse Reactions
Sulfonylureas[a]	Enhance pancreatic insulin release	Liver/kidney	Hypoglycemia
Meglitinide, repaglinide	Enhance pancreatic insulin release	Liver	Hyperglycemia; hypoglycemia
Metformin	Reduces endogenous glucose production; increases muscle glucose uptake; reduces insulin resistance	Kidney	Transient GI side effects; lactic acidosis (rare)
Acarbose	Reduces small bowel absorption of glucose via inhibition of α-glucosidase	Liver	GI side effects (flatulence, abdominal bloating); reversible elevation of liver enzymes at high doses
Troglitazone	Reduces insulin resistance via interactions with peroxisome proliferator – activated receptors in liver and muscle	Liver	Possible severe hepatic failure

[a] Chlorpropamide, tolbutamide, glyburide, glipizide, and glimepiride.

Directions: For each of the following questions, choose the **one best** answer.

1. Which of the following statements is correct?

(A) Calcitonin enhances bone remodeling.

(B) Estrogen increases bone resorption.

(C) Parathyroid hormone decreases bone remodeling.

(D) Vitamin D metabolites provide bone mineral from the diet.

2. A molecular target of corticosteroids is best described by

(A) membrane pores

(B) ligand-gated ion channels

(C) G-protein–coupled receptors

(D) cytoplasmic receptors and transcription

3. Continuous administration of GnRH agonists is used to treat

(A) dysfunctional labor

(B) endometriosis

(C) idiopathic hypogonadotropic hypogonadism

(D) polycystic ovary syndrome

(E) primary hypothalamic amenorrhea

4. Testosterone enanthate treatment of men with hypogonadotropic hypogonadism may result in

(A) increased plasma levels FSH and LH

(B) spermatogenesis

(C) increased plasma levels of 17α-hydroxyprogesterone

(D) polycythemia

(E) increased HDL-cholesterol levels

5. Beneficial effects of HRT in postmenopausal women include a decreased incidence of all of the following EXCEPT

(A) osteoporosis

(B) cardiovascular disease

(C) breast cancer

(D) vasomotor instability (hot flashes)

(E) urogenital atrophy

6. Which of the following statements regarding estrogen treatment is correct?

(A) Osteoblasts lack estrogen receptors.

(B) Osteoclasts lack estrogen receptors.

(C) A transdermal patch is available.

(D) Concurrent treatment with a progestin is contraindicated in women with a uterus.

7. Which of the following agents is used to terminate lactation in non-nursing postpartum women?

(A) Vasopressin

(B) Dopamine agonists

(C) Human menopausal gonadotropin

(D) Octreotide

(E) Oxytocin

8. Which of the following drugs enhances pancreatic insulin release?

(A) Acarbose

(B) Glyburide

(C) Metformin

(D) Troglitazone

9. The outcome of acute glucocorticoid therapy usually results in

(A) acne

(B) diabetes

(C) glaucoma

(D) puffiness of the face

(E) no adverse effect

10. Which of the following drugs is primarily eliminated only by the kidney?

(A) Acarbose

(B) Glyburide

(C) Metformin

(D) Troglitazone

11. An increase in IGF-1 leads to an increase in

(A) AVP

(B) GH

(C) GHRH

(D) SRIF

12. Medroxyprogesterone acetate is used on conjunction with estrogens in postmenopausal HRT because progestins

(A) improve lipoprotein profiles

(B) diminish thinning and atrophy of skin

(C) diminish alopecia

(D) decrease the incidence of endometrial carcinoma

(E) block osteoclast activation

13. The drug of choice for chronic thyroid-hormone replacement therapy is

(A) a preparation derived from animal thyroids

(B) a preparation derived from human thyroids

(C) levothyroxine sodium

(D) liothyronine sodium

14. Finasteride may be useful in the primary prevention of prostate cancer because it lowers the levels of

(A) IGF-1

(B) testosterone

(C) dihydrotestosterone

(D) epidermal growth factor

(E) GH

15. Tamoxifen has which of the following characteristics?

(A) It acts as a competitive antagonist at estrogen receptor sites in the breast.

(B) It decreases ovarian steroid production by inhibition of gonadotropin release.

(C) It prevents the development of endometrial cancers.

(D) It blocks the tyrosine kinase activity of peptide growth factors.

(E) It inhibits the aromatase-catalyzed conversion of androgens to estrogens.

16. In men, spironolactone may lead to which of the following conditions?

(A) Water retention

(B) Hypokalemia

(C) Gynecomastia

(D) Reduced plasma testosterone

(E) Hepatic failure

17. All of the following compounds are either direct or adjuvant antithyroid agents EXCEPT

(A) dexamethasone

(B) isoproterenol

(C) methimazole

(D) propylthiouracil

18. Adverse effects of combination oral contraceptives include all of the following EXCEPT

(A) venous thromboembolism

(B) ischemic heart disease

(C) stroke

(D) gallbladder disease

(E) ovarian cancer

PART VII: ANSWERS AND EXPLANATIONS

1. The answer is D.

Vitamin D and its metabolites stimulate the intestinal absorption of calcium and phosphate. Bone remodeling is controlled by the calciotropic hormones: parathyroid hormone stimulates bone remodeling, and calcitonin acts directly on osteoclasts to block their activity. Agents such as estrogen and bisphosphonates reduce bone resorption.

2. The answer is D.

Corticosteroids produce many of their regulatory effects through widely distributed glucocorticoid receptors, not membrane pores. The receptors are not members of ion-channel or G-protein–coupled receptor families. Instead, they are located within the cytoplasm. The binding of ligand to receptor disrupts the receptor heat shock protein 90 complex, which functions in the absence of ligand to keep the receptor within the cytoplasm and out of the nucleus. The ligand–receptor complex enters the nucleus and regulates transcription occurring at specific portions of the DNA molecule and, hence, the gene product (a protein) that brings about the observed corticosteroid response.

3. The answer is B.

The effects of GnRH depend on its method of administration, either pulsatile or continuous. Continuous administration of GnRH down-regulates its pituitary receptors and suppresses LH release, thereby suppressing gonadal hormones and decreasing the clinical symptoms of endometriosis. Pulsatile administration of GnRH stimulates LH release, thereby stimulating ovulation or spermatogenesis in cases of primary hypothalamic amenorrhea or idiopathic hypogonadotropic hypogonadism.

4. The answer is D.

Polycythemia sometimes occurs as a side effect of testosterone treatment especially in men predisposed to polycythemia, such as smokers with chronic lung disease. The mechanism may be via increased erythropoietin, but it is incompletely understood. Polycythemia is less common with transdermal than with intramuscular injections of testosterone, following which high plasma levels of testosterone often occur for 2–3 days. Testosterone will suppress, not increase, LH and FSH levels by inhibiting GnRH produced by the hypothalamus. Lower LH levels will result in decreased Leydig cell biosynthetic function and decrease the secretion of 17α-hydroxyprogesterone, a testosterone precursor steroid. Spermatogenesis is suppressed rather than stimulated. Replacement doses of testosterone may reduce HDL-cholesterol levels, or they remain unchanged; large doses of androgens sometimes used by athletes and body builders reduce HDL cholesterol.

5. The answer is C.

The prevention of bone loss is of primary importance in estrogen HRT in postmenopausal women. Estrogens act to prevent bone loss, not restore it, and their benefits in this regard require early and continuous use supplemented by an appropriate diet, adequate calcium intake, and weight-bearing exercise. Estrogens have also been demonstrated to reduce the risk of cardiovascular disease, presumably through their beneficial effects on plasma lipoprotein profiles. Cardiovascular disease is the leading cause of death in postmenopausal women. Postmenopausal women receiving estrogen, however, have a decreased incidence of coronary artery disease, and premenopausal women have a lower incidence of cardiovascular disease compared to age-matched men. Vasomotor instability (hot flashes) and vaginal wall dryness and atrophy are direct consequences of estrogen deficiency after menopause and are prevented by estrogen replacement. HRT does not lower the incidence of breast cancer, which now strikes 1 in 10 women. In fact, the concern has been that the estrogens in HRT or oral contraceptives may increase the risk of breast cancer. That question is under intense scrutiny and has not been resolved unequivocally.

6. The answer is C.

Estraderm is an example of a transdermal estrogen patch. Osteoclasts and osteoblasts have estrogen receptors and are responsive to estrogen. Women with a uterus should receive concurrent or cyclic treatment with a progestin such as medroxyprogesterone to block hyperproliferative changes in the uterus that might lead to endometrial cancer.

7. The answer is B.

Prolactin plays a major role in milk secretion. Dopamine agonists terminate postpartum physiologic hyperprolactinemia by suppressing prolactin release from the anterior pituitary. Oxytocin is also involved in lactation, but its role is stimulative: it triggers the milk ejection reflex in lactating women.

8. The answer is B.

Glyburide and other sulfonylureas (e.g., chlorpropamide, tolbutamide, glipizide, glimepiride) enhance insulin release from the pancreas. Acarbose reduces small bowel absorption of glucose. Metformin reduces glucose production, increases glucose uptake into muscle, and reduces insulin resistance. Troglitazone reduces insulin resistance.

9. The answer is E.

Acute treatment with even moderately high doses of glucocorticoids is generally well tolerated by most patients, although behavioral changes and acute peptic ulcer are possible. The other choices are possible adverse effects of glucocorticoid therapy, particularly during the chronic use of high doses. Excess glucocorticoid effects include puffiness of the face, fine hair growth, and acne, and more serious consequences of protein catabolism and gluconeogenesis. Some increase in intraocular pressure (glaucoma) and cataracts are relatively common with chronic treatment. Osteoporosis, not osteochondrosis, is a common complication of long-term treatment.

10. The answer is C.

Metformin is eliminated primarily by the kidney. Acarbose and troglitazone are eliminated primarily by the liver. Glyburide and other sulfonylureas are eliminated by both the liver and the kidney.

11. The answer is D.

Hypothalamic and pituitary hormones responsible for the release of IGF-1 interact in positive and negative feedback loops. IGF-1 suppresses GH release directly and by stimulating the GH suppressor, SRIF; the suppression of GH release results in a decrease in IGF-1. GHRH stimulates GH release and thus indirectly stimulates IGF-1.

12. The answer is D.

In the 1960s and 1970s, epidemiologic studies of HRT with estrogen alone revealed an increased incidence of endometrial carcinoma, presumably due to the continuous stimulation of endometrial hyperplasia by estrogen. Adding a progestin to the HRT significantly reduced the degree of endometrial hyperplasia. An estrogen-progesterone HRT is now recommended for most postmenopausal women with a uterus. Exceptions include women with an unfavorable lipoprotein profile and associated higher risk of cardiovascular disease, in whom estrogen only HRT may be preferable.

13. The answer is C.

Levothyroxine sodium (Synthroid, Levosyl, Euthyrox, Levothroid) is the drug of choice for chronic thyroid-hormone replacement therapy. Liothyronine sodium (Cytomel, Triostat) is more useful when a rapid onset is desired but less desirable for chronic treatment because of its requirement for more frequent dosing, its higher cost, and transient elevations of serum T_3 concentrations above normal. Extracts can have undesirable variability.

14. The answer is C.

Finasteride, approved for the treatment of benign prostatic hyperplasia and male pattern baldness, is a 5α-reductase inhibitor and blocks the bioconversion of testosterone to dihydrotestosterone in the prostate. It substantially lowers prostate and plasma levels of dihydrotestosterone.

15. The answer is A.

Tamoxifen is used for the treatment of breast cancers that express estrogen receptors as an adjuvant therapy to surgery, chemotherapy, and radiation. Tamoxifen competitively inhibits estrogen-induced proliferation of cultured human breast cancer cells and is an estrogen-receptor antagonist in breast tissue. However, tamoxifen stimulates the proliferation of endometrial cells and is an estrogen agonist in that tissue. Therefore, tamoxifen is frequently referred to as a mixed, estrogen-receptor agonist-antagonist, but its action in breast tissue specifically is competitive antagonism.

16. The answer is C.

As an antiandrogen, spironolactone blocks testosterone negative feedback inhibition of LH and FSH secretion. Plasma LH and FSH levels rise in spironolactone-treated men and thereby increase plasma levels of testosterone and estradiol. Elevated estradiol levels cause gynecomastia. Spironolactone is also an aldosterone antagonist, which promotes diuresis and lowers blood pressure. By blocking aldosterone action, it predisposes to hyperkalemia. Hepatic failure has occurred in men treated with the nonsteroidal antiandrogens flutamide and bicalutamide, but not with spironolactone.

17. The answer is B.

β-Adrenoceptor antagonists, not agonists, are useful adjunctive therapy in controlling some peripheral manifestations of thyrotoxicosis. Thioureylenes such as methimazole and propylthiouracil inhibit the enzyme thyroid peroxidase, which is required for the incorporation of iodine into tyrosyl residues. Dexamethasone inhibits peripheral T_4 to T_3 conversion.

18. **The answer is E.**

Oral contraceptives are associated with an increased incidence of venous thromboembolism and gallbladder disease. In women older than 35 years who smoke, oral contraceptives are associated with an increased incidence of myocardial infarction and stroke. However, combination oral contraceptives have actually been shown to decrease the incidence of ovarian and endometrial cancers by as much as 50% in some studies. The association between oral contraceptives and breast cancer is still debated. It should be noted that the doses of estrogen used in current oral contraceptives are significantly lower than the doses used in early oral contraceptives, for which most of the adverse effects have been described.

PART VIII
Adverse Reactions and Toxicology

67 Toxicology Basics
Robert B. Raffa, Ph.D.

Quantitative measure of toxic vs. therapeutic effects

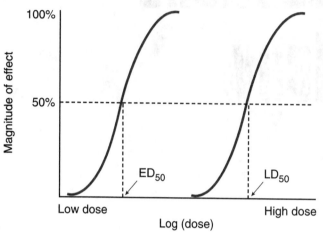

Parallel curves (might imply similar mechanisms)

$LD_{50}/ED_{50} > 1.0$

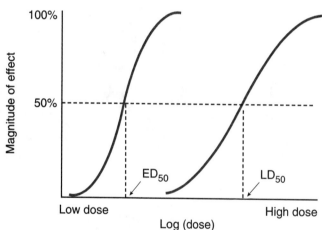

Nonparallel curves (might imply dissimilar mechanisms)

$LD_{50}/ED_{50} > 1.0$

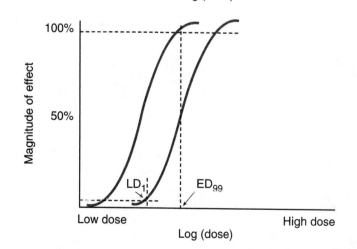

$LD_1/ED_{99} < 1.0$

OVERVIEW

- Toxicity can result from exposure to drugs or environmental chemicals.
- The sites of toxic actions can be local (e.g., caustic or corrosive effects) or systemic.
- The effects can be selective (i.e., related to the mechanism of action of a drug or the specific biochemical effect of an environmental toxin) or nonselective (i.e., indiscriminate destruction of all cells or cell components). Particular organs can be more susceptible than others to particular toxicants.
- The potency of a toxin can be expressed as an LD_{50} value. A drug's LD_{50} can be compared to its therapeutic ED_{50} value as some indication of the relative safety of the drug.
- In utero toxicity can be gross (e.g., teratogenicity) or subtle (e.g., learning defects).
- Drug toxicity is imperfectly predicted by tests in animals. Known toxicity of drugs is indicated on the package insert of each drug and in the *Physician's Desk Reference (PDR)*.

Terminology

In relation to pharmacotherapy, the following terminology is usually applicable. It should be noted that each term could have modifiers. For example, some toxic effects of chemicals are desirable (e.g., insecticides) and some "toxic" effects are extensions of a chemical's (drug's) mechanism of action, whereas other toxic effects are unrelated to the drug's mechanism of therapeutic action.

- Toxicology: the study of the harmful effects of chemicals, including drugs
- Acute: symptoms develop quickly and generally after only one exposure
- Subacute: frequent, repeated exposure over hours or days of a dose less than ("sub-") the acute toxic dose
- Chronic: repeated exposure over long periods, resulting in accumulation
- Poison: a substance that produces a toxic effect (usually without an obvious therapeutic effect)

Quantitative Measures

Median lethal dose (LD_{50}) is the dose of a drug that is lethal in exactly 50% of a group of test animals or accidentally exposed humans. The LD_{50} is determined from a plot of lethality versus dose or log (dose). When the drug is administered by inhalation, a median lethal concentration (LC_{50}) can be determined.

Therapeutic index is a ratio used to evaluate the safety of a drug in terms of the separation between the therapeutic dose and the lethal dose. In broader terms, it is a measure that describes quantitatively the relationship between doses of a drug that elicit undesired versus desired effects. A common therapeutic index (TI) is $TI = LD_{50}:ED_{50}$, where the ED_{50} is the dose of drug estimated to produce 50% effect (or effect in 50% of test subjects). Hence, larger values of TI indicate less toxicity (as defined by lethality). More conservative measures can be used, such as $LD_1:ED_{99}$.

Organ Sensitivity

Liver. The location of the liver in regard to the first-pass effect and the possible biotransformation of drugs to reactive (toxic) metabolites expose the liver to particular vulnerability. Toxicity occurs when the formation of reactive metabolites exceeds the detoxification capacity of the liver. Examples of hepatic toxins include solvents (e.g., carbon tetrachloride and halogenated benzenes), carcinogens (e.g., aflatoxin B and aromatic amines), and overdose of certain drugs (e.g., isoniazid or acetaminophen).

Lung. Through respiratory or systemic exposure, the lung becomes vulnerable. Gases can be corrosive or cytotoxic and some particulates can induce toxic reactions (e.g., asbestos). Pulmonary biotransformation can result in toxic metabolites (e.g., lung cancer is produced by reactive intermediates during the metabolism of benzo[a]pyrene or other polycyclic aromatic hydrocarbons). Pulmonary injury also can occur during exposure to systemic toxicants, such as reactive intermediates of the metabolism of paraquat (insecticide) or pyrrolidine alkaloids.

Kidney. Exposure of the kidney is high because it receives 25% of cardiac output and a high concentration of substances within the tubule as water is reabsorbed. Metabolism can result in toxicity (e.g., the proximal convoluted tubule damage caused by halogenated hydrocarbons such as carbon tetrachloride and chloroform).

CNS. High metabolic rate induces susceptibility to substances that interfere with oxidative metabolism (e.g., cyanide or dinitrophenol). Reliance on axonal transport induces vulnerability to interruption by acrylamide and diketone metabolites of *n*-hexane. Accumulated neurotoxicity might be a "normal" part of the aging process or lifetime exposure to environmental toxicants.

Management of Poisoning

- Reduction of exposure, supportive therapy, and antidotes (if available), are first-line treatment options.
- Induction of vomiting or gastric lavage is contraindicated when the toxicant is caustic (e.g., lye) or is a petroleum distillate (e.g., lighter fluid or gasoline), when the patient is comatose, or when there is a danger of convulsions.
- Antidotes can inhibit the absorption or distribution of the toxicant, increase its rate of elimination (via enhanced metabolism or excretion), or raise the threshold of toxicity. Antidotes have their own set of adverse effects and potential toxicity.

68 Drug-Drug Interactions

Philip D. Hansten, Pharm.D.

A Drug interaction mechanisms in the GI tract and liver

A Object drug alone: normal metabolism via CYP450 isozymes

B Object drug plus competitive inhibitor: reduced object drug metabolism and increased serum concentration of object drug

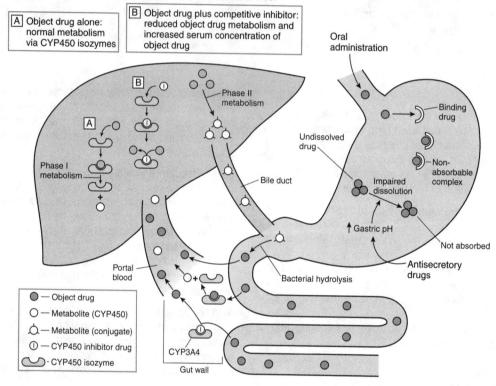

Phase II metabolism

Phase I metabolism

Oral administration

Binding drug

Undissolved drug

Non-absorbable complex

Bile duct

Impaired dissolution

↑ Gastric pH

Not absorbed

Portal blood

Antisecretory drugs

Bacterial hydrolysis

● — Object drug
○ — Metabolite (CYP450)
○ — Metabolite (conjugate)
① — CYP450 inhibitor drug
⬯ - CYP450 isozyme

CYP3A4

Gut wall

B Drug interaction mechanisms in the kidneys

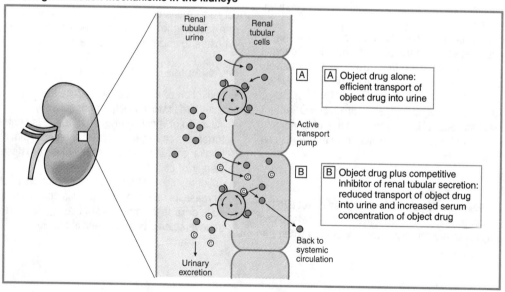

Renal tubular urine

Renal tubular cells

A Object drug alone: efficient transport of object drug into urine

Active transport pump

B Object drug plus competitive inhibitor of renal tubular secretion: reduced transport of object drug into urine and increased serum concentration of object drug

Back to systemic circulation

Urinary excretion

OVERVIEW

- Drug interactions occur by a wide variety of mechanisms involving the gut, liver, kidneys, and other tissues.
- Cytochrome P-450 isozymes in the gut wall and liver are involved in many clinically important drug interactions.
- Drug interactions usually result in an increase or decrease in the response of the affected drug.
- Many drug interactions can be predicted, based on the known interactive properties of the two drugs.
- Adverse drug interactions can almost always be prevented by making appropriate changes in drug therapy.

OBJECT DRUG: The drug whose response is affected by the drug interaction.

PRECIPITANT DRUG: The drug that causes the altered effect of the object drug.

Alteration in Drug Absorption

Drugs can be bound in the stomach and small intestine by precipitant drugs that attach to them, resulting in insoluble complexes that are not absorbed (Fig. A). A few drugs require a particular gastric or intestinal pH range to dissolve, and precipitant drugs that alter gut acidity can thus affect the absorption of other drugs.

Alteration in Intestinal Metabolism

The cells of the small intestine contain considerable amounts of a drug-metabolizing enzyme (CYP3A4), and many drugs are substantially metabolized by this enzyme during the absorption process. Many drugs (also grapefruit juice) can decrease the activity of intestinal CYP3A4, thus increasing the serum concentrations of object drugs metabolized by this enzyme.

Alterations in Distribution

Drugs in the blood are bound to serum proteins (primarily albumin) and highly bound drugs may displace other drugs from these binding sites. This potentially could increase the pharmacodynamic effect of the displaced drug.

Alterations in Hepatic Metabolism

The liver contains a number of drug-metabolizing enzymes, the most important of which are the cytochrome P-450 (CYP450) isozymes such as CYP1A2, CYP2C9, CYP2D6, and CYP3A4. These enzymes transform drug molecules (via phase I metabolism) to more polar (water-soluble) metabolites. This usually serves the dual purpose of inactivating the drug and allowing it to be eliminated by the kidneys. Many commonly used drugs can inhibit or compete for one or more of these isozymes, resulting in increased serum concentrations and response of the object drug. A small number of drugs called enzyme inducers have the opposite effect. They increase the synthesis of drug-metabolizing enzymes (especially CYP3A4) and thus tend to reduce the effect of object drugs metabolized by these isozymes. Compared to CYP450, relatively few drug interactions occur during the conjugation (phase II metabolism) of drugs. Examples of substrates and inhibitors for common cytochrome P-450 isozymes are given in Appendix, G.

Alterations in Renal Excretion

Although the liver and small intestine are the primary sites of drug inactivation, some drugs are eliminated (at least partially) as intact drug by the kidneys. Some drugs that are weak acids or weak bases are eliminated by a process termed *active renal tubular secretion*. When two drugs that both undergo this process are taken, one may inhibit the tubular secretion of the other, resulting in increased serum concentrations and response to the object drug (Fig. B).

Pharmacodynamic Drug Interactions

In addition to pharmacokinetic drug interactions, drugs can exhibit additive or antagonistic pharmacodynamic effects without affecting the pharmacokinetics of one another. Pharmacodynamic drug interactions can involve the same or different receptors and are largely predictable, if one knows the pharmacodynamic effects of the two drugs involved.

Clinical Risk Factors for Drug Interactions

The clinical outcome of drug interactions is highly variable from one patient to another, largely as a result of the presence or absence of predisposing patient or drug-administration factors. Attention to these factors can improve predictions of drug interaction risk in specific patients.

Patient Factors. These include diseases, genetic makeup, age, renal function, hepatic function, tobacco use, alcohol use, environmental exposures, and diet.

Drug Administration Factors. These include dose and duration of therapy for each drug, timing of administration of each drug relative to the other, sequence of administration of the two drugs, route of administration, and adherence to prescribed regimen.

PART VIII: QUESTIONS

Directions: For each of the following questions, choose the **one best** answer.

1. For most clinically used drugs, what is the relationship between the median lethal dose (LD_{50}) and the dose estimated to produce 50% effect (ED_{50})?

(A) $LD_{50} > ED_{50}$

(B) $LD_{50} < ED_{50}$

(C) $LD_{50} = ED_{50}$

(D) $LD_1 = ED_{50}$

2. Drug interactions involving inhibition or induction of metabolism are most likely to occur in which of the following locations?

(A) Plasma protein binding sites

(B) Renal tubular secretion sites

(C) Conjugation reactions in liver

(D) CYP450 enzymes in liver

(E) Enzymes in lung parenchyma

3. Which of the following statements regarding the therapeutic index (TI) of drugs is true?

(A) It gives a rule-of-thumb for a usable range of doses of a drug.

(B) It is the same for all drugs.

(C) It is the same for all drugs used to treat the same disorder.

(D) It is independent of the patient's condition (health, age).

4. Grapefruit juice can increase the serum concentration of drugs that are metabolized by which cytochrome P-450 isozyme?

(A) CYP1A2

(B) CYP2C9

(C) CYP2D6

(D) CYP3A4

(E) CYP2G19

PART VIII: ANSWERS AND EXPLANATIONS

1. **The answer is A.**

In the usual clinical situation, the dose of drug that would be lethal to 50% of treated patients (LD_{50}) is greater than the dose that is therapeutically effective in 50% of the patients (ED_{50}). Extreme conditions might warrant the limited use of drugs with therapeutic indices described by choice D or, rarely, even C or B.

2. **The answer is D.**

Many commonly used drugs can either inhibit or stimulate (less common) the activity of one or more cytochrome P-450 isozymes (located in high concentration in the liver and therefore part of the "first-pass" effect). The result is an increased or decreased serum concentration of the drug and, consequently, of the drug effect. The alteration in metabolizing activity can also affect the pharmacologic effect of other drugs metabolized by the same isozyme(s).

3. **The answer is A.**

The therapeutic index of a drug (commonly defined as $TI = LD_{50}:ED_{50}$) is a useful suggestion of the drug's relative safety (as defined by the unlikelihood of the dose being lethal). Clearly, different drugs have different TIs (except for coincidental equality) and the patient's condition affects both the therapeutic dose that is required and the patient's susceptibility to toxicity. For a particular drug, different disorders might require different doses, yielding different TIs.

4. **The answer is D.**

Considerable amounts of CYP3A4 are found in cells of the small intestine, and many drugs are metabolized to a significant extent by this isozyme. Grapefruit juice decreases the activity of intestinal CYP3A4, thus increasing the serum concentration of drugs metabolized by this enzyme.

PART IX
Special Topics

69 Vitamins and Nutritional Pharmacology

Thomas J. Lauterio, Ph.D., and Michael J. Davies, M.S.

VITAMIN METABOLISM, SOURCES, AND REQUIREMENTS

Vitamin	Sources	Symptoms of Deficiency	Functions	Antagonists	RDA[a]
Fat-soluble vitamins					
Vitamin A (retinol)	Milk, eggs, green leafy and yellow vegetables	Night blindness, itchy dry skin	Vision, cell growth and differentiation	Alcohol, coffee, cortisone	5000 IU
Vitamin D (cholecalciferol)	Milk, cod liver oil, tuna, eggs	Soft bones and teeth, spontaneous fractures	Calcium homeostasis	Mineral oil	400 IU
Vitamin E (α-tocopherol)	Vegetable oil, grains, wheat germ, lettuce	Poor circulatory and muscle performance	Antioxidant	Oral contraceptives, mineral oil	30 IU
Vitamin K (phylloquinone)	Green leafy vegetables, yogurt, alfalfa	Diarrhea, increased hemorrhaging	Blood clotting cofactor	Antibiotics, coumarin, mineral oil	N/A
Water-soluble vitamins					
Vitamin C (ascorbic acid)	Citrus fruits, vegetables	Bruising, poor wound healing, tooth or gum defects	Antioxidant	Antibiotics, aspirin, cortisone	60 mg
Vitamin B_1 (thiamin)	Cereals, fish, lean meat, milk	Fatigue, poor appetite, depression	Carbohydrate metabolism	Alcohol, coffee	1.5 mg
Vitamin B_2 (riboflavin)	Cereals, lean meat, yeast, green leafy vegetables	Light sensitivity, oral-buccal lesions	Redox reactions (i.e., FAD)	Alcohol, coffee	1.7 mg
Vitamin B_3 (niacin)	Cereals, lean meat, yeast, liver, eggs	Weakness, irritability, insomnia, memory loss	Redox reactions (i.e., NAD^+)	Alcohol, coffee	20 mg
Vitamin B_5 (pantothenic acid)	Most plants and animal foods	Increased susceptibility to infections, weakness	Fatty acid metabolism	Alcohol, coffee	10 mg
Vitamin B_6 (pyridoxine)	Cereals, wheat germ, egg yolk, lean meat	Fatigue, anemia, nerve dysfunction	Amino acid metabolism	Alcohol, coffee, hydralazine, isoniazid	2 mg
Vitamin B_7 (biotin)	Egg yolk, liver, kidney, green leafy vegetables	Dermatitis, muscle pains	Carboxylation	Alcohol, coffee, raw egg whites (avidin)	200 μg
Vitamin B_9 (folic acid)	Lean meat, yeast, green leafy vegetables	Anemia, leukopenia, GI problems	One-carbon metabolism	Alcohol, methotrexate, oral contraceptives	400 μg
Vitamin B_{12} (cobalamin)	Fish, lean meat, liver, milk	Anemia, fatigue, nerve degeneration, weakness	Methylmalonyl CoA isomerization	Alcohol, coffee, nitrous oxide, cimetidine	6 μg

[a]Recommended daily allowances (based on normal 70-kg man). Requirements may differ for women (including pregnant and lactating women) and children.

OVERVIEW

- An increased understanding of nutrition's role in the prevention and treatment of diseases along with heightened consumer awareness and advertising has resulted in a dramatic upswing in the pharmacologic use of vitamins.
- Unfortunately many claims have not been scientifically validated.
- There are many common therapeutic applications for vitamins in homeopathic medicine that are worth noting.
- See table (opposite) for information regarding vitamin metabolism, sources, and requirements.

Water-Soluble Vitamins

Vitamins in this category generally function as cofactors in metabolic processes. Their requirements increase with increased activity as well as during periods of elevated metabolism such as illness or stress. They are not stored to an appreciable degree, so toxicity is not a problem under most circumstances.

Vitamin B_6 (Pyridoxine). Because of the role this vitamin plays in transaminations and decarboxylations, requirements are usually adjusted with protein intake. Pharmacologic uses include treatment of sideroblastic anemia not responding to Fe^{2+} or B_{12} and to improve muscle tone in Parkinson's disease patients receiving levodopa.

Vitamin B_{12} (Cobalamin). Although this vitamin is frequently deficient in alcoholics, the most common therapeutic use is in the treatment of pernicious anemia. Gastric bypasses or other conditions that result in the loss of "intrinsic factor" essential for vitamin B_{12} absorption also necessitate B_{12} supplementation.

Niacin. Deficiency of niacin results in the classic symptoms of dementia, dermatitis, and diarrhea, often referred to as the three Ds. Since niacin is one of the vitamins that is usually fortified in common foods such as bread, these symptoms and the accompanying deficiency disease known as pellagra are rarely observed in Western societies. Furthermore, tryptophan may be converted to niacin at a 1:60 molar ratio of niacin per tryptophan. A common pharmacologic use of niacin is the treatment of hypercholesterolemia. Niacin, in doses ranging from 500 mg to 3 g a day is effective in reducing serum cholesterol levels in many individuals. High doses of niacin reduce levels of triglycerides, LDL-C, and lipoprotein (a), while elevating levels of HDL-C and the HDL_2-C variant known to be associated with decreased cardiovascular disease. Nicotinamide, the more commonly found form of niacin, does not exert these effects, although this form prevents pellagra. Both slow-acting and acute-release forms of niacin are available, with the former less likely to elicit flushing when compared at equal doses. Flushing is often eliminated by taking a "baby" aspirin along with the vitamin. As with other 3-hydroxy-3-methylglutaryl CoA reductase inhibitors, liver enzymes must be watched for signs of hepatotoxicity.

Vitamin C (Ascorbic Acid). Vitamin C has received much attention and use as a therapeutic agent since Nobel Laureate Linus Pauling championed its use to prevent the common cold. However, controlled studies have shown only marginal effects on cold symptoms. More recently, the antioxidant and reducing agent effects of vitamin C have been studied extensively. Vitamin C stimulates hydroxylation with Cu^{2+} or Fe^{2+} as cofactors. These actions of vitamin C have led to the speculation that it may be useful as an adjunct treatment for cancer or aging. Withdrawal from high doses of vitamin C may result in rebound scurvy.

Fat-Soluble Vitamins

Vitamins in this category are naturally acquired through dietary fat intake, and they are not readily excreted in the urine. Overuse of vitamin supplements may therefore result in toxic levels, whereas agents that interfere with fat absorption such as cholestyramine may result in a deficiency of vitamins A, D, E, and K.

Vitamin A. Retinoids, such as vitamin A, act directly in the nucleus to alter transcription of mRNA, and this has led to speculation as to their role in cellular growth and differentiation. Vitamin A has been highly touted as a means to prevent cancers, and an effect of retinoids in high doses has been substantiated for reducing the incidence of colon cancer. In addition, vitamin A has been shown to confer protection against carcinogen-induced vaginal, cervical, and intestinal cancers. β-Carotene provides the benefits of vitamin A without the associated toxicity and may be the preferable form for pharmacologic use.

Vitamin D. This vitamin has been prescribed with and without calcium supplementation for regulation of calcium levels in postmenopausal women, particularly those with additional intestinal or liver problems that exacerbate calcium loss. When administered therapeutically, vitamin D is usually prescribed in 2.5 mg doses (100,000 IU) in either capsule or oil form. Vitamin D has antiproliferative effects on tumor cell lines including those for breast cancer and melanomas. Moreover, vitamin D is effective in the treatment of the hyperproliferative epidermal disorder, psoriasis.

Vitamin E (Tocopherols). Increased intake of this vitamin has not been associated with decreased risk of cancers as originally thought. However, long-term studies have now demonstrated a beneficial effect of vitamin E on cardiovascular disease.

70 Drugs Used in Dentistry

Stephen A. Cooper, D.M.D., Ph.D.

A Sites of action for centrally acting narcotic analgesics, peripherally acting NSAID analgesics, and local anesthetics

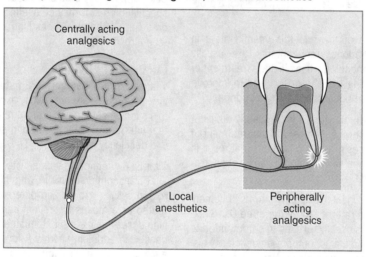

Centrally acting analgesics

Local anesthetics

Peripherally acting analgesics

B Mechanisms of action for major classes of antibiotics

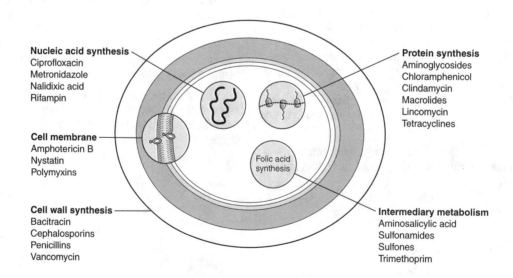

Nucleic acid synthesis
Ciprofloxacin
Metronidazole
Nalidixic acid
Rifampin

Cell membrane
Amphotericin B
Nystatin
Polymyxins

Cell wall synthesis
Bacitracin
Cephalosporins
Penicillins
Vancomycin

Protein synthesis
Aminoglycosides
Chloramphenicol
Clindamycin
Macrolides
Lincomycin
Tetracyclines

Folic acid synthesis

Intermediary metabolism
Aminosalicylic acid
Sulfonamides
Sulfones
Trimethoprim

- Dentists utilize a limited armamentarium of drug classes, and this usage varies widely according to specialty area.
- The vast majority of drugs fall into the general pharmacologic classes of analgesics (peripheral and central), antimicrobial (antibiotics and antifungals), antianxiety-sedative-hypnotics, and antisialogogues and anesthetics (mostly local anesthetics).
- There are also some drug products uniquely associated with dentistry such as fluorides and astringents.

Analgesics

The use of analgesics ranges from the more mild OTC agents to narcotic combinations. Single-entity narcotics and other Drug Enforcement Agency (DEA) Schedule II combinations are rarely indicated to treat dental pain.

Specific Agents (Not All-inclusive). OTC agents include acetaminophen (Tylenol), aspirin, ibuprofen (Advil), and naproxen sodium (Aleve). Prescription agents can be further classified as NSAIDs, such as diflunisal (Dolobid) and diclofenac (Voltaren, Cataflam), and narcotics combinations. The latter include acetaminophen with codeine, hydrocodone, or oxycodone (Tylenol with codeine, Vicodin, Percocet); acetaminophen combined with propoxyphene (Darvocet-N); and ibuprofen with hydrocodone (Vicoprofen).

Antimicrobials

Although a wide range of antimicrobials are used in dentistry, most oral bacterial infections are sensitive to the penicillins and oral fungal infections are sensitive to local application of nystatin (Mycostatin). Prophylaxis against bacterial endocarditis represents a major use of the penicillins. Culture sensitivity testing is recommended prior to using antibiotics for treating periodontal infections.

Specific Agents (Not All-inclusive). The penicillins include penicillin V (Pen•Vee K), amoxicillin (Amoxil), and cloxacillin (Tegopen, penicillinase-resistant). Some representative cephalosporins are cephradine (Velosef), cephalexin (Keflex), cefadroxil (Duricef), and cefaclor (Ceclor). The macrolides include erythromycin salts (E.E.S., Erythrocin, ERYC) and clarithromycin (Biaxin). Most commonly used tetracyclines are doxycycline (Vibramycin) and tetracycline HCl periodontal fiber (Actisite). Miscellaneous antibiotics include clindamycin (Cleocin) and metronidazole (Flagyl). The antifungals group includes nystatin (Mycostatin), ketoconazole (Nizoral), and fluconazole (Diflucan).

Antianxiety-Sedative-Hypnotics

As part of pain control regimens, a wide variety of antianxiety-sedative-hypnotics are used alone or in combination. Pedodontists and oral surgeons also may use general anesthetic agents.

Specific Agents (Not All-inclusive). Oral sedation agents include benzodiazepines such as diazepam (Valium), oxazepam (Serax), or lorazepam (Ativan); chloral hydrate; and hydroxyzine (Atarax). For intravenous sedation, diazepam (Valium), midazolam (Versed), and propofol (Diprivan) are used. Inhalation analgesia is obtained with nitrous oxide.

Antisialogogues

These anticholinergics are used to dry oral secretions, reducing the potential for contaminating the operative area. CNS toxicity and tachycardia are two potential side effects. These drugs are contraindicated with narrow-angle glaucoma.

Specific Agents. Agents include atropine, glycopyrrolate, and propantheline (Pro-Banthine).

Local Anesthetics

This is by far the most important group of drugs for the dentist. Local anesthetics are used to block nerve conduction of pain impulses. Many are combined with small amounts of a vasoconstrictor (e.g., 1/100,000 epinephrine) to enhance localization of drug and duration of effect.

Specific Agents. Injectable, short-acting agents are lidocaine (Xylocaine), mepivacaine (Carbocaine), and prilocaine (Citanest). Injectable, long-acting agents include bupivacaine (Marcaine) and etidocaine (Duranest). Topical agents used are benzocaine, lidocaine, and tetracaine.

Fluorides

Fluorides are used in toothpastes and applied by the dentist to strengthen the enamel structure of teeth. In most parts of the United States, fluoride is added as a supplement to the water supply.

Specific Agents for Professional Application. Included in this group are sodium fluoride 2%, stannous fluoride 8%, and acidulated phosphate fluoride 1.23%.

Toothpastes and Plaque Reducers

Toothpastes can contain various drugs to strengthen enamel, reduce tooth sensitivity, prevent plaque formation, or whiten teeth.

Specific Agents. To strengthen enamel, fluoride in the form of sodium monofluorophosphate 0.76% is most commonly used. For tooth sensitivity, strontium is the active agent in Sensodyne toothpaste. Tooth whiteners are offered as abrasives and in hydrogen-peroxide-containing toothpastes. To reduce plaque, commercial products are triclosan (Colgate Total toothpaste) and chlorhexidine rinse (Peridex, PerioGard).

71 Neuroactive Peptides

Robert B. Raffa, Ph.D.

A — Comparison of cellular processes of neuropeptide neurotransmitters with those of "classic" neurotransmitters

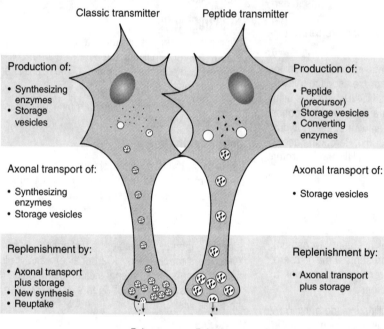

Classic transmitter

Peptide transmitter

Production of:
- Synthesizing enzymes
- Storage vesicles

Axonal transport of:
- Synthesizing enzymes
- Storage vesicles

Replenishment by:
- Axonal transport plus storage
- New synthesis
- Reuptake

Production of:
- Peptide (precursor)
- Storage vesicles
- Converting enzymes

Axonal transport of:
- Storage vesicles

Replenishment by:
- Axonal transport plus storage

Release   Release

B

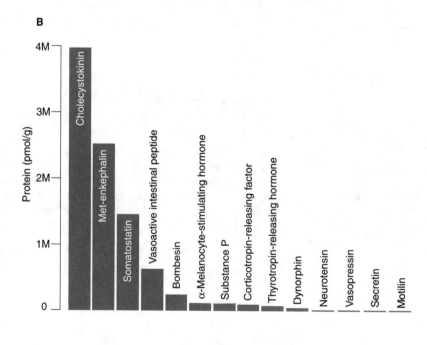

Protein (pmol/g)

- Cholecystokinin
- Met-enkephalin
- Somatostatin
- Vasoactive intestinal peptide
- Bombesin
- α-Melanocyte-stimulating hormone
- Substance P
- Corticotropin-releasing factor
- Thyrotropin-releasing hormone
- Dynorphin
- Neurotensin
- Vasopressin
- Secretin
- Motilin

C Diversity of effects possible with co-localization

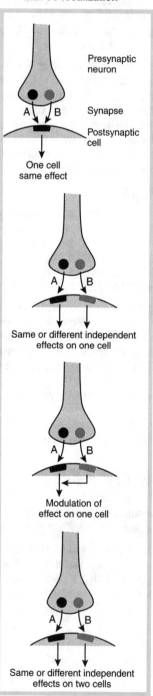

Presynaptic neuron

Synapse

Postsynaptic cell

One cell same effect

Same or different independent effects on one cell

Modulation of effect on one cell

Same or different independent effects on two cells

OVERVIEW

- Peptides consist of relatively short sequences of amino acids (50 is usually regarded as the cutoff). The C-terminus is typically amidated, along with posttranslational modifications of specific residues and, if present, intramolecular disulfide bonds can confer partial cyclic conformation.
- There are not many peptides in natural (plant) products, and most natural products do not interact with peptide signaling pathways.
- Peptides were recognized as being physiologic mediators in mammals in the 1930s, but structural elucidation and synthesis of a peptide was not accomplished until 1953 (du Vigneaud; oxytocin).
- The number of known endogenous peptide mediators and neurotransmitters now exceeds the number of known nonpeptide mediators (~60 versus ~10). The peptide neurotransmitters differ from the nonpeptide ones (such as ACh and NE) in being represented directly in the genome.
- Neuropeptides represent novel targets for therapeutic agents, and drug discovery efforts are directed at synthesizing nonpeptidic, small drug molecules that either mimic or antagonize the action of the endogenous neuropeptide. Such drugs offer the hope of therapeutic agents that might subtly affect or correct a host of vegetative, perceptual, and emotional functions of the CNS.

Peptide Signaling Systems

In general, peptide-mediated neurotransmission closely resembles transmission by nonpeptide mediators (vesicular storage, Ca^{2+}-activated release, binding to receptors, activation of second-messenger systems). Their effects can be pre- or postsynaptic, excitatory or inhibitory, and extend over short or long distances. Normally they are synthesized in the cell body (lack of ribosomes in nerve terminals); thus replenishment is slower. The peptide receptors are generally G-protein–coupled, not voltage- or ligand-gated ion channels, but peptides can act as modulators at ion-channel (ionotropic) receptors. Peptides are commonly co-localized in the same neurons as are nonpeptide neurotransmitters and are co-released with them in ratios sometimes determined by nerve activity.

Examples of Neuroactive Peptides

Cholecystokinin (CCK). CCK has a role in appetite, satiety, analgesia (modulation at level of spinal cord), and anxiety.

Calcitonin Gene-related Peptide (CGRF). CGRF is located in spinal motoneurons, sensory neurons of dorsal root ganglia (DRG), and amygdala (some aspects of social function).

Endogenous Opioids. Endogenous opioids bind to "morphine" receptors; mimic opioid action; and include endorphins, enkephalins, and dynorphins.

Endothelins. Endothelins are the most powerful vasoconstrictors (decrease cerebral blood flow). They increase cerebral metabolism; increase secretion of Glu, dopamine, and NO; are receptors in high concentration in the hypothalamus and the rest of the limbic system; and have a possible role in stress-related disorders (depression).

Neurotensin. Is found in largest amounts in hypothalamus, nucleus accumbens, septum; lowers body temperature; stimulates release of growth hormones and prolactin; is postulated as "endogenous antipsychotic peptide."

Neuropeptide Y (NPY). NPY has 36 amino acids, is released primarily in limbic system and cerebral cortex, is a powerful vasoconstrictor, potentiates NE, reduces anxiety, and stimulates appetite and weight gain.

Somatostatin. Somatostatin has 28 amino acids, is widely distributed in the GI tract, pancreas, hypothalamus (and other brain and spinal cord regions), enhances responsiveness to ACh, frequently coexists with GABA, inhibits growth hormone release, decreases spontaneous locomotor activity, reduces sensitivity to barbiturates, depresses REM sleep, and increases appetite. Somatostatin is reduced in certain types of Alzheimer's disease.

Substance P. Substance P was the first neuropeptide to be isolated and characterized. It is an undecapeptide (11 amino acids); is a member of "tachykinin" family of peptides; is present in hypothalamus and dorsal horn of spinal cord; is proposed as an excitatory transmitter of primary afferent neurons; and is a smooth muscle stimulant and vasodilator.

Vasopressin and Oxytocin. Vasopressin and oxytocin are the two main hormones produced by the posterior pituitary. Vasopressin is antidiuretic hormone (ADH). Oxytocin causes uterine contractions during labor and stimulates lactation in nursing mothers. It is involved in maternal behavior, raises libido (male and female), and is involved in social behavior and in memory.

Vasoactive Intestinal Peptide (VIP). VIP stimulates production of nerve-growth factors, NO, and interleukins. It is necessary for survival of neurons, is involved in induction of sleep, and potentiates Glu in maintaining circadian rhythms.

72 Immunopharmacology

Toby K. Eisenstein, Ph.D.

A Cells of the immune system

Cells	Surface markers	Function	Site
B cells	Surface IgM or IgG	Make antibodies	Lymph nodes, lamina propria of the GI tract, and blood
T cells	CD3		Lymph nodes and blood
T-helper 1 cells (Th-1)	CD4	Release interferon-γ to stimulate monocytes and macrophages	
T-helper 2 cells (Th-2)	CD4	Help B cells make antibody	
T-cytotoxic cells	CD8	Kill tumor cells, virus-infected cells, and transplanted tissue	
Monocytes and macrophages	CD14	Ingest and kill microbes	Blood, peritoneal cavity, lung, and Kupffer cells of liver
Dendritic cells	CD1	Present antigen	Lymph nodes
Granulocytes			
Polymorphonuclear neutrophils (PMNs)		Ingest and kill microbes	Blood
Eosinophils	CD23	Kill parasites by antibody-dependent cytotoxicity	Blood
Basophils	Surface IgE	Release histamine Mediate anaphylaxis	Blood (basophil) and tissue (mast cell)
Natural killer (NK) cells	CD56	Kill tumor cells Antiviral activity	Blood and spleen

B

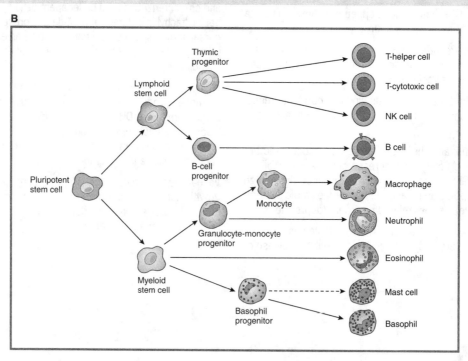

Functions of the Immune System

The function of the immune system is to recognize foreignness or non-self. An antigen is a molecule recognized by the immune system. Antigens include microbes and microbial antigens, such as toxins, capsular polysaccharides, and microbial proteins. Plant products can be antigenic and induce allergic rhinitis (hay fever) or skin reactions (e.g., poison ivy). Tumor cells that acquire new surface molecules not present on normal tissue can be recognized by the immune system. Tissue that is engrafted and is not sufficiently histocompatible is recognized as foreign, and the body mounts an immune response, leading to rejection.

Types of Immune Responses

The immune response can be humoral or cellular. Humoral immune responses result in the formation of antibody that is released into the blood and lymph. Cellular immune responses result in activated macrophages or cytotoxic T cells, which have the capacity to kill many types of microbes and tumor cells, respectively.

Vaccines

Attenuated microbes or microbial products, such as toxoids or capsular polysaccharides, can be injected or given orally to induce an active immune response that will protect the host against subsequent exposure to the infectious agent. Examples include:

- DPT = Diphtheria, pertussis, tetanus
- MMR = Measles, mumps, rubella
- Hib = *Haemophilus influenzae*, type B
- Hep B = Hepatitis B
- Varicella = Chicken pox

Immunoglobulins

Passive antibody can be given to produce immunity for several months.

Tetanus Immune Globulin. It contains antibodies to tetanus toxoid that also bind and neutralize tetanus toxin.

Pooled Gamma Globulin. Pooled gamma globulin protects against hepatitis A (HAV) and other infectious agents to which the general population has been exposed.

Rh(D) Immune Globulin. This immunoglobulin recognizes Rh-positive cells from the fetus in the circulation of an Rh-negative mother and removes them so that the mother will not make anti-Rh(D) antibodies and endanger a subsequent fetus with erythroblastosis fetalis.

Transplant Rejection

Cyclosporine and FK506 (tacrolimus) are both microbial products that inhibit T-cell activation through inhibition of calcineurin activity. These drugs prevent rejection of transplanted organs by interfering with the cellular immune response.

Treatment of Asthma

Cromolyn Sodium. Cromolyn inhibits mast cell degranulation and release of histamine. It is used prophylactically to prevent an asthma attack.

Glucocorticoids. The glucocorticoids inhibit cellular inflammation and are used chronically to treat asthma.

Epinephrine. Is used to relieve bronchospasm and is used acutely for relief of an asthma attack.

Autoimmune Diseases

Glucocorticoids are used to suppress inflammatory reactions associated with autoimmune phenomena.

Cytokines and Immunostimulation

Cytokines are small proteins that communicate signals between cells of the immune system. They can enhance or depress immune responses. Cytokines currently used for therapy are immunostimulants.

Interferon-α and Interferon-β. Interferon-α and -β are a family of proteins that have antiviral and antiproliferative properties. Interferon-α-2a (Roferon-A) and interferon-α-2b (Intron A) are used to treat chronic hepatitis B and C, hairy cell leukemia, chronic myelogenous leukemia, AIDS-related Kaposi's sarcoma, genital warts, and malignant melanoma. Interferon-α-n3 (Alferon N) is used to treat genital warts. Interferon-β-1a (Avonex) and interferon-β-1b (Betaseron) are used to treat relapsing multiple sclerosis.

Interleukin-2 (IL-2). IL-2 activates T cells and NK cells and is used to boost antitumor cellular immune responses.

Granulocyte Colony–Stimulating Factor (G-CSF). G-CSF is used to treat and prevent neutropenia resulting from chemotherapy.

Granulocyte-Macrophage Colony–Stimulating Factor (GM-CSF). GM-CSF is used to enhance bone marrow transplantation.

New-Drug Approval Process

Gary E. Stein, Pharm.D.

New-drug development and approval process

| | Early research/preclinical testing | Clinical trials | | | FDA | Phase IV |
		Phase I	Phase II	Phase III		
Years	6.5	1.5	2	3.5	1.5 Total 15	
Test population	Laboratory and animal studies	20–80 healthy volunteers	100–300 patient volunteers	1000–3000 patient volunteers	Review process and approval	Additional post-marketing testing required by FDA
Purpose	Assess safety and biologic activity	Determine safety and dosage	Evaluate effectiveness, look for side effects	Confirm effectiveness, monitor adverse reactions from long-term use		
Success rate	5000 compounds evaluated		5 drugs enter trials		1 drug approved	

(Between preclinical and Phase I: "File IND at FDA"; between Phase III and FDA: "File NDA at FDA")

Source. Pharmaceutical Research and Manufacturers of America (PhRMA), Washington, D.C.

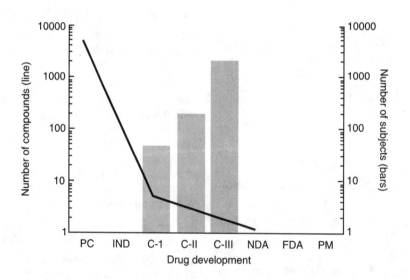

PC   = discovery and preclinical testing for efficacy and safety
IND   = investigational new-drug application to FDA
C-I   = phase I of clinical trials on healthy volunteers to determine safety and dose
C-II = phase II of clinical trials to evaluate efficacy and side effects in patient population
C-III = phase III of clinical trials to assess safety and efficacy in larger patient population
NDA   = new-drug application to FDA
FDA   = Food and Drug Administration
PM   = postmarketing testing, also called phase IV

OVERVIEW

- All compounds for which a medical claim is made must undergo a vigorous review and approval process by the FDA.
- The compound first must be shown to be safe enough to test in humans. Preclinical data (in vitro and animal testing) is submitted in an investigational new drug (IND) application.
- Phase I clinical trials evaluate dose range and safety in a small number of healthy volunteers.
- Phase II clinical trials test therapeutic efficacy in a small population of patients.
- Phase III clinical trials test safety and efficacy in a large population of patients.
- The results of the clinical trials are submitted to the FDA in a new-drug application (NDA) for approval of specific dose(s) and medical indication(s).
- If the compound has abuse potential, it must also be assigned a Schedule (I-V), with input from the FDA, the Drug Enforcement Agency (DEA), and other agencies and organizations.
- Phase IV (postmarketing) clinical trials may be desired or required for approval of new indications or to further assess adverse effects.

Before initiating a study in humans, an investigator must obtain approval from an Institutional Review Board (IRB). The IRB is responsible for ensuring the ethical acceptability of the proposed research. The IRB must determine that the research design and procedures are sound and that the risk to subjects is minimized. The IRB also approves an informed consent document that is signed by the study subjects. This document explains the purposes and procedures of the research, foreseeable risks, expected benefits, confidentiality of records, and subjects' rights.

If acceptable clinical findings are obtained, the sponsor can submit an NDA to the FDA. In approving the NDA, the FDA ensures the drug's safety and effectiveness for each use. Postapproval research may be requested by the FDA as a condition of new-drug approval. This additional research may be used to speed drug approval, to uncover unexpected adverse drug reactions, and to define the incidence of known drug reactions under actual clinical use.

The post-NDA approval or postmarketing period (phase IV) involves monitoring new drug safety during clinical use. Postmarketing surveillance is important to define the true side-effect profile of a new drug. New safety information obtained during this period is used to update the current NDA and to make changes on the drug's label.

74 Scheduling and Prescription Writing

Gary E. Stein, Pharm.D.

No. 7147
Clinic or physician's name
Address
Phone

Date

Patient

Address

R_x Drug name and strength
Quantity to dispense
Directions for administration

☐ Label

No safety cap ☐
Refill ___ times
☐ No refill

Dr. signature _____
Printed name _____
DEA no. _____

OVERVIEW

- Prescriptions are written communications directing the dispensing and proper use of medications for a diagnosed medical condition.
- Prescription accuracy can affect the safe and effective use of medications, and patient compliance to the proper dosage regimen.
- Government regulations and agencies specify and enforce the schedule of CNS-active agents, from I (compounds with greatest abuse potential and least medical utility) to V (least restrictions).
- Controlled substances are labeled with a large 'C' followed by the Roman numeral schedule designation on with the Roman numeral within the 'C'.

Prescriptions are written by a prescriber (physician, dentist, veterinarian) to instruct the pharmacist regarding preparation and dispensation of a specific medication for a specific patient or client. It is important that a prescription communicate clearly and exactly what medication is needed and how the medication is to be used by the patient or client. Compliance is often related to the clarity of directions on the prescription. Many drugs have similar proprietary names, so both the generic and brand names should be written on the prescription to avoid confusion.

Prescriptions contain certain elements to facilitate interpretation by the pharmacist (see Fig.). Both apothecary and metric systems are utilized to indicate weights and measures. Patient instructions (signature) on the prescription can be written with Latin abbreviations (e.g., PO = by mouth) as shorthand for prescribers to give instructions to the pharmacist on how and when the patient is to take the medication. The prescriber also may instruct the pharmacist to place an additional label on the prescription container (e.g., may cause drowsiness).

Those drugs that are called scheduled drugs have abuse potential, and special requirements control their use. Schedule I substances have high abuse potential. Less abuse potential and greater medical utility are designated by progression from Schedule I to Schedule V.

Many prescribed drugs are available from several different manufacturers. Pharmacists receiving prescriptions for brand-name products may dispense a bioequivalent generic drug without prescriber approval and pass on the savings to the patient. Many states have mandatory substitution laws, and the brand-name product is dispensed only when "dispense as written" is stated on the prescription.

SCHEDULE DESIGNATION OF CONTROLLED SUBSTANCES

Category	Condition of Use	Exmaples
I	Restricted to research use	Hallucinogens (LSD, mescaline, peyote, ibogaine, psilocybin, PCP); marijuana; methaqualone; heroin; and "date rape" drugs such as flunitrazepam
II	Refills on a prescription are not allowed, nor are telephone prescriptions	Opium and many medically used opioids (morphine, codeine, methadone, fentanyl and analogs, etc.); coca leaves and cocaine; potent amphetamines; some barbiturates and the cannabinoid dronabinol
III	Restricted to 5 refills or 6 months without a new prescription	Certain opioid formulations and combination products; some amphetamine analogs; some barbiturates and combination products; anabolic steriods, in some states
IV	Similar to schedule IV, but monitoring and penalties are somewhat less severe	Weaker opioids such as propoxyphene; some amphetamine analogs; some barbiturates (e.g., phenobarbital); most benzodiazepines
V	Similar to controls on other prescription drugs or can be dispensed without prescription if not restricted by state regulations	Combination products containing limited amounts of opioids (diphenoxylate with atropine, codeine with acetaminophen, etc.); drugs with some, but limited, abuse potential

Directions: For each of the following questions, choose the **one best** answer.

1. Which is the neuroactive peptide that inhibits the release of growth hormone?

(A) NPY

(B) Somatostatin

(C) Substance P

(D) Vasopressin or oxytocin

(E) VIP

2. A patient taking megadoses of vitamins (several times the RDA) on a daily basis for several years is likely to accumulate toxic levels of which nutrient?

(A) Vitamin B_6

(B) Vitamin C

(C) Folic acid

(D) Vitamin A

(E) β-Carotene

3. Which of the following acronyms is defined correctly?

(A) FDA = Federal Drug Administration

(B) IND = investigational new drug

(C) IRB = International Regulatory Board

(D) NDA = National Drug Advisory Committee

4. A prescription form omits which of the following information?

(A) Date of the prescription

(B) Patient's name

(C) Cost of the medication

(D) Directions to the patient

(E) Physician's signature

5. Which of the following situations will occur in an individual who consumes 3 g of niacin daily?

(A) Blood total cholesterol will decrease, with increased triglycerides.

(B) Blood total cholesterol will decrease while HDL_2-C cholesterol increases.

(C) Blood test cholesterol will increase while LDL-C cholesterol increases.

(D) Blood total cholesterol will increase along with HDL cholesterol levels.

(E) Dementia, dermatitis, and diarrhea will be observed.

6. Which of the following agents can be used to treat sensitive teeth?

(A) Triclosan

(B) Benzocaine

(C) Vitamin E

(D) Strontium

7. Which of the following neuroactive peptides is most closely related to a role in appetite and satiety?

(A) CCK

(B) CGRF

(C) Endogenous opioids

(D) Endothelins

(E) Neurotensin

8. Which clinical trial phase involves healthy volunteers?

(A) Phase I

(B) Phase II

(C) Phase III

(D) Phase IV

9. Which of the following statements regarding vitamins is true?

(A) Mineral oil will increase the efficacy of dietary vitamin E.

(B) Vitamin B_{12} excess is a primary cause of pernicious anemia in the United States.

(C) Vitamin B_6 supplementation is recommended in individuals receiving isoniazid treatment for tuberculosis.

(D) The body has a greater capacity to store water-soluble vitamins compared to fat-soluble vitamins.

(E) Individuals increasing their activity level should reduce their intake of vitamins B_1 and B_2.

10. Which one of the following agents is a long-acting local anesthetic?

(A) Bupivacaine (Marcaine)

(B) Lidocaine (Xylocaine)

(C) Mepivacaine (Carbocaine)

(D) Prilocaine (Citanest)

11. Which of the following agents contains passive antibody that can be given to produce immunity for a short period of time?

(A) DPT

(B) Varicella vaccine

(C) Hep B vaccine

(D) Tetanus immune globulin

12. Antisialogogues should not be used in patients with

(A) liver disease

(B) diabetes

(C) narrow-angle glaucoma

(D) high blood pressure

13. Which of the following is a small protein that communicates signals between cells of the immune system?

(A) Glucocorticoid

(B) Cyclosporine

(C) Polio

(D) Cytokine

14. Which schedule designates the lowest abuse potential for a medically useful drug?

(A) I

(B) II

(C) III

(D) IV

(E) V

PART IX: ANSWERS AND EXPLANATIONS

1. The answer is A.

NPY is released primarily in the limbic system and cerebral cortex, is a powerful vasoconstrictor, potentiates norepinephrine, reduces anxiety, and stimulates appetite and weight gain. Somatostatin is widely distributed in the GI tract, pancreas, hypothalamus (and other brain and spinal cord regions) and frequently coexists with GABA. It inhibits the release of GH and is reduced in certain types of Alzheimer's disease. Substance P was the first neuropeptide isolated and characterized. It is present in the hypothalamus and the dorsal horn of the spinal cord and is proposed as a transmitter in primary afferent neurons. Vasopressin and oxytocin are the two main hormones produced by the posterior pituitary. Vasopressin is ADH. Oxytocin stimulates uterine contraction during labor and stimulates lactation in nursing mothers. At the CNS level, it is involved in libido (male and female), social behavior, and memory. VIP stimulates production of nerve-growth factors, NO, and interleukins. It is necessary for neuron survival, is involved in induction of sleep, and potentiates Glu in maintaining circadian rhythms.

2. The answer is D.

Vitamin A accumulates in fat depots and in the liver. In fact, consumption of liver enriched with vitamin A has been known to be lethal in humans. Vitamins B_6, C, and folic acid are all water-soluble vitamins that are excreted from the body when consumed in excessive quantities. β-Carotene is fat-soluble, but it is nontoxic when consumed in doses many times those required by the body, although accumulation of carotenoids can occur in the fat.

3. The answer is B.

An IND must be submitted to the FDA (Food and Drug Administration) and approval of the appropriate IRB (Institutional Review Board) must be obtained before initiating clinical trials. The NDA (new-drug application) is submitted to the FDA, summarizing all of the preclinical and clinical findings.

4. The answer is C.

The cost of medication does not appear on the prescription form. The date of the prescription (and a stated or implied duration of acceptability), the patient's name, and the physician's signature help validate the prescription and ensure that the proper medication is given to the intended patient. The directions to the patient assist compliance.

5. The answer is B.

Blood cholesterol should decrease when niacin is consumed in large doses, especially in individuals with familial hypercholesterolemia. Therefore answers C and D are incorrect. Dementia, diarrhea, and dermatitis are signs of deficiency, not toxicity. Triglycerides also decrease with niacin, while HDL_2-C levels are specifically elevated.

6. The answer is D.

Toothpastes can contain various agents that strengthen enamel (e.g., fluorides), reduce tooth sensitivity (e.g., strontium), reduce plaque formation (e.g., triclosan), or whiten teeth (e.g., abrasives or hydrogen peroxide).

7. The answer is A.

In addition to a role in regulating appetite and satiety, CCK has roles in analgesia (modulation at spinal cord level) and anxiety. CGRF is located in spinal motoneurons, sensory neurons of dorsal root ganglia, and the amygdala (responsible for some aspects of social function). Endogenous opioids bind to "morphine" receptors and mimic opioid actions. Endothelin receptors are present in high concentration in the hypothalamus and the rest of the limbic system and have possible roles in stress-related disorders. Neurotensin lowers body temperature, stimulates the release of GH and prolactin, and has been postulated to be an endogenous antipsychotic peptide.

8. The answer is A.

Phase I studies are conducted in healthy volunteers to determine a safe dose range and pharmacokinetic parameters. Phases II and III are conducted in patients. Phase IV consists of special (postmarketing) studies.

9. The answer is C.

Mineral oil causes a loss of vitamin E as well as other fat-soluble vitamins. Vitamin B_{12} deficiency, not excess, may be a causative factor in pernicious anemia, and vitamin B_{12} is frequently used to treat it. The body has no capacity to store water-soluble vitamins. Vitamin B intake requirements increase with increased activity because the need for them is tied to the number of metabolic processes a body undertakes. Isoniazid is an antagonist of vitamin B_6 and depletes the available vitamin if it is not supplemented.

10. The answer is A.

The amide-linkage local anesthetics are metabolized mainly in the liver by the microsomal cytochrome P450 system. There is considerable variation in the rate of metabolism of these amide-linked anesthetics. This and other factors lead to the general order of duration: prilocaine (fastest) lidocaine > mepivacaine > bupivacaine (slowest).

11. The answer is D.

DPT, varicella, and Hep B are vaccines that induce active immune response and protect against subsequent exposure. Tetanus immune globulin is an antibody that neutralizes a toxin.

12. The answer is C.

Antisialogogues are used to dry oral secretions to reduce the potential for contamination of the operative area. The commonly used agents are anticholinergics (i.e., cholinergic antagonists). Hence, anti-sialogogues are contraindicated with narrow-angle (closed-angle) glaucoma because the use of drugs in acute narrow-angle glaucoma is limited mainly to cholinergic *agonists* and osmotic agents prior to surgical intervention. Therefore, anticholinergics would aggravate, not alleviate, the problems associated with narrow-angle glaucoma.

13. The answer is D.

Glucocorticoid is used to treat asthma by inhibiting cellular inflammation. Cyclosporine is used to prevent transplant rejection by inhibiting T-cell activation. Polio is the name of either a disease or a vaccine. Cytokine modulates immune responses, that is, they are clinically used as immunostimulants.

14. The answer is E.

The least abused, medically useful drugs are placed on schedule V (e.g., acetaminophen plus codeine combinations). Abused drugs with little medical use (e.g., LSD) are placed on schedule I. Descending abuse potential (with medical utility) determines the placement of a drug into the intermediate schedules II (most abuse) through V (least abuse).

Appendix

A SUMMARY OF ANTIARRHYTHMIC DRUG PROPERTIES

Drug Class	Drug Names	Primary Target	Action	Conditions Treated Effectively
IA	Quinidine Procainamide	Na^+ channels	Prolong action potential duration, depress excitability; reduce pacemaker activity	Premature atrial and ventricular contractions; ventricular tachycardia
IB	Lidocaine Mexiletine	Na^+ channels	Shorten action potential duration, slight decrease in excitability; reduce pacemaker activity	Ventricular tachycardia; fibrillation
IC	Flecainide Propafenone	Na^+ channels	Little change in action potential duration, decrease excitability; reduce pacemaker activity	Supraventricular and ventricular tachycardia
II	Propranolol Sotalol	β-Adrenergic receptors	Blockade of sympathetic tone; also some direct membrane actions	Premature atrial and ventricular contractions; atrial and ventricular tachycardia
III	Amiodarone Bretylium	Na^+, Ca^{2+}, K^+ channels	Prolong action potential duration, decrease excitability; reduce pacemaker activity	Premature atrial and ventricular contractions; supraventricular and ventricular tachycardias
IV	Verapamil Diltiazem Bepridil	Ca^{2+} channels	Block Ca^{2+} channels in AV node, reduce impulse conduction and transmission	Supraventricular tachycardias, atrial flutter, and fibrillation (reduce ventricular rate)

B SPECIFIC DIURETIC AGENTS

CA inhibitors
Acetazolamide (most frequently used of this group)
Dichlorphenamide
Methazolamide

Na^+-K^+-$2Cl^-$ symport inhibitors (loop diuretics or high-ceiling diuretics)
Bumetanide
Ethacrynic acid (higher ototoxicity potential; use only if other loop diuretics not tolerated)
Furosemide (most frequently used of this group)
Torsemide

Na^+-Cl^- symport inhibitors (thiazide diuretics)
Derivatives of 1,2,4-benzothadiazine-1,1-dioxide (chemically are thiazides)
Bendroflumethiazide
Benzthiazide
Chlorothiazide
Hydrocholorothiazide (most frequently used of this group)
Hydroflumethiazide
Methylclothiazide
Polythazide
Trichlormethiazide

(thiazide diuretics, cont'd)
Others (chemically are not thiazides, but often called thiazide or thiazide-like diuretics)
Chlorthalidone
Indapamide
Metolazone (most frequently used of this group)
Quinethazone

Renal epithelial Na^+-channel inhibitors (potassium-sparing diuretics)
Amiloride
Triamterene

Mineralocorticoid receptor antagonists (aldosterone antagonists or potassium-sparing diuretics)
Spironolactone

Osmotic diuretics
Glycerin
Isosorbide
Mannitol (most frequently used of this group)
Urea

C   CHOLINERGIC AND ADRENERGIC AGENTS AND THEIR THERAPEUTIC USE

Class	Drug	Ophthalmic Use (Mechanism of Action)
Cholinergic, muscarinic antagonist	Atropine, scopolamine, homatropine, cyclopentolate, tropicamide	Mydriasis (pupillary dilation via relaxation of iris circular muscle), cycloplegia (relaxation of ciliary smooth muscle and blockage of lens accommodation), uveitis
Cholinergic, direct muscarinic agonist	Pilocarpine, carbachol, acetylcholine	Glaucoma (enhance aqueous humor "outflow"), miosis (pupillary constriction via contraction of iris circular muscle), diagnosis of anisocoria or unequal pupils
Cholinergic, indirect muscarinic	Echothiophate iodide, demecarium	Glaucoma (enhance aqueous humor "outflow")
α_1-Adrenergic agonist	Phenylephrine	Mydriasis (pupillary dilation via contraction of iris radial dilator muscle)
α_1-Adrenergic antagonist	Dapiprazole	Miosis (antagonizes α_1-adrenergic receptors in iris dilator smooth muscle)
α_2-Adrenergic agonist	Brimonidine, apraclonidine	Glaucoma (decrease aqueous humor "inflow")
β-Adrenergic agonist	Epinephrine, dipivefrin	Glaucoma (enhance aqueous humor "outflow")
β-Adrenergic antagonist	Timolol, betaxalol, carteolol, levobunolol, metipranolol	Glaucoma (decrease aqueous humor "inflow")

D   SPECIFIC AGENTS FOR THE TREATMENT OF ASTHMA

Sympathomimetics
Nonselective
   Ephedrine (generic)
   Epinephrine (generic)
β-Selective
   Isoproterenol (generic, Isuprel, others)
β_2-Selective
   Albuterol (Proventil, Ventolin, generic)
   Terbutaline (Brethine, Bricanyl)

Antimuscarinics
Ipratropium (Atrovent)

Mast cell stabilizers
Cromolyn sodium (Intal)
Nedocromil sodium (Tilade)

Corticosteroids
Beclomethasone (Beclovent, others)
Dexamethasone (Decadron)
Flunisolide (AeroBid)
Triamcinolone (Azmacort)

Xanthines
Theophylline
Aminophylline (79% theophylline)

Leukotriene synthesis inhibitor
Zileuton (Zyflo)

Leukotriene receptor antagonists
Zafirlukast (Accolate)
Montelukast sodium (Singulair)

E   SPECIFIC ANTIDEPRESSANT AGENTS

TCAs
Amitriptyline (Elavil)
Amoxapine (Asendin)
Chlordiazepoxide and amitriptyline (Limbitrol)
Clomipramine (Anafranil)
Desipramine (Norpramin)
Doxepin (Dinequan)
Imipramine (Tofranil)
Maprotiline (Ludiomil)
Nortriptyline (Pamelor)
Perphenazine and amitriptyline (Etrafon and Triavil)
Protriptypline (Vivactil)

SNRIs
Milnacepran (Ixel)
Nefazodone (Serzone)
Venlafaxine (Effexort)

SSRIs
Fluoxetine (Prozac)
Fluvoxamine (Luvox)
Paroxetine (Paxil)
Sertraline (Zoloft)

MAOIs
Phenelzine (Nardil)
Tranylcypromine (Parnate)

Miscellaneous
Buproprion (Wellbutrin)
Mirtazepine (Remeron)

CNS

- Analgesia—dose-related increase in pain threshold (objective); decrease in the emotional reaction to pain (subjective)
- Euphoria—individual- and situation-dependent; first experience often dysphoric in persons not in pain
- Sedation—species dependent; drowsiness and mental clouding in humans (no effect on memory); potentiation with CNS depressants
- Respiratory depression—inhibition of brainstem respiratory center
- Cough suppression—codeine is the most widely used opioid antitussive
- Miosis—distinguishing feature of opioid overdose
- Nausea and vomiting—activation of brainstem chemoreceptor trigger zone; relatively common adverse effect, particularly in persons not in pain; accentuated during ambulation
- Truncal rigidity—uncommon adverse effect, but can occur with high doses of very lipid-soluble opioids, such as the fentanyl series

Peripheral

- CV—generally no significant effect (some bradycardia)
- GI tract—constipation, with central and peripheral components; opioids used to manage diarrhea
- Biliary tract—constriction, possible reflux of contents (pain of renal or biliary colic may increase following low doses of morphine; alleviated by higher dose)
- GU tract—depressed renal function; possible urinary retention postoperatively
- Uterus—possible prolongation of labor
- Neuroendocrine—usually not clinically significant
- Miscellaneous—flushing and warming of skin at therapeutic doses, sometimes sweating and itching (due to histamine release?); psychotomimetic effects (nightmares, hallucinations, anxiety) reported with pentazocine

Other

- Acute pulmonary edema—mechanism unknown
- Cough—action on brainstem at doses lower than analgesic
- Diarrhea—both CNS and peripheral actions
- Anesthesia—preoperative sedation and "preemptive" analgesia.

Note. All opioid-receptor-mediated effects are reversed by naloxone (Narcan).

SPECIFIC OPIATES AND OPIOIDS

Full agonists (μ receptor)

- Codeine sulfate or phosphate (generic)—opiate; metabolizes to morphine in brain
- Morphine sulfate (generic)—prototypic opiate
- Hydromorphone (generic; Dilaudid)
- Oxymorphone (Numorphan)
- Heroin—semisynthetic opioid; rapidly passes BBB (favors its abuse); metabolized to morphine in brain
- Meperidine (generic; Demerol)—different chemical class from morphine; little antitussive activity
- Methadone (generic; Dolophine)—synthetic, different chemical class from morphine; used to treat opiate "addicts"; good oral absorption (decreases needle use); long duration
- Fentanyl (Sublimaze)—highly potent, high lipid solubility; available as patch and "lollipop"
- Alfentanil (Alfenta) and sufentanil (Sufenta)—related to fentanyl
- Oxycodone (generic) and hydrocodone (generic)—efficacy nearly equals codeine; adverse effects limit dose to about morphine efficacy
- D-Propoxyphene (generic; Darvon; others)—chemically related to methadone; weak alone, so often used in combinations

Agonist and antagonists

- Pentazocine (Talwin)
- Butorphanol (Stadol)

Partial agonist

- Buprenorphine (Buprenex)

Antagonists

- Naloxone (Narcan) and naltrexone (Trexan)

Combinations

- Tylenol w/ codeine, others—acetaminophen and codeine
- Empirin with codeine—codeine and aspirin
- Vicodin, others—hydrocodone and acetaminophen
- Percocet, others—oxycodone and acetaminophen
- Percodan, others—oxycodone and aspirin
- Darvon Compound–65—propoxyphene and aspirin

Antidiarrheals

- Diphenoxylate + atropine (Lomotil)—atropine added to limit abuse
- Loperamide (Imodium)—limited BBB passage

Antitussive

- Dextromethorphan (generic)—modest analgesic effect

Miscellaneous

- Tramadol (Ultram)—for mild to moderate persistant pain; dual mechanism (μ agonist plus inhibitor of NE and 5-HT reuptake)

CYP1A2		CYP2C9		CYP2D6		CYP3A4	
Substrates	**Inhibitors**	**Substrates**	**Inhibitors**	**Substrates**	**Inhibitors**	**Substrates**	**Inhibitors**
Caffeine	Cimetidine	Diclofenac	Amiodarone	Codeine	Amiodarone	Cisapride	Clarithromycin
Clomipramine	Ciprofloxacin	Flurbiprofen	Cimetidine	Desipramine	Chloroquine	Cyclosporine	Cyclosporine
Clozapine	Enoxacin	Fluvastatin	Cotrimoxazole	Flecainide	Cimetidine	Diltiazem	Diltiazem
Imipramine	Fluvoxamine	Ibuprofen	Dislufiram	Haloperidol	Fluoxetine	Ergotamine	Erythromycin
Olanzapine	Isoniazid	Indomethacin	Fluconazole	Hydrocodone	Haloperidol	Felodipine	Indinavir
Tacrine	Mexiletine	Losartan	Fluvoxamine	Metoprolol	Mibefradil	Lovastatin	Itraconazole
Theophylline	Tacrine	Naproxen	Isoniazid	Mexiletine	Paroxetine	Rifabutin	Ketoconazole
Zileuton	Zileuton	Phenytoin	Metronidazole	Perphenazine	Propafenone	Saquinavir	Grapefruit juice
		Piroxicam	Sulfinpyrazone	Propafenone	Propoxyphene	Sildenafil	Mibefradil
		Tolbutamide	Zafirlukast	Propranolol	Quinacrine	Simvastatin	Nefazodone
		Torsemide		Risiperidone	Quinidine	Triazolam	Ritonavir
		Warfarin		Tramadol	Ritonavir	Verapamil	Verapamil
				Venlafaxine	Thioridazine	Vincristine	Zafirlukast

References

Chapter 8

Conley EC, Brammer WJ (eds): *The Ion Channel, Intracellular Ligand-Gated Channels*, vol. 2. San Diego, CA: Academic Press, 1966.

Hardie G, Hanks S (eds): *The Protein Kinase, Protein-Tyrosine Kinases.* San Diego, CA: Academic Press, 1995.

Hobbs WR, Rall TW, Verdoorn TA: Hypnotics and sedatives: ethanol. In *Goodman and Gilman's The Pharmacological Basis of Therapeutics*, 9th ed. Edited by Hardman JG, Limbird LE, Molinoff PB, et al. New York, NY: McGraw-Hill, 1996, pp 361–398.

Michelangeli F, Mezna M, Tovey S, et al: Pharmacological modulators of the inositol 1,4,5-triphosphate receptor. *Neuropharmacol* 34:111–112, 1995.

North RA (ed): *Ligands and Voltage-Gated Ion Channels.* Boca Raton, FL: CRC Press, 1995.

Reisine T, Pasternak G: Opioid analgesics and antagonists. In *Goodman and Gilman's The Pharmacological Basis of Therapeutics*, 9th ed. Edited by Hardman JG, Limbird LE, Molinoff PB, et al. New York, NY: McGraw-Hill, 1996, pp 521–556.

Robertson RM, Robertson D: Drugs used for the treatment of myocardial ischemia. In *Goodman and Gilman's The Pharmacological Basis of Therapeutics*, 9th ed. Edited by Hardman JG, Limbird LE, Molinoff PB, et al. New York, NY: McGraw-Hill, 1996, pp 759–780.

Schimmer BP, Parker KL: Adrenocorticotropic hormone; adrenocortical steroids and their synthetic analogs; inhibition of the synthesis and actions of adrenocortical hormone. In *Goodman and Gilman's The Pharmacological Basis of Therapeutics*, 9th ed. Edited by Hardman JG, Limbird LE, Molinoff PB, et al. New York, NY: McGraw-Hill, 1996, pp 1459–1488.

Watson S, Arkinstall A: *The G-Protein–Linked Receptor.* San Diego, CA: Academic Press, 1994.

William CL, Stancel GM: Estrogens and progestins. In *Goodman and Gilman's The Pharmacological Basis of Therapeutics*, 9th ed. Edited by Hardman JG, Limbird LE, Molinoff PB, et al. New York, NY: McGraw-Hill, 1996, pp 1411–1440.

Chapter 14

Silverman, DG: *Neuromuscular Block.* Philadelphia, PA: J.B. Lippincott, 1994.

Chapter 17

Nickerson M: The pharmacology of adrenergic blockade. *Pharmacol Rev* 1:27–101, 1949.

Powell CE, Slater IH: Blocking of inhibitory adrenergic receptors by a dichloro analogue of isoproterenol. *J Pharmacol Exp Ther* 122:480–488, 1958.

Chapter 20

Borda I, Slone DH: Assessment of adverse reactions within a drug surveillance program. *J Am Med Assoc* 205:645, 1968.

Gell P, Coombs R: Classification of allergic reactions responsible for clinical hypersensitivity and disease. In *Clinical Aspects of Immunology.* Edited by Gell P, Coombs R, Hachmann P. New York, NY: Blackwell, 1975, pp 761–781.

Patterson R. Diagnosis and treatment of drug allergy. *J Allergy Clin Immunol* 81:380–384, 1988.

Recchia A, Shear N: Organization and functioning of an adverse drug reaction clinic. *J Clin Pharmacol* 34:68–79, 1994.

Weiss M: Drug allergy. *Med Clin N Am* 76:857–882, 1992.

Chapter 21

Grant AO: Mechanisms of action of antiarrhythmic drugs: from ion channel blockage to arrhythmia termination. *PACE* 20:432–444, 1997.

Hondeghem LM, Roden DM: Agents used in cardiac arrhythmias. In *Pharmacology.* Edited by Katzung BG. Norwalk, CT: Appleton and Lange, 1995, pp 205–229.

Nattel S: Comparative mechanisms of action of antiarrhythmic drugs. *Am J Cardiol* 72:13F–17F, 1993.

Chapter 28

Moroi SE, Lichter, PR: Ocular pharmacology. In *Goodman and Gilman's The Pharmacological Basis of Therapeutics*, 9th ed. Edited by Hardman JG, Limbird LE, Molinoff PB, et al. New York, NY: McGraw-Hill, 1996, pp 1619–1645.

Zimmerman TJ, Kooner KS, Sharir M, et al: *Textbook of Ocular Pharmacology.* Philadelphia, PA: Lippincott-Raven, 1997.

Chapter 30

Awouters F, Megens A, Verlinden M, et al: Loperamide: survey of studies on mechanism of its antidiarrheal activity. *Dig Dis Sci* 38:977–995, 1993.

Garcia Compean D, Ramos Jimenez J, Guzman de la Garza F, et al: Octreotide therapy of large-volume refractory AIDS-associated diarrhea: a randomized controlled trial. *AIDS* 8:1563–1567, 1997.

Scarpignato C, Rampal P: Prevention and treatment of traveler's diarrhea: a clinical pharmacological approach. *Chemotherapy* 41 (Suppl 1):48–81, 1995.

Schiller LR: Anti-diarrheal pharmacology and therapeutics. *Aliment Pharmacol Ther* 9:87–106, 1995.

Chapter 31

Dunnick JK, Hailey JR: Phenolphthalein exposure causes multiple carcinogenic effects in experimental model systems. *Cancer Res* 56:4922–4926, 1996.

Ewe K, Ueberschaer B, Press AG, et al: Effect of lactose, lactulose and bisacodyl on gastrointestinal transit studied by metal detector. *Aliment Pharmacol Ther* 9:69–73, 1995.

Gaginella TS, Mascolo N, Izzo AA, et al: Nitric oxide as a mediator of bisacodyl and phenolphthalein laxative action: induction of nitric oxide synthase. *J Pharmacol Exp Ther* 270:1239–1245, 1994.

Gattuso JM, Kamm MA: Adverse effects of drugs used in the management of constipation and diarrhea. *Drug Safety* 10:47–65, 1994.

Izzo AA, Sautebin L, Rombola L, et al: The role of constitutive and inducible nitric oxide synthase in senna- and cascara-induced diarrhea in the rat. *Eur J Pharmacol* 323:93–97, 1997.

Muller-Lissner SA: Adverse effects of laxatives: fact and fiction. *Pharmacology* 47 (Suppl 1):138–145, 1993.

Chapter 33

Baird DT: Clinical use of mifepristone (RU 486). *Ann Med* 25:65–69, 1993.

Bolton TB, Kitamura K: Evidence that ionic channels associated with the muscarinic receptor of smooth muscle may admit calcium. *J Pharmacol* 78:405–416, 1983.

Bulbring E, Tomita T: Catecholamine action on smooth muscle. *Pharmacol Rev* 39:49–96, 1987.

Carsten ME, Miller JD: *Uterine Function: Molecular and Cellular Aspects.* New York, NY: Plenum Press, 1990.

Ichida S, Hayashi T, Kita T, et al: Estradiol-induced increase of specific ^{3}H-ketanserin binding sites on rat uterine membranes. *Eur J Pharmacol* 108:257–264, 1985.

Marshall JM: Adrenergic innervation of female reproductive tract: anatomy, physiology and pharmacology. *Ergeb Physiol* 62:6–67, 1970.

Perusquía M, Hernández R, Jasso-Kamel J, et al: Relaxing effect of progestins on spontaneous contractile activity of gravid human uterus. *Med Sci Res* 25:585–587, 1997.

Chapter 41

American Psychological Association: *Diagnostic and Statistical Manual of Mental Disorders*, 4th ed. Washington, DC: American Psychological Association, 1996.

Benet LZ, Oie S, Schwartz JB: Design and optimization of dosage regimens: pharmacokinetic data. In *Goodman and Gilman's The Pharmacological Basis of Therapeutics*, 9th ed. Edited by Hardman JG, Limbird LE, Molinoff PB, et al. New York, NY: McGraw-Hill, 1996, pp 1707–1792.

Goldin SM: Depression: etiology, advances in pharmacotherapy and worldwide socioeconomic factors. *Drug Mark Dev* 8:182–189, 1997.

Chapter 42

Fisher RS: Emerging antiepileptic drugs. *Neurology* 43 (Supp 5):S12–S20, 1993.

Loscher W, Schmidt D: Strategies in antiepileptic drug development: is rational drug design superior to random screening and structural variation? *Epilepsy Res* 17:95–134, 1994.

Rogawski MA, Porter RJ: Antiepileptic drugs: pharmacological mechanisms and clinical efficacy with consideration of promising developmental stage compounds. *Pharmacol Rev* 42:223–286, 1990.

Chapter 61

Braverman LE: Iodine and the thyroid: 33 years of study. *Thyroid* 4:351–356, 1994.

Braverman LE, Utiger RD (eds): *Werner and Ingbar's The Thyroid.* Philadelphia, PA: Lippincott-Raven, 1996, p 112.

Brent GA: The molecular basis of thyroid hormone action. *N Engl J Med* 331:847–853, 1994.

Evans RM: The steroid and thyroid hormone superfamily. *Science* 241:889–895, 1988.

Farwell AP, Braverman LE: Thyroid and antithyroid drugs. In *Goodman and Gilman's The Pharmacological Basis of Therapeutics*, 9th ed. Edited by Hardman JG, Limbird LE, Molinoff PB, et al. New York, NY: McGraw-Hill, 1996, pp 1383–1410.

Glinoer D: Maternal thyroid function in pregnancy: *J Endocrinol Invest* 16(5):374–378, 1993.

Hays MT: Localization of human thyroxine absorbtion. *Thyroid* 1:241–248, 1991.

Leonard JL, Koehrle J: Intracellular pathways of iodothyronine metabolism. In *Werner and Ingbar's The Thyroid.* Edited by Braverman LE, Utiger RD. Philadelphia, PA: Lippincott-Raven, 1996, pp 125–161.

Mendel CM: The free hormone hypothesis: a physiologically based mathematical model. *Endocr Rev* 10:232–274, 1989.

Meyer-Gessner M, Benker G, Lederbogen S, et al: Antithyroid drug-induced agranulocytosis: clinical experience with ten patients and a review of the literature. *J Endocrinol Invest* 17:29–36, 1994.

Porterfield SP, Hendrich CE: The role of thyroid hormones in prenatal and neonatal development: current perspectives. *Endocr Rev* 14:94–106, 1993.

Ross DR (ed): Subclinical thyrotoxicosis. *Advances in Endocrinology and Metabolism*, vol. 2. St. Louis, MO: C.V. Mosby, 1991, pp 89–103.

Taurog A: Hormone synthesis. In *Werner and Ingbar's The Thyroid.* Edited by Braverman LE, Utiger RD. Philadelphia, PA: Lippincott-Raven, 1996, pp 47–81.

Wolff J: Perchlorate and the thyroid gland. *Pharmacol Rev.* In press, 1998.

Chapter 63

Williams CL, Stancel GM: Estrogens and progestins. In *Goodman and Gilman's The Pharmacological Basis of Therapeutics*, 9th ed. Edited by Hardman JG, Limbird LE, Molinoff PB, et al. New York, NY: McGraw-Hill, 1996, pp 1411–1440.

Chapter 66

Bailey CJ: Biguanides and NIDDM. *Diabetes Care* 15:755, 1992.

Chiasson J-L, Josse RG, Hunt JA, et al: The efficacy of acarbose in the treatment of patients with non-insulin-dependent diabetes mellitus: a multicenter controlled clinical trial. *Ann Intern Med* 121:928, 1994.

Defronzo RA, Goodman AM: The multicenter metformin study group: efficacy of metformin in patients with non-insulin-dependent diabetes. *N Engl J Med* 333:541, 1995.

Howey DC, Bowsher RR, Brunell RL, et al: Lys (B28) pro (B29)—human insulin: a rapidly absorbed analog of human insulin. *Diabetes* 43:396, 1996.

Mathews DR, Riddle MC: International Glimepiride Symposium. *Horm Metab Res* 28:403, 1996.

Saltiel AR, Olefsky JR: Thiazolidinediones in the treatment of insulin resistance and type II diabetes. *Diabetes* 45:1661, 1996.

Chapter 68

Bertz RJ, Granneman GR: Use of in vitro and in vivo data to estimate the likelihood of metabolic pharmacokinetic interactions. *Clin Pharmacokinet* 32:210, 1997.

Hansten PD: Understanding drug interactions. *Sci Med* 5(1):16, 1998.

Levy RH, Bajpai M: Phenytoin: interactions with other drugs: mechanistic aspects. In *Antiepileptic Drugs*, 4th ed. Edited by Levy RH, Mattson RH, Meldrum BS. New York: Raven Press, 1995.

Quinn DI, Day RO: Drug interactions of clinical importance. *Drug Saf* 12:393, 1995.

Rizack MA: *The Medical Letter Handbook of Adverse Drug Interactions—1997.* New Rochelle, NY: The Medical Letter, 1997.

Chapter 70

Cooper SA: Narcotic analgesics in dental practice. *Compend Contin Educ Dent* 14: 1061–1068, 1993.

Cooper SA: New peripherally-acting oral analgesics. *Ann Rev Pharmacol Toxicol* 23:617–647, 1983.

Cooper SA: Treating acute pain: do's and don't's, pros and cons. *J Endocrinol* 16:85–91, 1990.

deJong RH: *Local Anesthetics.* St. Louis, MO: Mosby–Year Book, 1994.

Hardman JG, Limbird LE, Molinoff PB, et al (eds): *Goodman and Gilman's The Pharmacological Basis of Therapeutics*, 9th ed, New York, NY: McGraw-Hill, 1996.

Hersh EV: Local anesthetics in dentistry: clinical considerations, drug interactions, and novel formulations. *Compend Contin Educ Dent* 14:1020–1028, 1993.

Jastak JT, Yagiela JA, Donaldson D: *Local Anesthesia of the Oral Cavity.* Philadelphia, PA: W.B. Saunders, 1995.

Malamed SF: *Sedation: A Guide to Patient Management*, 3rd ed. St. Louis, MO: Mosby–Year Book, 1995.

Yagiela JA, Neidle EA, Dowd FJ: *Pharmacology and Therapeutics for Dentistry*, 4th ed. St. Louis, MO: Mosby–Year Book, 1998.

Index

An "f" after a page number denotes a figure; a "t" after a page number denotes a table.